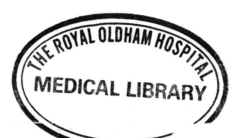

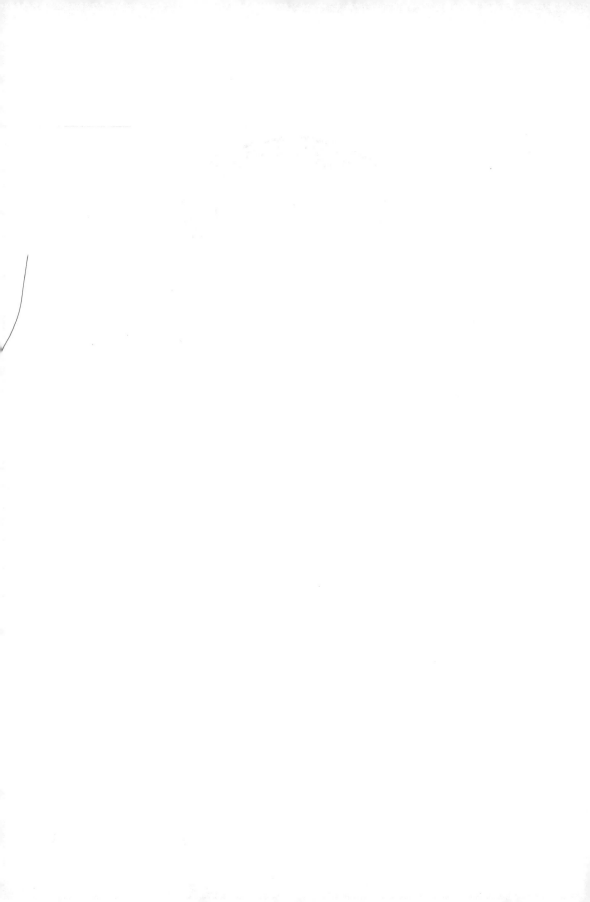

Fatigue in Cancer

Fatigue in Cancer

Edited by

Jo Armes
Department of Palliative Care and Policy
Guy's, King's and St Thomas' School of Medicine
Kings College London

Meinir Krishnasamy
Peter MacCallum Cancer Centre
Melbourne, Australia

and

Irene J. Higginson
Department of Palliative Care and Policy
Guy's, King's and St Thomas' School of Medicine
Kings College London

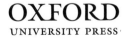

OXFORD
UNIVERSITY PRESS

OXFORD

UNIVERSITY PRESS

Great Clarendon Street, Oxford OX2 6DP

Oxford University Press is a department of the University of Oxford.
It furthers the University's objective of excellence in research, scholarship,
and education by publishing worldwide in

Oxford New York

Auckland Bangkok Buenos Aires Cape Town Chennai
Dar es Salaam Delhi Hong Kong Istanbul Karachi Kolkata
Kuala Lumpur Madrid Melbourne Mexico City Mumbai Nairobi
São Paulo Shanghai Taipei Tokyo Toronto

Oxford is a registered trade mark of Oxford University Press
in the UK and in certain other countries

Published in the United States
by Oxford University Press Inc., New York

A catalogue record for this title is available from the British Library

ISBN 0 19 263094 6

10 9 8 7 6 5 4 3 2 1

Typeset by Cepha Imaging Pvt. Ltd, Bangalore, India
Printed in Great Britain
on acid-free paper by Biddles Ltd., King's Lynn

Foreword

The nineteenth century American neurologist George Beard once remarked that 'fatigue is the Central Africa of medicine, an unexplored territory which few men enter' (Beard 1880). Beard himself made the journey by inventing the illness he called 'neurasthenia', the forerunner of our modern fatigue syndromes, but it remains true even today that fatigue is regarded with a certain suspicion by doctors and health professionals.

One can understand why we as a profession are wary of fatigue; it is, after all, an elusive concept. During our training we are taught the importance of elucidating symptoms that help the diagnostic process. Physicians become alert when a patient mentions coughing blood, since this immediately narrows down the diagnostic possibilities and almost mandates the investigative sequence required. Psychiatrists can endlessly debate the significance of second versus third person auditory hallucinations, since their presence has considerable diagnostic significance. But fatigue lacks any of this specificity. The list of conditions featuring fatigue encompasses most of the *Oxford Textbook of Medicine*, with the equivalent title in *Psychiatry* added for good measure. We can't measure it either – a hundred years' attempts to do so have resulted in failure (Muscio 1921). And it is also true that it is far from easy to treat. So it is understandable that generations of professionals have preferred to simply ignore the problem.

That however, would be a mistake. The problem with fatigue is that it may be all of the above – non-specific, difficult to measure, and difficult to treat – but it is also a major source of morbidity to our patients. Hence, when an American epidemiological study asked lay people and doctors to rate symptoms in order of importance, the professionals placed fatigue at the bottom of the list (as expected), while the public ranked it at the top (Dohrenwend and Crandell 1970).

So far I have been describing fatigue as a general symptom in the population. But all of the above applies in equal measure to fatigue associated with cancer. As this book will amply confirm, study after study shows that fatigue is a critical symptom of neoplastic disease. Yet, it also can have many overlapping causes. Medical factors such as infection, anaemia, and metabolic or endocrine disruption all may be contributing. Physiological disruptions from sleep disturbance and lack of exercise may figure prominently. And of course depression remains a powerful association. It is not true that every fatigued patient is depressed, but it is true that virtually every depressed patient is fatigued.

The current volume is therefore more than welcome, and represents a 'coming of age' of writing on cancer and fatigue. In particular, the editors are to be congratulated on understanding just how wide is the scholarship relevant to cancer and fatigue. George Beard thought that fatigue was a matter for neurologists, an organic condition. His narrow view was largely repudiated, but an equally monolithic view of fatigue as a psychological problem, dominated thinking for the next few decades. Now we appreciate the breadth that is necessary if we are to grasp the problem. We need to understand both the metabolic and endocrine markers of fatigue, and how fatigue affects mental functioning and *vice versa*. What is the physiology of fatigue, and why do physiological interventions such as exercise benefit? How do people talk about fatigue? There are several different conceptualizations of fatigue even within medicine – a neurologist's fatigue is not the same as a psychologist's, for example – let alone the many nuances of fatigue in lay language and concepts. And finally we need to think about how fatigue affects well being, and what we can do about it.

It is a pleasure to commend this multi-author volume which addresses all of these issues. I have been thinking and researching fatigue now for some fifteen years (Wessely *et al.* 1998); this has also meant fifteen years of being asked if I have yet become tired of it. But just when I think the answer is finally affirmative, along comes another fresh look at the subject which rekindles my interest and excitement. This is such a book.

Professor Simon Wessely
London
November 2003

References

Beard, G. (1880) A practical treatise on nervous exhaustion (neurasthenia): its symptoms, nature, sequences, treatment. William Wood, New York.

Dohrenwend, B. and Crandell, D. (1970) Psychiatric symptoms in community, clinic and mental hospital groups. *American Journal of Psychiatry*, **126**, 1611-21.

Muscio, B. (1921) Is a fatigue test possible? *British Journal of Psychology*, **12**, 31-46.

Wessely, S., Hotopf, M., and Sharpe, M. (1998) Chronic fatigue and its syndromes. Oxford University Press, Oxford.

Preface

Fatigue has been identified as one of the most common and distressing problems for people with cancer. Depending on treatment modality, 65-100% of patients will experience fatigue at some stage during their illness. Fatigue is often the first sign of ill health and so it may be perceived as a potent indicator of disease status throughout the illness and, for some, on into survivorship. Whilst health professionals increasingly recognize the impact of cancer-related fatigue on patients' lives, fatigue continues to be poorly defined and inadequately understood, despite a growth in the number of research studies addressing this issue. As a result, the development of appropriate measurement tools and effective interventions has been severely hampered. Nevertheless current evidence suggests that fatigue transcends symptom boundaries, affecting all aspects of patients' lives.

Much of the work undertaken has been carried out by discrete professional groups, and, to date, there is no comprehensive text which draws together current basic research and clinician perspectives for the many disciplines involved in working towards a better understanding of fatigue. The impetus behind this book came from a desire to bring together the views and experiences of some of those most prominent in the field of fatigue research from across Europe and North America. In doing so, it aims to provide those interested in the management of fatigue within cancer populations with a source of expert knowledge to guide their practice, irrespective of professional group or specific area of interest.

The need for a shift away from conceptualizing fatigue as a discrete symptom entity underlies the approach to the book, as does the notion that future developments in its management will only be fully realized through an integrated and multi-professional approach. This will not only need to be guided by research-based evidence, but also patients' experiences. As a result, this book addresses essential domains that require further conceptual development, scientific, and clinical evaluation. Consideration is given to the complexity of definition, along with a review of existing and emergent models of cancer-related fatigue. The text critically appraises factors associated with fatigue, such as multiple treatment modalities, pain, anxiety and depression, breathlessness, weight loss, and existential crises. The instruments available to measure fatigue are assessed. Drawing on insights gained from qualitative research, the evidence surrounding 'living with fatigue throughout the cancer illness' is debated, and consideration given to the place of fatigue within the wellness/illness trajectory. The impact of fatigue on quality of life is a recurring concept, culminating with an evaluation of pharmacological and non-pharmacological interventions targeted at minimising its potential to negatively influence individuals' lives.

Our aim has been to stimulate professional colleagues of whatever discipline to re-evaluate the importance of this complex and distressing problem, and to engage in innovative research to enhance the fatigue knowledge base. The book is intended for specialist oncology and palliative care practitioners, researchers, and primary health care professionals, whilst also being appropriate for diploma, degree, and postgraduate students who have a prior knowledge of basic cancer biology, cancer treatments, side-effects, and physical, psychological, and social consequences of a cancer diagnosis. We hope that you find the book relevant, thought provoking, and stimulating.

We owe a debt of gratitude to the authors of the chapters for their forbearance with the ponderous gestation of this book. It has been a great pleasure working with them all. Each of us has people whom we would like to thank. JA is grateful to Jon for his unfailing encouragement and support and Stevie for her fun, laughter, and ability to rise early - the latter has provided a taster of what it means to be fatigued. For Kumar – thanks for making it all possible, and to Nia, Rhys, and Carys, for giving life such meaning (MK). IJH would like to thank her co-editors; and the patients and families over the years with whom she has worked, who first made her interested in fatigue in cancer.

Jo Armes
Meiner Krishnasamy
Irene J. Higginson

Contents

List of Contributors

Patricia Alcoser
Clinical Instructor
Department of Pediatrics
Baylor College of Medicine, Houston
Texas, USA

Paul Andrews
Professor of Comparative Physiology
Department of Basic Medical Sciences
St George's Hospital Medical School
Cranmer Terrace
London, UK

Jo Armes
Cancer Research UK Nursing Research
Fellow
Department of Palliative Care
and Policy
Guy's, King's and St Thomas' School of
Medicine
London, UK

Patrick Barrera
Research Coordinator
Department of Pediatrics
Baylor College of Medicine, Houston
Texas, USA

Sarah Bottomley
Clinical Instructor
Department of Pediatrics
Baylor College of Medicine, Houston
Texas, USA

Eduardo Bruera
Professor and Chair
Department of Palliative Care and
Rehabilitation Medicine (Unit 008)
UT MD Anderson Cancer Center
1515 Holcombe Boulevard, Houston
Texas, USA

Cindy Burleson
Nursing Director
St Jude Children's Research Hospital
Memphis, Tennessee, USA

David Cella
Professor, Psychiatry and Behavioral
Science
Research Professor, Institute for Health
Services Research and Policy Studies
Northwestern University
and
Director, Center on Outcomes Research
and Education
Evanston Northwestern Healthcare
Evanston, Illinois, USA

Mónica Castro
Clinical Research Physician of the
Supportive Care Division and
Translational Research
Unit
Angel H. Roffo Cancer Institute
University of Buenos Aires, Argentina

David Field
Department of Epidemiology and
Public Health
University of Leicester
Leicester, UK

Mei Fu
Ph.D Student, MU Sinclair School of
Nursing
University of Missouri—Columbia
Columbia, Missouri, USA

Jami Gattuso
Nursing Research Specialist
St Jude Children's Research Hospital
Memphis, Tennessee, USA

Jane T. Hickok
Research Assistant Professor of
Oncology in Community and Preventive
Medicine
University of Rochester James P. Wilmot
Cancer Center
Rochester, New York, USA

Irene Higginson
Professor of Palliative Care and Policy
Department of Palliative Care and Policy
Guy's, King's and St Thomas' School of
Medicine
London, UK

Pamela Hinds
Director of Nursing Research
St Jude Children's Research Hospital
Memphis, Tennessee USA

Marilyn Hockenberry
Professor of Pediatrics
Baylor College of Medicine
Director of Pediatric Nurse Practitioner
Services
Texas Children's Hospital
Cancer Center
Houston, Texas, USA

Matthew Hotopf
Reader in Psychological Medicine
Department of Psychological Medicine,
Institute of Psychiatry
Kings College London
London, UK

Paul Jacobsen
Professor of Psychology
University of South Florida
USA

Nancy Kline
Director
Center for Clinical Innovation and
Scholarship
Children's Hospital Boston
Brookline, Massachussetts, USA

Meinir Krishnasamy
Research Fellow, Peter MacCallum
Cancer Centre
Melbourne, Victoria, Australia

Trudy Mallinson
Clinical Research Scientist
Center for Rehabilitation Outcomes
Research
Rehabilitation Institute of Chicago
Research Assistant Professor
Feinberg School of Medicine
Northwestern University
Evanston, Illinois, USA

Maryellen McSweeney
Professor Emerita
School of Nursing
St Louis University
St. Louis, Missouri, USA

Christina A. Meyers
Professor of Neuropsychology
Department of Neuro-Oncology
The University of Texas MD Anderson
Cancer Center
Houston, Texas, USA

Gary R. Morrow
Professor of Radiation Oncology and
Professor of Psychiatry
Director, URCC CCOP Research Base
University of Rochester Cancer Center
Rochester, New York, USA

Jill Brace O'Neill
Pediatric Nurse Specialist
Dana-Farber Cancer Institute
Boston, Massachussets, USA

Hilary Plant
Practice Development Nurse
Cancer and Haematology Services
Guys and St Thomas' Hospital NHS Trust
Guy's Hospital
London, UK

Davina Porock
Associate Professor in Gerontology
Oncology
MU Sinclair School of Nursing
University of Missouri—Columbia
Columbia, Missouri, USA

Emma Ream
Senior Lecturer
Florence Nightingale School of Nursing
and Midwifery
Kings College London
London, UK

Alison Richardson
Professor of Cancer and Palliative
Nursing Care
Florence Nightingale School of Nursing
and Midwifery
Kings College London
London, UK

Joseph A. Roscoe
Research Assistant Professor
Behavioral Medicine Unit
University of Rochester Cancer Center
Rochester, New York, USA

Paddy Stone
Senior Lecturer and Honorary
Consultant in Palliative Medicine
Department of Psychiatry
St George's Hospital
London, UK

Michael Weitzner
Professor of Interdisciplinary Oncology
University of South Florida
USA

Horng-Shiuann Wu
Assistant Professor
St Louis University
Community and Family Medicine
St Louis, Missouri, USA

Introduction

Irene J. Higginson, Jo Armes, and
Meinir Krishnasamy

Why consider fatigue in cancer?

In Western societies one in three people will experience cancer at some point in their lifetime, and one in four will die from it (Higginson 1997). In England and Wales there are 220 000 new cases of cancer per year, and around 140 000 deaths from cancer. Cancer accounts for around 22% of all deaths within developed countries and 9.5% of deaths within developing countries (Stjernsward and Pampallona 1998).

In the future cancer is predicted to increase worldwide, with cancer of the lung, trachea and bronchus alone rising to the fifth most common form of death globally in 2020 (Murray and Lopez 1997*a,b*, 2000). In 2015 predictions estimate that almost 14% of deaths in developed countries and around 28% in developing countries will be due to cancer (Stjernsward and Pampallona 1998). Cancer affects people of all ages, from children and adolescents through to the very old, although most people who suffer cancer are in the older age groups, over 65 or 75 years of age (Higginson 1997).

Cancer is characterized by multiple symptoms, caused by the primary tumour, metastasis, and the side-effects of treatment, be it surgery, radiotherapy, or chemotherapy. Symptoms also result from the emotional, social, and spiritual effects of cancer and its treatment. They can also be caused by, or exacerbate, pre-existing illness, especially in older people who may have other chronic conditions. Sometimes symptoms can be devastating. Suffering can extend beyond the person directly affected to family members, friends, and anyone involved in caring for the person.

It is in this context that this book considers an important symptom—that of fatigue. Patients, caregivers, and oncology health professionals now are realizing a consensus that fatigue is one of the most important symptoms of cancer today (Curt 2001). In advanced cancer, many studies have found that fatigue (or weakness, or asthenia) is the most common symptom (Coyle *et al.* 1990; Edmonds *et al.* 1998; Connill *et al.* 1997). This is consistent in different cultures (Koffman *et al.* 2003).

Cancer-related fatigue is emerging now partly because the management of many other symptoms, particularly pain, nausea, and vomiting, has improved, and partly because until recently cancer-related fatigue was something to be endured rather than a symptom amenable to differential diagnosis and treatment. Only recently has the problem been considered as real, and still it is too seldom discussed and treated (Curt 2001).

This book challenges this relative neglect, and gathers together the main evidence regarding the epidemiology, pathophysiological mechanisms, associated factors and symptoms, meaning, assessment, and treatment options of fatigue in cancer.

What is fatigue and what causes it?

What is meant by fatigue? Fatigue can be defined in different ways. The term originates from the Latin *fatigare*, meaning tired out. The *Oxford English Dictionary*'s main definitions of fatigue are: (1) extreme tiredness after exertion and (2) a reduction in the efficiency of a muscle. One common definition is 'a subjective state of overwhelming, sustained exhaustion and decreased capacity for physical and mental work that is not relieved by rest' (Piper *et al*. 1989). In some medical texts fatigue is likened or considered equivalent to asthenia. Asthenia is taken from the Greek word *asthenos*, meaning absence or loss of strength.

Fatigue can be considered as behaviour or a feeling state (see Chapter 1), and it is the latter on which we mainly concentrate. But terms such as feeling tired, feeling sleepy, lacking motivation, feeling weak or washed out are part of everyday conversation. Indeed, most people in society will have experienced fatigue at some time. Studies within family practice populations found the prevalence of fatigue ranged around 10 to 35%. Prevalence is higher in people with a health problem (see Chapters 1 and 2). This book, therefore, considers the epidemiology of fatigue in the general population as well as among cancer patients, and some of the differences. Who gets fatigue, what precipitates it, who is disposed to it, and what affects the reported prevalence are all important if we are to understand fatigue, manage it well in practice, and research effective solutions.

The aetiology, pathophysiology, and mechanisms of fatigue are complex. There are many inter-related symptoms, in particular cachexia, anorexia, depression, and anxiety (see Chapters 2–5). Fatigue may be caused by direct effects of the cancer and by tumour-induced products, particularly on muscle and the central nervous system. It may also be caused, or increased, by accompanying factors such as infection, anaemia, metabolic disorders, dehydration, lack of sleep because of uncontrolled pain or worry, or simply interruptions, and a whole host of other potential mediators. Understanding these mechanisms suggests useful lines of enquiry for the future assessment, prevention, and treatment of fatigue in cancer.

How important is fatigue in cancer?

Fatigue is important for patients with cancer at all stages of their illness, for some at diagnosis and for many during treatment. It occurs 80% to 99% of those receiving chemotherapy, radiotherapy, or both (Curt *et al*. 2000) and in 20% to 90% as the disease progresses. In the last week of life it is the most common symptom (Coyle *et al*. 1990; Edmonds *et al*. 1998; Connill *et al*. 1997). These variations in prevalence exist because epidemiological information about cancer fatigue is often poor. A previous lack of a consensus around the definition of fatigue and very varied methods of detection, assessment, and monitoring of fatigue, as well as the different populations studied, means that very different levels of fatigue are reported.

Fatigue: a complex symptom with wide-reaching effects

Fatigue is associated with increased distress due to some other symptoms, including pain. It often clusters with cachexia and anorexia, and is difficult to distinguish between them (see Chapter 5). It has profound effects on everyday functioning and, perhaps consequently, service use. It reduces quality of life and increases suffering. Fatigue has been associated with hospital admission and increased stress to caregivers (Hinton 1994; Robinson and Posner 1992). The needs of lay caregivers in this context are often overlooked (see Chapter 9). A deeper comprehension of these factors is important in assessing patients, planning care, and in designing and testing future treatments for fatigue.

But do the effects of fatigue stretch even wider, reaching well beyond traditional symptom boundaries? Having energy and vitality is an important part of self-image. Fatigue is often seen as a sign of impending deterioration. So if doctors and nurses are to discuss fatigue with patients, grasping their interpretation and understanding of fatigue is essential (see Chapter 7). Fatigue can have a profound meaning for patients living with fatigue, and for their carers or family, which also need to be considered and assessed.

Uncertainties regarding assessment, treatment, and future care

The complexity of fatigue in cancer and the wide range of different mechanisms means that accurate assessment, with an understanding of the likely cause(s) and associated factors, is critical to considering treatment options. There has been a lack of information on this in the past, often leading doctors and nurses to feel hopeless in the face of fatigue. But some possible methods of assessing fatigue and monitoring progress are now available. Measuring the severity and consequences of fatigue is complex; fatigue is difficult to measure, because of the different ways in which it is interpreted and understood. Yet this is vital if treatments and their outcomes are to be monitored over time.

Treatment options are varied, depending on the likely cause. The evidence base for treatments is only now developing; studies are often lacking and are difficult to conduct. However, correction of simple causes, such as sleep interruption or anaemia, if identified, is a common first step. There are also general non-pharmacological measures such as adapting activities of daily living and occupational therapy to help match clinical function and symptom status with the expectation of patients and families. There is a wide range of pharmacological and non-pharmacological interventions available.

Corticosteroids have been proposed as a treatment, and are often used. It is argued that they may decrease fatigue, either by inhibiting the release of tumour-induced substances or by a central euphoria effect. Amphetamines have been favoured in some settings, in particular in North American countries. Many other pharmacological treatments are emerging for the treatment of fatigue and its related symptoms. Counselling, gentle activity, physiotherapy, and multifactorial interventions have also been proposed. The evidence for these varied approaches is appraised in more detail in the chapters of this book.

Because of the lack of concentration of research and clinical effort in cancer-related fatigue some aspects the findings are preliminary and in some areas they contradict. Here we have sought to present the best knowledge and to debate opposing evidence, in the hope that it will provide doctors, nurses, and all those involved in caring for patients and families with mechanisms for improving care, as well as identifying important future lines of enquiry through research. The appraisals may begin to break the past, sometimes nihilistic, attitude to the assessment, discussion, and treatment of fatigue and encourage future trials and investigation, so that ultimately the effects of this most common and neglected symptom may be reduced.

References

Connill, C., Verger, E., Henriquez, I., Saiz, N., Espier, M., Lugo, F., *et al.* (1997) Symptom prevalence in the last week of life. *Journal of Pain and Symptom Management,* **14**, 328–31.

Coyle, N., Adelhardt, J., Foley, K.M., and Portenoy, R.K. (1990) Character of terminal illness in the advanced cancer patient: pain and other symptoms during the last four weeks of life. *Journal of Pain and Symptom Management,* **5**, 83–93.

Curt, G.A. (2001) Fatigue in cancer. *British Medical Journal,* **322**, 1560.

Curt, G.A., Breitbart, W., Cella, D., Groopman, J.E., Horning, S.L., Itri, L.M., *et al.* (2000) Impact of cancer-related fatigue on the lives of patients: new findings from the Fatigue Coalition. *Oncologist,* **5**, 353–60.

Edmonds, P.M., Stuttaford, J.M., Penny, J., Lynch, A.M., and Chamberlain, J. (1998) Do hospital palliative care teams improve symptom control? Use of modified STAS as an evaluative tool. *Palliative Medicine,* **12**, 345–51.

Higginson, I.J. (1997) Health care needs assessment: palliative and terminal care. In: *Health Care Needs Assessment* (eds. A. Stevens, and J. Raftery), pp. 183–260. Wessex Institute of Public Health Medicine, Oxford.

Hinton, J. (1994) Which patients with terminal cancer are admitted from home care? *Palliative Medicine,* **8**, 197–210.

Koffman, J., Higginson, I.J., and Donaldson, N. (2003) Symptom severity in advanced cancer assessed in two ethnic groups by interviews with bereaved family members and friends. *Journal of the Royal Society of Medicine,* **96**, 10–16.

Murray, C.J.L. and Lopez, A.D. (1997*a*) Alternative projections of mortality and disability by cause 1990–2020: Global Burden of Disease Study. *The Lancet,* **349**, 1498–504.

Murray, C.J.L. and Lopez, A.D. (1997*b*) Mortality by cause for eight regions of the world: Global Burden of Disease Study. *The Lancet,* **349**, 1269–76.

Murray, C.J.L. and Lopez, A.D. (2000) Progress and directions in refining the global burden of disease approach: a response to Williams. *Health Economics,* **9**, 69–82.

Piper, B.F., Lindsey, A.M., Dodd, M.J., Ferketich, S., Paul, S.M., and Weller, S. (1989). The development of an instrument to measure the subjective dimension of fatigue. In: Key Aspects of Comfort: Management of Pain, Fatigue, and Nausea (eds. S.G. Funk, E.M. Tornquist, M.T. Champagne, L.A. Copp, and R.A. Wiess), p. 199. Springer, New York.

Robinson, K.D. and Posner, J.D. (1992) Patterns of self-care needs and interventions related to biologic response modifier therapy: fatigue as a model. *Seminars in Oncology Nursing* **8**, 17–22.

Stjernsward, J. and Pampallona, S, (1998), Palliative medicine—a global perspective. In: *Oxford Textbook of Palliative Medicine* (eds. D. Doyle, G.W.C. Hanks, and N. MacDonald), pp. 1227–45. Oxford University Press, Oxford.

Part 1

The nature and pathophysiology of fatigue

Chapter 1

Definitions, epidemiology, and models of fatigue in the general population and in cancer

Matthew Hotopf

Introduction

Fatigue is a universal experience and a common symptom. Most people experiencing fatigue do not see it as anything unusual, but instead put it down to the toils of normal life (David *et al.* 1990). In some individuals fatigue can become chronic and disabling. Fatigue is rated by patients as an especially alarming and difficult symptom, whereas doctors—who are perhaps aware of its non-specific nature—tend to underestimate its importance (Dohrenwend and Crandell 1970).

Fatigue is a common and important symptom of cancer. However, in order to understand and manage fatigue in cancer patients, it is worth exploring the nature of fatigue in the general population and identifying areas of overlap. There is, perhaps, a temptation to view the symptoms of cancer patients as totally different from those of individuals without cancer, and to view them in isolation. Researchers investigating cancer-related pain have been criticised for doing just that (Turk and Fernandez 1990), so this chapter starts with a summary of some of the literature on the epidemiology of non-cancer fatigue. Over the past 20 years there has been a growth in research on chronic fatigue syndrome (also known as 'myalgic encephalomyelitis' or ME) following the increasingly high profile of this condition. This has included a number of epidemiological studies which have looked at the distribution of fatigue within the population. This chapter will describe the main features of these studies, and point to some of the other key aspects of research in chronic fatigue syndrome, before describing the smaller literature on fatigue in cancer.

Definitions

Fatigue has numerous meanings in the scientific literature, as well as to lay people. Wessely *et al.* (1998) defined four components of fatigue, but for the purposes of this discussion, the essential distinction is between fatigue as a behaviour and fatigue as a feeling state.

Fatigue as a behaviour

In the physiological literature, fatigue has a specific meaning relating to a decrement in performance of either physical or psychological tasks (Sharpe *et al.* 1991). Research subjects when asked to perform a repeated task involving either physical or mental exertion will show fatigue over time. Their performance will deteriorate, and the pattern in which this happens has been widely studied.

Fatigue as a feeling state

Fatigue can also be used to describe the *symptom* of feeling tired. No matter how universal such a feeling may be, it has numerous connotations including:

- lack of energy
- weakness
- fatigability
- effort, in relation to a task
- sleepiness
- tiredness
- desire for rest
- lack of motivation
- lassitude
- boredom.

Despite the range of meanings in circulation, the symptom can be simplified into three main components: a sensory quality (the feeling of a lack of energy); the affective component (lack of motivation); and a cognitive component (the meaning the individual attaches to the symptom). It is particularly fatigue as a feeling state which we shall focus on in this chapter.

'Chronic fatigue' describes persistent fatigue, present at least 50% of the time over a period of at least 6 months (Wessely *et al.* 1999). Chronic fatigue syndrome (CFS) describes chronic fatigue which is associated with significant disability, and is not associated with physical diseases which can cause fatigue (such as anaemia, cancer, or endocrine complaints) or with major psychiatric disorders such as schizophrenia, eating disorders, and substance misuse (Pawlikowska *et al.* 1994). As such chronic fatigue syndrome is best viewed as a medically unexplained syndrome akin to fibromyalgia, irritable bowel syndrome, or atypical chest pain (Wessely *et al.* 1997).

Epidemiology of fatigue in the general population

Fatigue is a continuum

A number of epidemiological studies have shown that fatigue is distributed continuously throughout populations (David *et al.* 1990; Lewis *et al.* 1992; Ozguler *et al.* 2000).

This has two consequences. Firstly, most people report at least some fatigue, and those who report none are unusual. Thus a study based on a consecutive sample of primary care patients showed that only 18% reported no fatigue at all (David *et al.* 1990). Secondly, there is no 'point of rarity' in the frequency distribution. In other words, it is not possible to distinguish one group with 'normal' fatigue from another with 'abnormal' fatigue. Any definition of 'pathological' fatigue is therefore arbitrary. This is a familiar problem in epidemiology—most symptoms, illnesses, or diseases are on a continuum of severity, and the same applies to physiological variables such as blood pressure and serum cholesterol. One consequence of this is that researcher may use different thresholds for defining 'cases', and different risk factors may be involved in the definition of the level of severity, chronicity, or disability used to identify such cases—a point powerfully made in the literature on low back pain (Ozguler *et al.* 2000).

Fatigue is common

Most community studies which have asked about fatigue report it as being among the top ten most common symptoms. In the UK a recent study on the prevalence of psychiatric symptoms found fatigue (measured on the Revised Clinical Interview Schedule (Lewis *et al.* 1992)) was the most common symptom present in one-third of women and a fifth of men (Meltzer *et al.* 1995). The Health and Lifestyles Survey (Cox *et al.* 1987) asked 9003 subjects 'within the last month have you suffered from any problems of feeling tired?' Tiredness was the second commonest symptom after headache, with a prevalence of approximately 20% for men and 30% for women. Similar prevalence rates have been derived in the USA from the Epidemiologic Catchment Area Study (Kroenke and Price 1993). This survey also estimated that in at least 60% of subjects with significant fatigue the cause was unexplained by medical disease.

Fatigue in primary care

Studies have shown that fatigue is also prevalent in general practice patients. In an American study (Bates *et al.* 1993) 1000 primary care attenders were assessed and 32% ($n = 323$) reported fatigue. Of these, 271 (27%) reported chronic fatigue defined as at least 6 months of unusual fatigue which interfered with daily life. In the UK, David *et al.* (1990) found that 10.2% of men and 10.6% of women attending primary care reported substantial fatigue for 1 month or more. Cathebras *et al.* (1992) found that 13.6% of GP attenders presented with fatigue, and in 6.7% fatigue was the main complaint. An Israeli study assessed GP notes over a 10-year period and found that approximately 32% of 508 patients' records had entries regarding fatigue during that period, and in 9% of these the symptom appeared to be persistent (Shahar and Lederer 1990). Kroenke *et al.* (1990) found that fatigue was the most common symptom reported among 410 ambulatory medical outpatients in the USA.

Unsurprisingly, as more stringent criteria are used to diagnose fatigue the prevalence falls. In community samples 8–19% of adults surveyed meet criteria for chronic fatigue

(Buchwald *et al.* 1995; Lawrie and Pelosi 1995; Fukuda *et al.* 1997; Wessely *et al.* 1997). For idiopathic chronic fatigue, the figure drops to between 6 and 9% (Buchwald *et al.* 1995; Wessely *et al.* 1997;) and for chronic fatigue syndrome estimates range from 0.3–2.8% (Bates *et al.* 1993; Buchwald *et al.* 1995; Lawrie and Pelosi 1995; Wessely *et al.* 1997). The incidence of chronic fatigue is estimated at 370/100 000 per year (Lawrie *et al.* 1997) and that of CFS at 180/100 000 per year (Reyes *et al.* 2003).

Who gets the most fatigue?

We have already seen from community studies that fatigue is more common in women than men, with women reporting it approximately one and a half to two times more commonly than men. Children very rarely experience fatigue, but the symptom becomes increasingly prevalent in adolescence and early adulthood, rising to a peak in the late 20s and early 30s (Meltzer *et al.* 1995; Fukuda *et al.* 1997). If anything, the prevalence then tends to decline with advancing age, despite the growing prevalence of medical ailments in this group (Meltzer *et al.* 1995; Fukuda *et al.* 1997). There is an inverse relationship between socioeconomic status and fatigue, with more deprived groups having slightly higher rates of the symptom (Meltzer *et al.* 1995; Lawrie and Pelosi 1995). Despite this patients presenting for investigation or treatment of CFS tend to come from higher socioeconomic groups (Euba *et al.* 1996). This almost certainly reflects referral bias—with patients from professional backgrounds tending to label their symptoms as chronic fatigue syndrome and being more effective at seeking specialist help for it.

Fatigue is associated with psychiatric disorders and psychological distress

There is considerable evidence that patients who report fatigue are more likely to suffer with the common psychological disorders of depression and anxiety. This relationship exists no matter what setting fatigue is studied in. In population surveys there is a striking and powerful correlation between increased fatigue and increasing psychological distress on measures such as the General Health Questionnaire (GHQ-12) (Pawlikowska *et al.* 1994; Buchwald *et al.* 1995; Lawrie and Pelosi 1995; van der Linden *et al.* 1999). In primary care, patients presenting with fatigue have much higher rates of psychological distress than their non-fatigued counterparts (Cathebras *et al.* 1992), and in secondary or tertiary care settings up to 75% of patients with CFS have been found to suffer from depression, anxiety, or other operationally defined psychiatric disorders (Wessely *et al.* 1998). In studies which have compared CFS sufferers with medically ill controls (in order to control for the possible effects on mood of having a disabling physical illness), patients with CFS still seem to be especially prone to psychiatric disorder, with a two- to seven-fold increase in rates over the physically ill controls

(Wessely and Powell 1989; Katon *et al.* 1991; Wood *et al.* 1991; Pepper *et al.* 1993; Fischler *et al.* 1997).

Fatigue is associated with disability

Although fatigue is sometimes thought of as a trivial symptom, it is associated with considerable disability. Studies that have assessed the levels of disability in CFS sufferers suggest profound deficits. Two prevalence surveys (Buchwald *et al.* 1995; Wessely *et al.* 1997) used quality of life questionnaires and found a stepwise increase in disability from healthy subjects to those with chronic fatigue and those with CFS. Role performance (the ability to fulfil occupational or household functioning) was especially impaired. Patients with CFS have disabilities comparable to, or worse than, patients with many common medical illnesses such as heart disease, diabetes, or arthritis (Wells *et al.* 1989). This applies both to cases seen in clinical settings and those who do not consult. Patients with CFS who also suffer from psychological distress or depression have particularly severe impairments. Wessely *et al.* (1997) demonstrated a striking gradient of decreasing function in subjects with chronic fatigue according to the severity of psychological morbidity. Individuals with the worst function were those with chronic fatigue and high psychological morbidity. Whilst these findings do not indicate whether patients with chronic fatigue become disabled due to the presence of psychological distress, or become distressed due to the presence of disability, they make the important clinical point that those with the worst disability are also those most likely to have a psychiatric disorder.

Precipitating factors for fatigue

There are a number of increasingly recognized acute triggers for the onset of CFS. Most widely studied are viral infections. Whilst there is no evidence that minor viral infections presenting to GPs are associated with subsequent chronic fatigue (Wessely *et al.* 1995), more severe illnesses such as glandular fever, hepatitis A, and viral meningitis probably are associated with a considerably increased risk of subsequent chronic fatigue (Berelowitz *et al.* 1995; Hotopf *et al.* 1996; White *et al.* 1998). The risk does not appear to be specifically associated with any one severe viral infection, but may be related to non-specific behavioural factors such as the duration of time the individual has off work following the illness (Hotopf *et al.* 1996). The risk is not associated solely with viral infections—other acute physical insults such as surgical procedures and trauma are recognized as being associated with fatigue, even in the absence of an ongoing active disease process (Wessely *et al.* 1998).

If acute physical illness can cause prolonged fatigue states, what about acute psychological stressors—the traditional life events of the social psychiatry literature? There is a vast literature on the role of life events in the onset of depression and anxiety disorders, which shows an undisputed relationship (Brown and Harris 1978). The literature for fatigue is much slimmer, but there is some evidence. Bruce-Jones *et al.* (1994)

followed up individuals who had suffered acute glandular fever, and found a modest association between life events and fatigue, but (as expected) a stronger one between life events and depression. Chalder (1998) has assessed the relationship with a cohort of GP attendees and found that there was also an association. She showed that severity of fatigue was predicted by negative life events, perceived discrepancy in emotional support, and breathlessness (used as a proxy for physical deconditioning). Chronicity of fatigue was better predicted by low practical support. Thus unfit individuals with low emotional support who experience a negative life event may be at risk of developing acute fatigue, which may then become chronic in the absence of practical support. It is therefore possible that life events are a contributory factor in the development of fatigue, as well as being a sufficient explanation for CFS in its own right.

Predisposing factors

It is difficult to design good studies to investigate the relationship between predisposing factors and fatigue in the general population, and the evidence in the main is weak. The strongest evidence comes from cohort studies of infection (Wessely *et al.* 1995; Hotopf *et al.* 1996). These demonstrate that the individuals at greatest risk of developing subsequent fatigue are those with a past history of unexplained symptoms. Genetic markers of fatigue have been examined in adults and children. In an Australian twin study a genetic influence was found (Hickie *et al.* 1999), which suggested that although fatigue and depression were strongly correlated, they may have separate genetic determinants. In a study of twin children the heritability (that is, the proportion of variance explained) of fatigue was estimated at between 0.42 and 0.83. This indicates a potentially strong genetic component (Farmer *et al.* 1999). There is also a growing literature on early experience and subsequent development of medically unexplained symptoms (Hotopf *et al.* 1999*a*,*b*, 2000). This demonstrates powerful associations between chronic illness in parents and later symptoms in their children. Thus it may be that those exposed to illness early in life react differently when they subsequently get ill themselves and this acts as a predisposing factor for more chronic problems.

Perpetuating factors for fatigue

Once an individual has developed fatigue, what factors are associated with it getting better or remaining bad? Sharpe *et al.* (1992) assessed patients presenting to an infectious disease specialist with fatigue. The patients were followed up and the strongest risk factors for fatigue remaining chronic were (a) psychiatric disorder, (b) attributions that the individual was suffering from a physical disorder, and (c) behavioural change, such as changing or stopping work and joining a patient support group. Other studies reviewed in a systematic review by Joyce *et al.* (1997) found broadly similar results. These studies of the prognosis of chronic fatigue consistently show that patients who have prominent psychological distress or clear psychiatric disorder do less well (Wilson *et al.* 1994; Bombardier and Buchwald 1995; Clark *et al.* 1995). Behavioural change and attributions that the fatigue has an underlying organic basis are also important (Wilson *et al.* 1994; Chalder *et al.* 1996). Many of the studies examined the effects of various hypothesized physical correlates of fatigue on prognosis, and in general found little evidence that they are related to prognosis. So, for example, there is no association between recovery from fatigue and viral titres, leukocyte levels, or liver function in patients with fatigue associated with coxsackie B virus infection (Calder *et al.* 1987); no association between recovery from CFS and viral antibodies (Hellinger *et al.* 1988), and no evidence that cell-mediated immunity has any impact on recovery (Wilson *et al.* 1994). These three groups of risk factors for fatigue in non-cancer patients are discussed further in the section on models of fatigue.

The epidemiology of fatigue in cancer

Prevalence: how common is fatigue in cancer?

The simple answer to this question is 'very'. However, there are a number of important obstacles to determining the prevalence of fatigue in cancer patients. In part it is difficult to gain a reliable picture of the prevalence of fatigue in cancer because most studies which look at fatigue in cancer assess the symptom in special groups. Table 1.1 describes some of the factors which might lead to variation in rates of fatigue in cancer patients. It is likely that the prevalence of fatigue in cancer patients varies significantly according to site and type of cancer, stage of disease, presence of medical co-morbidity (anaemia, infection, metabolic disturbance), and psychiatric disorders (especially depression and anxiety).

Treatment is also likely to be a major contributing factor. Another problem in summarizing this growing literature is that a wide variety of different measures are used to assess fatigue and many of these are reported as continuous as opposed to binary outcomes. Whilst this reflects the continuous spread of fatigue within the population,

Table 1.1 Factors likely to affect the prevalence of fatigue reported in cancer patients

Disease factors	Stage of disease
	Site of cancer
	Type of cancer
	Release of cytokines
Consequences of disease	Medical complications of cancer—anaemia, infection, metabolic disturbance, malnutrition
	Presence of psychiatric disorder—anxiety, depression etc.
	Inactivity and deconditioning
Treatment factors	Radiotherapy
	Chemotherapy
	Surgery
	Opiates

it makes the results difficult to interpret except to those familiar with the question-naires involved.

Taking these considerations into account, Table 1.2 describes some of the studies which provide clear prevalence estimates of the symptom of fatigue. Apart from stud-ies of survivors of lymphoma (Loge *et al.* 1999) it is hard to find any studies with prevalence estimates of fatigue, however defined, below 30%.

Some studies have assessed the prevalence of fatigue against other common symp-toms: Ng and von Gunten (1998) found that fatigue and weakness were the two com-monest symptoms in hospice patients, with a prevalence of over 80%, whereas pain was only present in approximately half. Despite the almost universal presence of fatigue in this population, it was relatively infrequently rated as the 'main symptom'—only being reported by 6%, as opposed to 11% for pain (the most common 'main symptom' was respiratory problems, present in 22%). Other studies which have assessed multiple symptoms also point to fatigue being the most common symptom of cancer irrespective of diagnosis or stage (Kurtz *et al.* 1994; Savage *et al.* 1997; Newell *et al.* 1998), except where the symptom was ascertained from case notes (Savage *et al.* 1997), implying that medical staff tend not to question patients about it, or ignore the symptom if it is spontaneously reported.

Relatively few studies have attempted to compare patients with cancer and other control populations: Mendoza *et al.* (1999) and Stone *et al.* (1999) (see Table 1.2) are exceptions and took healthy controls as comparison groups. Both studies found very significant differences in prevalence rates of severe fatigue between these groups. There can be little doubt that cancer is strongly associated with fatigue when healthy control populations are used. In contrast Andrykowski *et al.* (1998) compared levels of fatigue in 88 women with breast cancer and a similar number of women who had attended a breast clinic for benign breast disease. Whilst the women with breast cancer had more fatigue than those with benign disease the difference was slight and not statistically sig-nificant on several of the fatigue scales used. This may say more about their control group of symptomatic women consulting for a breast problem than about the cancer patients.

Two studies (Mendoza *et al.* 1999; Stone *et al.* 1999) looked at the distribution of fatigue among patients with cancer. In the general population the distribution is strongly skewed, with a long tail going to the right of the distribution. These studies indicate that the entire distribution is shifted to the right in cancer patients. Hence the increased prevalence of fatigue in cancer patients is not due to a relatively few sufferers who are very fatigued, but to a general shift in the population's experience of the symptom.

Risk factors for fatigue in cancer

If fatigue is strongly related to cancer, are there other risk factors among cancer patients which predict who is most likely to suffer from fatigue? The literature here

Table 1.2 Key studies assessing prevalence of fatigue in cancer patients

Study	Population	Prevalence of fatigue
Ashbury et al. (1998)	913 cancer patients recruited by advertisements. Had to have received treatment for cancer in previous 2 years	Fatigue most common symptom affecting 78%. Fatigue rated as causing difficulties with functional activities in 71% of sample
Bladé et al. (1996)	72 patients under age 40 presenting to Mayo Clinic (USA) with multiple myeloma	'One-third' complained of weakness and fatigue—from case note review
Degner and Sloan (1995)	434 newly diagnosed patients with lung cancer. Consecutive sample from two tertiary referral clinics in Manitoba, Canada	Fatigue present in 39% (defined as high score on a symptom distress inventory). Fatigue was most common of 13 symptoms
Donnelly et al. (1995)	Consecutive sample of 1000 advanced cancer patients (mixed diagnoses) referred to a palliative care services in Cleveland, Ohio	48% with 'clinically important' fatigue; 47% with; clinically important' weakness
Glaus (1998)	499 mixed cancer patients identified from inpatients and outpatients in four Swiss hospitals	Loss of energy reported in 53%; weakness in 49% on fatigue assessment questionnaire
Hickok et al. (1996)	50 consecutive patients receiving radiotherapy for lung cancer in a cancer centre in Rochester, USA	78% experienced fatigue at some point during radiotherapy
Hopwood and Stephens (1995)	650 patients entering a UK multicentre randomized trial into the treatment of lung cancer	'Tiredness' and 'loss of energy' were the two most common symptoms, present in over 80% of patients
Irvine et al. (1994)	Convenience sample of 104 patients with mixed cancer diagnoses (mainly breast) about to undergo radiotherapy (55) or chemotherapy (49) in a Canadian hospital	39% fatigued (score >25 on Pearsons Byars Fatigue Feeling Checklist) pretreatment. Post-treatment 61%—similar figures for chemotherapy and radiotherapy
Kurtz et al. (1994)	208 mixed cancer (solid tumour and lymphoma) patients undergoing treatment for new disease or recurrence. All with caregiver prepared to participate	Fatigue reported by 78.4% who survived >1 year, 77.1% who survived 6 months–1 year and 83.9% who survived less than 6 months
Loge et al. (1999)	557 Hodgkin disease survivors identified from cancer centres in Norway	26% of survivors were fatigue cases (<4 on Chalder questionnaire with at least 6 month duration

(continued)

Table 1.2 (continued) Key studies assessing prevalence of fatigue in cancer patients

Study	Population	Prevalence of fatigue
Mendoza et al. (1999)	305 consecutive inpatients and outpatients with cancer presenting to cancer centre in Texas, USA	35% of patients but 5% of controls had 'severe fatigue' (7–10 on Brief Fatigue Inventory)
Nail et al. (1991)	49 patients with cancer receiving chemotherapy in Rochester, USA. Used a self-care diary to report symptoms	2 days after treatment, fatigue was reported in 81%, and was most common symptom
Newell et al. (1998)	204 mixed cancer patients attending outpatients in a medical oncology unit in Australia	66.4% reported fatigue in past week
Ng and von Gunten (1998)	100 consecutive hospice patients admitted acutely to a US teaching hospital	83% weakness, 81% fatigue. Fatigue 'main complaint' in 6%
Richardson and Ream (1996)	109 patients undergoing chemotherapy for mixed cancers in UK. Patients were asked to keep a symptom diary during treatment	90% reported fatigue at some point during diary keeping period
Savage et al. (1997)	430 patients with new onset chronic myeloid leukaemia identified from a UK cancer centre	33.5% had fatigue or lethargy recorded as clinical feature in case notes at presentation
Smets et al. (1998a)	154 consecutive disease-free patients recruited 9 months post radiotherapy	In first 3 months post radiotherapy 32% had moderate fatigue and 19% very much
Smets et al. (1996)	141 patients in Holland in last week of radiotherapy. 134 cancer patients in Scotland undergoing radiotherapy	Dutch sample: 54% moderate or severe tiredness; 31% lack of energy. Scotland: 40% and 35% respectively
Smets et al. (1998b)	250 patients undergoing radiotherapy for various cancers with curative intent interviewed before and 2 weeks after completion of radiotherapy	After treatment: 40% reported feeling tired most of the time during treatment. 44% experienced increase in fatigue, 26% a decrease and 30% no change
Stone et al. (1999)	95 patients with advanced cancer from palliative care services in UK	'Severe subjective fatigue' defined as score of greater than the 95% percentile for a control population present in 75% of patients
Vainio and Auvinen (1996)	1840 mixed cancer patients from seven hospices in USA, Europe and Australia	No direct questions on fatigue. Weakness present in 35–75% of sample depending on site of cancer. Weakness and pain most common two symptoms
Vogelzang et al. (1997)	419 cancer patients who had received chemo- or radiotherapy	78% experienced fatigue during course of disease and treatment. 32% experienced fatigue on daily basis

becomes very complex, but for simplicity we will group the risk factors into sociodemographic factors, disease-specific risk factors, and depression, pain, and disability.

Sociodemographic risk factors for fatigue in cancer

The pattern of increased risk of fatigue among women which was so clearly demonstrated in population-based studies of healthy individuals is not so obvious in cancer-related fatigue. Of nine studies identified which assessed the relationship, five found no difference between men and women (Hickok *et al.* 1996; Smets *et al.* 1998*a*; Glaus 1998; Donnelly *et al.* 1995; Stone *et al.* 1999), whilst the remaining four (Vogelzang *et al.* 1997; Smets *et al.* 1998*b*; Loge *et al.* 1999; Akechi *et al.* 1999) showed that women had more fatigue than men. The key difference between papers which appear to show a difference and those which do not is the disease stage or time from treatment—those that found a difference in rates between men and women tended to have taken samples with earlier disease or 'survivors' in whom the disease had remitted. It may be that with less aggressive or remitted disease, the pattern of fatigue becomes closer to that of the general population.

The pattern of fatigue in cancer according to age is confusing. There might be an expectation that younger cancer patients suffer less fatigue, but Hickok *et al.* (1996) found a U-shaped distribution of fatigue in cancer patients according to age, with fatigue symptoms at their highest in relatively young adults (aged less than 50) and the over 70s. Glaus (1998) found a slightly more complex biphasic relationship, with younger patients having more affective symptoms of fatigue whilst the older group had more physical symptoms of fatigue. Two other studies reported a relationship between age and fatigue—Loge *et al.* (1999) found that older patients were more fatigued and Vogelzang *et al.* (1997) found younger patients were more fatigued. The remaining studies showed no relationship (Andrykowski *et al.* 1998; Smets *et al.* 1998*a*; Stone *et al.* 1999; Cimprich 1999; Hann *et al.* 1999).

One other remaining sociodemographic characteristic was widely studied, namely educational status. Here there appears to be a consistent association, with most studies reporting greater fatigue in the less well educated (Irvine *et al.* 1994; Mast 1998; Loge *et al.* 1999) although, as ever, there are exceptions, with one study (Akechi *et al.* 1999) describing the opposite relationship.

Physical associations with fatigue

Site and stage of disease

Perhaps surprisingly, very few studies have reported associations between site of primary disease and fatigue. One exception is an important study by Glaus (1998) who performed a cross-sectional study on 583 inpatients and outpatients attending a Swiss cancer centre. Lung cancer, melanoma, and ovarian cancer had the highest rates of fatigue, whereas testicular cancer and breast cancer had the lowest. This may be due to the stage of disease— lung cancer, for example, may present later than breast cancer. The same study found a strong association between stage of disease and fatigue, with patients in remission having much less fatigue than those with localized disease, who in turn had less than those with metastatic disease. Glaus' study aimed to address the importance of stage of disease more specifically than many others, but it is none the less worth noting that much of the remaining literature failed to find any relationship between stage of disease and fatigue (Irvine *et al.* 1994; Hickok *et al.* 1996; Loge *et al.* 1999; Stone *et al.* 1999; Hann *et al.* 1999).

Disease activity

Several studies have attempted to link fatigue to other markers of disease activity. These include general measures of nutritional status such as weight and albumin, and tumour-specific markers of disease. In general these studies show disappointingly few clear associations: Mendoza *et al.* (1999) showed a relationship between albumin levels and fatigue for both solid and haematological malignancy, but Monga *et al.* (1999) found no association between fatigue and haematocrit or body weight in patients with carcinoma of the prostate. Monga's study also did not find any association between prostate-specific antigen and fatigue in this group. Similarly Stone *et al.* (1999) found no association between subjective fatigue and malnutrition.

Should we be surprised by the somewhat unspectacular associations between disease activity and fatigue? In a review of the literature Wessely *et al.* (1998) assessed the association between many different physical diseases and fatigue and in general found a consistent lack of association between disease severity and fatigue. This held for renal failure (Brunier and Graydon 1993), heart failure (Wilson *et al.* 1995), Parkinson's disease (Friedman and Friedman 1993), and rheumatoid arthritis (Belza *et al.* 1993; Belza 1995). Whilst all these diseases are *in themselves* powerful risk factors for the development of disabling fatigue, there is little association between disease severity and severity of fatigue, or indeed other important symptoms.

There are probably a number of reasons for this failure to find an association between disease severity and symptom severity. Firstly, it may be an artefact of study design. Many studies selected homogeneous populations of patients among whom the disease status may not vary sufficiently to demonstrate the importance of severity as a risk factor for the symptom. Secondly, most studies are cross-sectional, and a true relationship between disease severity and fatigue may get lost in the 'noise' of interindividual differences. If longitudinal studies were used to follow patients across the course of their illnesses these might demonstrate rather more convincing associations. Thirdly, it may simply be that any association is overwhelmed by the importance of psychological and behavioural factors—the presence of depression, interindividual differences in terms of self-efficacy, the effects of behavioural change and deconditioning, and so on. These factors are addressed later in this chapter.

Anticancer treatments as risk factors for fatigue

Treatment variables have been widely studied and are addressed in greater detail later in this book. Here, a more consistent relationship emerges. Most studies which have followed patients having chemotherapy or radiotherapy throughout the course of their treatment have found that there was a clear association between fatigue symptoms and each cycle of treatment. It is also probably true that chemotherapy is the treatment most strongly associated with fatigue (Mast 1998; Woo *et al.* 1998). Glaus (1998) also noted that patients receiving treatments for other non-cancer ailments had more fatigue, although whether this is due to the treatment *per se* or the presence of co-morbidity is unclear. Where studies have taken groups of cancer patients who have undergone a variety of treatments, perhaps some time before assessment, the pattern with treatment becomes less clear—hence cytotoxic treatments have a clear relationship with acute fatigue, but may be less important as determinants of chronic fatigue (Irvine *et al.* 1994; Andrykowski *et al.* 1998).

Cancer-related fatigue and psychological distress, depression, and disability

Whereas physical markers of fatigue in cancer patients have been difficult to demonstrate consistently, the evidence for an association with depression and anxiety (reviewed in Chapter 10) is overwhelming. Indeed, it is difficult to find studies which have measured cancer-related fatigue and any measure of psychological distress which do *not* report an association. Thus Fulton (1997) reported an association between fatigue and anxiety and depression measured on the Hospital Anxiety and Depression Scale (Zigmond and Snaith 1983), Irvine *et al.* (1994) and Cimprich (1999) found associations with low mood and fatigue, Schneider (1998) found an association with fatigue and depression on the Beck Depression Inventory (Beck *et al.* 1961) and Broeckel *et al.* (1998) showed a strong association between fatigue and common psychiatric diagnoses such as depression and anxiety. Other studies showed similar associations on a variety of measures (Smets *et al.* 1996, 1998*a,b*; Akechi *et al.* 1999; Cimprich 1999). Fatigue is also strongly associated with sleep disturbance (Smets *et al.* 1998*a,b*; Broeckel *et al.* 1998). There has been less written about the role of patients' beliefs and behaviour as risk factors for perpetuating fatigue in cancer, but one study (Broeckel *et al.* 1998) found that in women undergoing chemotherapy for breast cancer, those who had the highest fatigue scores tended to use more 'catastrophizing' coping strategies. This finding might fit into a model of fatigue that suggests that patients' reactions to symptoms are crucial in terms of how disabling such symptoms become.

From a clinical viewpoint, the lack of association (or at least weak association) between disease activity and fatigue and the much stronger association between fatigue and psychological distress suggests that when a patient diagnosed with cancer presents with severe fatigue, an exhaustive physical assessment should be balanced with a detailed psychological one. Naturally the clinician will want to rule out a few specific and readily remedial physical causes of fatigue (such as anaemia); however, a detailed psychosocial assessment should then attempt to rule out the presence of depression and to tease out the patient's view of the meaning behind his or her symptom, and what it stops them from doing. As shown later in this book (Chapter 12) the best approach in patients whose disease status is relatively stable may share much with the cognitive behaviour therapy and graded exercise used in CFS.

Problems with interpretation

Most of the studies reporting associations between fatigue and other variables are cross sectional, so it is usually impossible to determine which comes first. It is also important to consider the range of participants in these studies. As previously noted, there is likely to be considerable heterogeneity in terms of stage and site of disease, treatments received, co-morbidity, and so on. Studies which try to control for this by choosing a single group of patients with a specific severity of disease are unlikely to be able to demonstrate relationships between disease severity and fatigue because there is too little variation of the variables under study. This may in part account for some of the negative finding discussed above, and the studies with the widest range of cancer patients have tended to find greater associations between fatigue and markers of disease severity.

A further problem of interpretation comes from the inter-relatedness of many of the variables. Pain, fatigue, and depression are all strongly associated in the general population (Hotopf *et al.* 1998). Disability, activity levels, quality of life, and physical markers of disease activity also strongly covary. It is therefore difficult to extract a single specific variable which is particularly associated with fatigue, and the strong association between variables may limit the usefulness of observational studies. Instead the future may lie in intervention studies which aim to modify specific risk factors (such as depression or inactivity) to determine whether such interventions have useful effects on fatigue.

Models of fatigue

Models have been developed for the development of fatigue in non-cancer and cancer patients. Our review of fatigue unrelated to cancer indicates that predisposed individuals (perhaps with a genetic vulnerability, previous experience of ill-health in childhood, or a past psychiatric disorder) who are confronted by an acute stressor (for example a serious viral illness, surgery, or stress from a life event) may develop fatigue, and this fatigue is more likely to become chronic if they respond by changing their lifestyle to avoid activities, become depressed, or harbour strong beliefs that the fatigue is due to a defined physical process (Fig. 1.1). Such behaviours and beliefs may lead to worsening inactivity and deconditioning, with the consequence that further attempts at resuming activity lead to worsening fatigue. The key points here are that the precipitating event may very well be a defined physical illness, but the perpetuating factors may be cognitive, behavioural, and emotional.

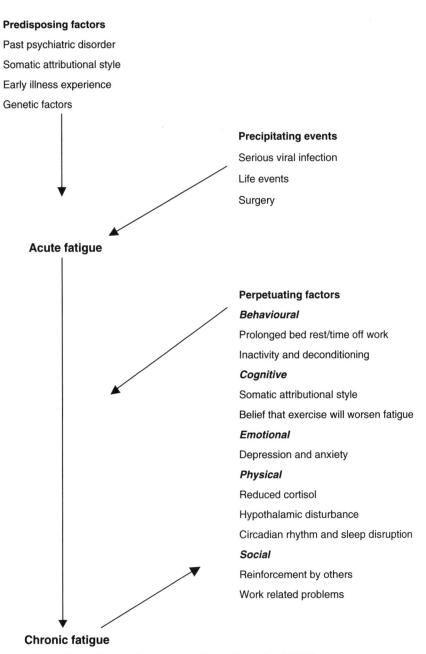

Predisposing factors

Past psychiatric disorder

Somatic attributional style

Early illness experience

Genetic factors

Precipitating events

Serious viral infection

Life events

Surgery

Acute fatigue

Perpetuating factors

Behavioural

Prolonged bed rest/time off work

Inactivity and deconditioning

Cognitive

Somatic attributional style

Belief that exercise will worsen fatigue

Emotional

Depression and anxiety

Physical

Reduced cortisol

Hypothalamic disturbance

Circadian rhythm and sleep disruption

Social

Reinforcement by others

Work related problems

Chronic fatigue

Fig. 1.1 Scheme for understanding fatigue (adapted from Fox (1998)).

This model predicts that it may be possible to ameliorate the fatigue by changing perpetuating factors, and two treatments which do this have now been shown to be effective. Graded exercise has been demonstrated to be effective in two randomized controlled trials (Fulcher and White 1997; Wearden *et al.* 1998). Cognitive behaviour therapy (CBT) also aims to change the cycle of perpetuating factors by encouraging increases in activity, and randomized trials have now found that it is more effective than 'usual care' (Sharpe *et al.* 1996) or relaxation (Deale *et al.* 1997).

In cancer there have also been theoretical models. Piper *et al.* (1987) suggested that there were a number of objective (physiological, biochemical, and behavioural) indicators of fatigue which would be determined by a wide range of different factors (Fig. 1.2). This has much in common with the biopsychosocial approach beloved by psychiatrists. Thus 'accumulation of metabolites', 'sleep–wake patterns', 'psychological patterns', and 'life event patterns', are all factors which might influence one or other of the fatigue manifestations at the centre of the model. The model has the advantage of being inclusive, but it is perhaps over-inclusive in its range and insufficiently specific in its predictions for these to be readily tested.

Winningham *et al.* (1994) describe previous models of fatigue before discussing their psychobiological entropy model. This is more explicit than Piper's model, and therefore provides a more readily testable framework (Fig. 1.3). It views decreases in activity as central in determining whether 'primary symptoms' lead to what is viewed as 'secondary fatigue'. Secondary fatigue then leads to decreased functional status and disability. Disease and treatments for the disease are viewed as two main contributors to both primary symptoms and decreased functional activity.

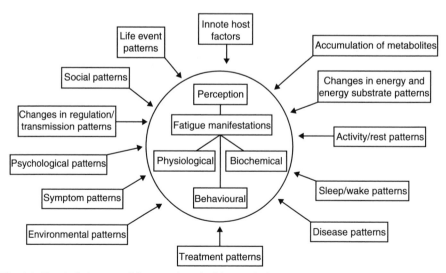

Fig. 1.2 Piper's fatigue model. Reproduced with permission.

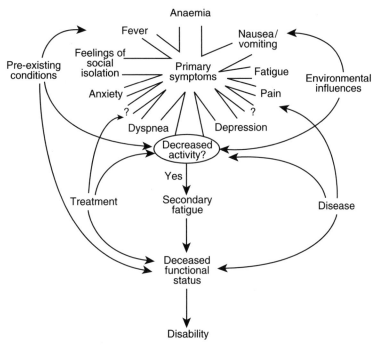

Fig. 1.3 Winningham's fatigue model. Permission sought.

Wessely *et al.* (1998) provided a general model for understanding the interdependences of different factors which might lead to fatigue in physical illness. This model (Fig. 1.4) views physical illness as acting on four main pathways which lead to fatigue. These include:

- via treatment (which we have seen is an important mechanism in cancer);
- via direct physical mechanisms of the illness;
- via depression; and
- via pain.

Sleep disturbance and behavioural avoidance and deconditioning are mediating factors between the latter two factors and fatigue. This model suggests that whilst some of the fatigue of physical illness may be essentially immutable unless the disease activity can be modified, interventions which have an impact on pain and depression might modify fatigue symptoms.

Are these models useful? To be helpful models need to have predictive validity—in other words, there needs to be evidence that one 'upstream' component of the model has an effect on 'downstream' components, and that this effect is reproducible in different settings. So far the predictive validity of the cancer models is questionable. To be helpful models also need to generate testable hypotheses regarding the relationship

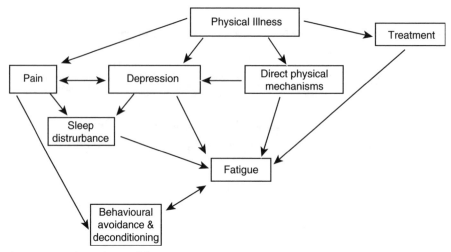

Fig. 1.4 Wessely *et al.*'s model.

between variables, and these are insufficiently explicit in most models we have reviewed. Finally models should be parsimonious—in other words involve the fewest possible variables to explain the most fatigue. Research into fatigue is too limited so far to allow such parsimony, but this should be an aspiration.

Future research

Future research into the epidemiology and causes of fatigue in cancer should be informed by progress in the non-cancer population. There are often multiple candidate variables in assessing the cause of fatigue. Should researchers be reductionist and focus on relatively few variables, perhaps ones they understand best, and risk missing other important pathways? Or should researchers risk being over-inclusive and being unable to sift out key predictors from the confusing morass of candidates? There is no easy answer to this, but researchers need to examine the existing literature closely, and decide whether their inclusion of a variable is in order to test or replicate a previous finding or to generate novel hypotheses. When there is such a risk of data overload, and candidate variables may covary considerably, one approach is to use an experimental rather than an observational approach, and attempt to alter a single specific variable. Thus, if we thought that fatigue was primarily caused by physical deconditioning, it would be reasonable to test the effects of interventions which sought to reverse this process. Box 1.1 summarizes the situation.

Conclusions

What conclusions can be drawn from this brief synopsis of the epidemiology and models for cancer and non-cancer-related fatigue? Firstly, fatigue is common and is

Box 1.1 Future areas for research

◆ Longitudinal research on fatigue in cancer is required in order to determine the natural history and course of the symptom.

◆ Research should reflect the multiple causes of fatigue by measuring a range of biological, psychological, and social variables simultaneously.

◆ Where there may be multiple candidate causes of fatigue, intervention studies which aim to alter one specific component can give useful information on the aetiology of fatigue as well as its treatment.

best viewed as a continuum. Secondly, fatigue is an especially troublesome symptom—which in the cancer literature is frequently described as similar to pain in terms of the level of distress it can cause. Thirdly, there are relatively few consistent physical determinants of fatigue in cancer—in particular, disease severity is surprisingly weakly linked with fatigue, and although cancer treatments have relatively powerful associations with acute fatigue, these associations tend to decrease over time. Fourthly, depression and anxiety are strongly associated with fatigue in cancer patients, as indeed they are in the general population. The literature on chronic idiopathic fatigue suggests that intermediary factors such as fear of activities worsening fatigue and physical deconditioning may be important, and may also be ameliorated with behavioural interventions. A key question for researchers and clinicians is whether such interventions can help cancer patients with debilitating fatigue. Above all, fatigue is an integrative phenomenon—many factors probably act and interact to cause the symptom. The key clinical corollary of this is that most of the time, for most patients, fatigue is unlikely to be explained by a single underlying cause. Box 1.2 summarizes our discussions.

Box 1.2 Summary points

◆ Fatigue may be viewed either as a decrement in performance or a feeling state.

◆ Fatigue is a common symptom in the general population, which is best viewed as a continuum.

◆ Fatigue is nearly always multifactorial.

◆ There are many different candidate causes for fatigue in cancer; disease activity is a relatively weak predictor, whereas fatigue is strongly associated with depression in cancer.

◆ Models of fatigue have weak predictive validity.

References

Akechi, T., Kugaya, A., Okamura, H., Yamawaki, S., and Uchitomi, Y. (1999) Fatigue and its associated factors in ambulatory cancer patients: a preliminary study. *Journal of Pain and Symptom Management*, **17**, 42–8.

Andrykowski, M.A., Curran, S.L., and Lightner, R. (1998) Off-treatment fatigue in breast cancer survivors: a controlled comparison. *Journal of Behavioral Medicine*, **21**, 1–18.

Ashbury, F.D., Findlay, H., Reynolds, B., and McKerracher, K. (1998) A Canadian survey of cancer patients' experiences: are their needs being met? *Journal of Pain and Symptom Management*, **16**, 298–306.

Bates, D.W., Schmitt, W., Buchwald, D., Ware, N.C., Lee, J., Thoyer, E. *et al.* (1993) Prevalence of fatigue and chronic fatigue syndrome in a primary care practice. *Archives of Internal Medicine*, **153**, 2759–65.

Beck, A.T., Ward, C.H., and Mendelson, M. (1961) An inventory for measuring depression. *Archives of General Psychiatry*, **4**, 561–71.

Belza, B.L. (1995) Comparison of self report fatigue in rheumatoid arthritis and controls. *Journal of Rheumatology*, **22**, 639–43.

Belza, B.L., Henke, C.J., Yelin, E.H., Epstein, W.V., and Gilliss, C.L. (1993) Correlates of fatigue in older adults with rheumatoid arthritis. *Nursing Research*, **42**, 93–9.

Berelowitz, G.J., Burgess, A.P., Thanabalasingham, T., Murray-Lyon, I.M., and Wright, D.J.M. (1995) Post-hepatitis syndrome revisited. *Journal of Viral Hepatitis*, **2**, 133–8.

Bladé, J., Kyle, R.A., and Greipp, P.R. (1996) Presenting features and prognosis in 72 patients with multiple myeloma who were younger than 40 years. *British Journal of Haematology*, **93**, 345–51.

Bombardier, C.H. and Buchwald, D. (1995) Outcome and prognosis of patients with chronic fatigue vs chronic fatigue syndrome. *Archives of Internal Medicine*, **155**, 2105–10.

Broeckel, J.A., Jacobsen, P.B., Horton, J., Balducci, L., and Lyman, G.H. (1998) Characteristics and correlates of fatigue after adjuvant chemotherapy for breast cancer. *Journal of Clinical Oncology*, **16**, 1689–96.

Brown, G.W. and Harris, T.O. (1978) *Social Origins of Depression: a Study of Psychiatric Disorder in Women*. Tavistock Publications, London.

Bruce-Jones, W.D.A., White, P.D., Thomas, J.M., and Clare, A.W. (1994) The effect of social adversity on the fatigue syndrome, psychiatric disorders and physical recovery, following glandular fever. *Psychological Medicine*, **24**, 651–9.

Brunier, G.M. and Graydon, J. (1993) The influence of physical activity on fatigue in patients with ESRD on hemodialysis. *ANNA Journal*, **20**, 457–61.

Buchwald, D., Umali, P., Umali, J., Kith, P., Pearlman, T., and Kormaroff, A.L. (1995) Chronic fatigue and the chronic fatigue syndrome: prevalence in a Pacific Northwest Health Care System. *Annals of Internal Medicine*, **123**(2), 81–8.

Calder, B.D., Warnock, P.J., McCartney, R.A., and Bell, E.J. (1987) Coxsackie B viruses and the post viral fatigue syndrome: a prospective study in general practice. *Journal of the Royal College of General Practitioners*, **37**, 11–14.

Cathebras, P.J., Robbins, J.M., Kirmayer, L.J., and Hayton, B.C. (1992) Fatigue in primary care: prevalence, psychiatric comorbidity, illness behaviour and outcome. *Journal of General Internal Medicine*, **7**, 276–86.

Chalder, T. (1998) *Factors Affecting the Development and Maintenance of Fatigue in Primary Care*. University of London.

Chalder, T., Power, M.J., and Wessely, S. (1996) Chronic fatigue in the community: 'A question of attribution'. *Psychological Medicine*, **26**, 791–800.

Cicchetti, D.V. and Prussoff, B.A. (1983) Reliability of depression and associated clinical symptoms. *Archives of General Psychiatry*, **40**, 987–90.

Cimprich, B. (1999) Pretreatment symptom distress in women newly diagnosed with breast cancer. *Cancer Nursing*, **22**, 185–94.

Clark, R.R., Katon, W., Russo, J., Kith, P., Sintay, M., and Buchwald, D. (1995) Chronic fatigue: risk factors for symptom persistence in a 2 1/2 year follow-up study. *American Journal of Medicine*, **98, 187–95.**

Cox, B., Blaxter, M., and Buckle, A. (1987) *The Health and Lifestyle Survey*, 1st edn. Health Promotion Research Trust, London.

David, A., Pelosi, A., McDonald, E., Stephens, D., Ledger, D., Rathbone, R. *et al.* (1990) Tired, weak or in need of rest: fatigue among general practice attenders. *British Medical Journal*, **301**, 1199–202.

Deale, A., Chalder, T., Marks, I., and Wessely, S. (1997) A randomised controlled trial of cognitive behaviour versus relaxation therapy for chronic fatigue syndrome. *American Journal of Psychiatry*, **154**, 408–14.

Degner, L.F. and Sloan, J.A. (1995) Symptom distress in newly diagnosed ambulatory cancer patients and as a predictor of survival in lung cancer. *Journal of Pain and Symptom Management*, **10**, 423–31.

Dohrenwend, B.P. and Crandell, D.L. (1970) Psychiatric symptoms in community, clinic and mental hospital groups. *American Journal of Psychiatry*, **126**(11), 87–94.

Donnelly, S., Walsh, D., and Rybicki, L. (1995) The symptoms of advanced cancer: identification of clinical and research priorities by assessment of prevalence and severity. *Journal of Palliative Care*, **11**, 27–32.

Euba, R., Chalder, T., Deale, A., and Wessely, S. (1996) A comparison of the characteristics of chronic fatigue syndrome in primary and tertiary care. *British Journal of Psychiatry*, **168**, 121–6.

Farmer, A., Scourfield, J., Martin, N., Cardno, A., and McGuffin, P. (1999) Is disabling fatigue in childhood influenced by genes? *Psychological Medicine*, **29**, 279–82.

Fischler, B., Cluydts, R., De Gucht, V., Kaufman, L., and De Meirleir, K. (1997) Generalized anxiety disorder in chronic fatigue syndrome. *Acta Psychiatrica Scandinavica*, **95**, 405–13.

Fox, R. (1998) *A Research Portfolio on Chronic Fatigue*, 1st edn. London: Royal Society of Medicine Press.

Friedman, J. and Friedman, H. (1993) Fatigue in Parkinson's disease. *Neurology*, **43**, 2016–19.

Fukuda, K., Dobbins, J.G., Wilson, L.J., Dunn, R.A., Wilcox, K., and Smallwood, D. (1997) An epidemiologic study of fatigue with relevance to the chronic fatigue syndrome. *Journal of Psychiatric Research*, **31**, 19–29.

Fulcher, K.Y. and White, P.D. (1997) A randomised controlled trial of graded exercise therapy in patients with the chronic fatigue syndrome. *British Medical Journal*, **314**, 1647–52.

Fulton, C.L. (1997) The physical and psychological symptoms experienced by patients with metastatic breast cancer before death. *European Journal of Cancer Care (English Language Edition)*, **6:4**, 262–6.

Gandevia, S.C., Enoka, R.M., McComas, A.J., Stuart, D.G., and Thomas, C.K. (1996) *Fatigue: Neural and Muscular Mechanisms*. Plenum Press, New York.

Glaus, A. (1998) Fatigue in patients with cancer. *Recent Results in Cancer Research*, **145**, 105–50.

Hann, D.M., Garovoy, N., Finkelstein, B., Jacobsen, P.B., Azzarello, L.M., and Fields, K.K. (1999) Fatigue and quality of life in breast cancer patients undergoing autologous stem cell transplantation: a longitudinal comparative study. *Journal of Pain and Symptom Management*, **17**, 311–19.

Hellinger, W.C., Smith, T.F., Van Scoy, R.E., Spitzer, P.G., Forgacs, P., and Edson, R.S. (1988) Chronic fatigue syndrome and the diagnostic utility of antibody to Epstein–Barr virus early antigen. *Journal of the American Medical Association*, **260**, 971–3.

Hickie, I., Kirk, K., and Martin, N. (1999) Unique genetic and environmental determinants of prolonged fatigue: a twin study. *Psychological Medicine*, **29**, 259–68.

Hickok, J.T., Morrow, G.R., McDonald, S., and Bellg, A.J. (1996) Frequency and correlates of fatigue in lung cancer patients receiving radiation therapy: implications for management. *Journal of Pain and Symptom Management*, **11**, 370–7.

Hopwood, P. and Stephens, R.J. (1995) Symptoms at presentation for treatment in patients with lung cancer: implications for the evaluation of palliative treatment. *British Journal of Cancer*, **71**, 633–6.

Hotopf, M.H., Noah, N., and Wessely, S. (1996) Chronic fatigue and psychiatric morbidity following viral meningitis: a controlled study. *Journal of Neurology Neurosurgery and Psychiatry*, **60**, 504–9.

Hotopf, M., Mayou, R., Wadsworth, M.E.J., and Wessely, S. (1998) Temporal relationships between physical symptoms and psychiatric disorder. Results from a national birth cohort. *British Journal of Psychiatry*, **173**, 255–61.

Hotopf, M., Mayou, R., Wadsworth, M., and Wessely, S. (1999*a*) Psychosocial and developmental antecedents of chest pain in young adults. *Psychosomatic Medicine*, **61**, 861–7.

Hotopf, M., Mayou, R., Wadsworth, M., and Wessely, S. (1999*b*) Childhood risk factors for adult medically unexplained symptoms: results of a national birth cohort study. *American Journal of Psychiatry*, **156**, 1796–800.

Hotopf, M., Wilson-Jones, C., Mayou, R., Wadsworth, M., and Wessely, S. (2000) Childhood predictors of adult medically unexplained hospitalisations. Results from a national birth cohort study. *British Journal of Psychiatry*, **176**, 273–80.

Irvine, D., Vincent, L., Graydon, J.E., Bubela, N., and Thompson, L. (1994) The prevalence and correlates of fatigue in patients receiving treatment with chemotherapy and radiotherapy. *Cancer Nursing*, **17**, 367–78.

Joyce, J., Hotopf, M., and Wessely, S. (1997) The prognosis of chronic fatigue and chronic fatigue syndrome: a systematic review. *Quarterly Journal of Medicine*, **90**, 223–33.

Katon, W., Buchwald, D., Simon, G., Russo, J., and Mease, P. (1991) Psychiatric illness in patients with chronic fatigue and rheumatoid arthritis. *Journal of General Internal Medicine*, **6**, 277–85.

Kroenke, K. and Price, R.K. (1993) Symptoms in the community: prevalence, classification, and psychiatric comorbidity. *Archives of Internal Medicine*, **153**, 2474–80.

Kroenke, K., Arrington, M.E., and Mangelsdorff, A.D. (1990) The prevalence of symptoms in medical outpatients and the adequacy of therapy. *Archives of Internal Medicine*, **150**, 1685–9.

Kurtz, M.E., Given, B., Kurtz, J.C., and Given, C.W. (1994) The interaction of age, symptoms, and survival status on physical and mental health of patients with cancer and their families. *Cancer*, **74**, 2071–8.

Lawrie, S.M. and Pelosi, A.J. (1995) Chronic fatigue syndrome in the community: prevalence and associations. *British Journal of Psychiatry*, **166**, 793–7.

Lawrie, S.M., Manders, D.N., Geddes, J.R., and Pelosi, A.J. (1997) A population-based incidence study of chronic fatigue. *Psychological Medicine*, **27**, 343–53.

Lewis, G., Pelosi, A.J., Araya, R., and Dunn, G. (1992) Measuring psychiatric disorder in the community: a standardised assessment for lay interviewers. *Psychological Medicine*, **22**, 465–86.

Loge, J.H., Abrahamsen, A.F., Ekeberg, O., and Kaasa, S. (1999) Hodgkin's disease survivors more fatigued than the general population. *Journal of Clinical Oncology*, **17**, 253–61.

Mast, M.E. (1998) Correlates of fatigue in survivors of breast cancer. *Cancer Nursing*, **21**, 136–42.

Meltzer, H., Gill, B., and Petticrew, M. (1995) The prevalence of psychiatric morbidity among adults aged 16–64, living in private households, in Great Britain. *OPCS Surveys of Psychiatric Morbidity in Great Britain 1995*, Bulletin 1.

Mendoza, T.R., Wang, X.S., Cleeland, C.S., Morrissey, M., Johnson, B.A., Wendt, J.K. *et al.* (1999) The rapid assessment of fatigue severity in cancer patients: use of the brief fatigue inventory. *Cancer*, **85**, 1186–96.

Monga, U., Kerrigan, A.J., Thornby, J., and Monga, T.N. (1999) Prospective study of fatigue in localized prostate cancer patients undergoing radiotherapy. *Radiation Oncology Investigations*, **7**, 178–85.

Nail, L.M., Jones, L.S., Greene, D., Schipper, D.L., and Jensen, R. (1991) Use and perceived efficacy of self-care activities in patients receiving chemotherapy. *Oncology Nursing Forum*, **18**, 883–7.

Newell, S., Sanson-Fisher, R.W., Girgis, A., and Bonaventura, A. (1998) How well do medical oncologists' perceptions reflect their patients' reported physical and psychosocial problems? *Cancer*, **83**, 1640–51.

Ng, K. and von Gunten, C.F. (1998) Symptoms and attitudes of 100 consecutive patients admitted to an acute hospice/palliative care unit. *Journal of Pain and Symptom Management*, **16**, 307–16.

Ozguler, A., Leclerc, A., Landre, M.-F., Pietri-Taleb, F., and Niedhammer, I. (2000) Individual and occupational determinants of low back pain according to various definitions of low back pain. *Journal of Epidemiology and Community Health*, **54**, 215–20.

Pawlikowska, T., Chalder, T., Hirsch, S.R., Wallace, P., Wright, D.J.M., and Wessely, S.C. (1994) Population based study of fatigue and psychological distress. *British Medical Journal*, **308**, 763–6.

Pepper, C.M., Krupp, L.B., Friedberg, F., Doscher, C., and Coyle, P.K. (1993) A comparison of neuropsychiatric characteristics in chronic fatigue syndrome, multiple sclerosis, and major depression. *Journal of Neuropsychiatry*, **5**(2), 200–5.

Piper, B.F., Lindsey, A.M., and Dodd, M.J. (1987) Fatigue mechanisms in cancer patients: developing nursing theory [Review with 60 references]. *Oncology Nursing Forum*, **14**(6), 17–23.

Reyes, M., Nisenbaum, R., Hoaglin, D.C., Unger, E.R., Emmons, C., Randall, B. *et al.* (2003) Prevalence and incidence of chronic fatigue syndrome in Wichita, Kansas. *Archives of Internal Medicine*, **163:13**, 1530–6.

Richardson, A. and Ream, E. (1996) The experience of fatigue and other symptoms in patients receiving chemotherapy. *European Journal of Cancer Care*, **5**(Supplement 2), 24–30.

Savage, D.G., Szydlo, R.M., and Goldman, J.M. (1997) Clinical features and diagnosis in 430 patients with chronic myeloid leukaemia seen at a referral centre over a 16-year period. *British Journal of Haematology*, **96**, 111–16.

Schneider, R.A. (1998) Concurrent validity of the Beck Depression Inventory and the Multidimensional Fatigue Inventory-20 in assessing fatigue among cancer patients. *Psychological Reports*, **82**, 883–6.

Shahar, E. and Lederer, J. (1990) Asthenic symptoms in a rural family practice. *Journal of Family Practice*, **31**(2), 257–62.

Sharpe, M., Archnard, L.C., and Banatvala, J.E. (1991) A report—chronic fatigue syndrome, guidelines for research. *Journal of the Royal Society of Medicine*, **84**, 118–21.

Sharpe, M., Hawton, K., Seagroatt, V., and Pasvol, G. (1992) Follow up of patients presenting with fatigue to an infectious diseases clinic. *British Medical Journal*, **305**, 147–52.

Sharpe, M., Hawton, K., Simkin, S., Surawy, C., Hackmann, A., Klimes, I. *et al.* (1996) Cognitive therapy for chronic fatigue syndrome, a randomized controlled trial. *British Medical Journal*, **312**, 22–6.

Smets, E.M.A., Garssen, B., Cull, A., and de Haes, H.C.J.M. (1996) Application of the multidimensional fatigue inventory (MFI-20) in cancer patients receiving radiotherapy. *British Journal of Cancer*, **73**, 241–5.

Smets, E.M.A., Willems-Groot, A.F.M.N., Garssen, B., Oldenberger, F., van Tienhoven, G., and de Haes, H.C.J.M. (1998a) Fatigue and radiotherapy, (A) experience in patients undergoing treatment. *British Journal of Cancer*, **78**, 899–906.

Smets, E.M.A., Willems-Groot, A.F.M.N., Schuster-Uitterhoeve, A.L.J., and de Haes, J.C.J.M. (1998b) Fatigue and radiotherapy, (B) experience in patients 9 months following treatment. *British Journal of Cancer*, **78**, 907–12.

Stone, P., Hardy, J., Broadley, K., Tookman, A.J., Kurowska, A., and Ahern, R. (1999) Fatigue in advanced cancer: a prospective controlled cross-sectional study. *British Journal of Cancer*, **79**, 1479–86.

Turk, D.C. and Fernandez, E. (1990) On the putative uniqueness of cancer pain: do psychological principles apply? *Behaviour Research and Therapy*, **28**, 1–13.

Vaino, A. and Auvinen, A. (1996) Prevalence of symptoms among patients with advanced cancer: an international collaborative study. *Journal of Pain and Symptom Management*, **12**, 3–10.

van der Linden G, Chalder T, Hickie I, Koschera A, Sham PC, Wessely S. (1999) Fatigue and psychiatric disorder: different or the same? *Psychological Medicine*, **29**, 863–8.

Vogelzang, N.J., Breitbart, W., Cella, D., Curt, G.A., Groopman, J.E., Horning, S.J. *et al.* (1997) Patient, caregiver, and oncologist perceptions of cancer-related fatigue: results from a tripart assessment survey. *Seminars in Hematology*, **34**, 4–12.

Wearden, A., Morriss, R., Mullis, R., Strickland, P., Pearson, D., Appleby, L. *et al.* (1998) Randomised, double-blind, placebo-controlled treatment trial of fluoxetine and graded exercise for chronic fatigue syndrome. [comment] [erratum appears in Br J Psychiatry 1998, **173**, 89]. *British Journal of Psychiatry*, **172**, 485–90.

Wells, K.B., Stewart, A., Hays, R.D., Burman, A., Rogers, W., Daniels, M. *et al.* (1989) The functioning and well-being of depressed patients: results from the medical outcomes study. *Journal of the American Medical Association*, **262**, 914–19.

Wessely, S. and Powell, R. (1989) Fatigue syndromes: a comparison of chronic 'postviral' fatigue with neuromuscular and affective disorders. *Journal of Neurology, Neurosurgery and Psychiatry*, **52**, 940–8.

Wessely, S., Chalder, T., Hirsch, S., Palikowska, T., Wallace, P., and Wright, D.J.M. (1995) Post-infectious fatigue: prospective cohort study in primary care. *The Lancet*, **345**, 1333–8.

Wessely, S., Chalder, T., Hirsch, S., Wallace, P., and Wright, D. (1997) The prevalence and morbidity of chronic fatigue and chronic fatigue syndrome: a prospective primary care study. *American Journal of Public Health*, **87**, 1449–55.

Wessely, S., Hotopf, M., and Sharpe, M. (1998) *Chronic Fatigue and its Syndromes*, 1st edn. Oxford University Press, Oxford.

Wessely, S., Nimnuan, C., and Sharpe, M. (1999) Functional somatic syndromes:one or many? *The Lancet*, **354**, 936–9.

White, P.D., Thomas, J.M., Amess, J., Crawford, D.H., Grover, S., Kangro, H. *et al.* (1998) Incidence, risk and prognosis of acute and chronic fatigue syndromes and psychiatric disorders after glandular fever. *British Journal of Psychiatry*, **173**, 475–81.

Wilson, A., Hickie, I., Lloyd, A., Hadzi-Pavlovic, D., Boughton, C., Dwyer, J. *et al.* (1994) Longitudinal study of outcome of chronic fatigue syndrome. *British Medical Journal*, **308**, 756–9.

Wilson, J.R., Rayos, G., Gothard, P., and Bak, K. (1995) Dissociation between exertional symptoms and circulatory function in patients with heart failure. *Circulation*, **92**, 47–53.

Winningham, M.L., Nail, L.M., Burke, M.B., Brophy, L., Cimprich, B., Jones, L.S. *et al.* (1994) Fatigue and the cancer experience: the state of the knowledge [Review with 45 references]. *Oncology Nursing Forum*, **21**(1), 23–36.

Woo, B., Dibble, S.L., Piper, B.F., Keating, S.B., and Weiss, M.C. (1998) Differences in fatigue by treatment methods in women with breast cancer. *Oncology Nursing Forum*, **25**, 915–20.

Wood, G.C., Bentall, R.P., Gopfert, M., and Edwards, R.H.T. (1991) A comparative psychiatric assessment of patients with chronic fatigue syndrome and muscle disease. *Psychological Medicine*, **21**, 619–28.

Zigmond, A.S. and Snaith, R.P. (1983) The Hospital Anxiety and Depression Scale. *Acta Psychiatrica Scandinavica*, **67**, 361–70.

Chapter 2

A critical appraisal of the factors associated with fatigue

Alison Richardson

Introduction

The factors that cause fatigue and the exact mechanisms responsible for its production, sustenance, or amelioration are not well understood. However, multiple correlates and mechanisms have been proposed in the literature and integrated within models of cancer-related fatigue. These were introduced and discussed in Chapter 1. Such models have been developed by nurse scientists and scholars from complementary disciplines whilst attempting to understand the fatigue experienced by both healthy and acutely or chronically ill client populations. Based on these models, multiple causative factors or correlates of fatigue have been suggested. In this chapter a review of the pattern of fatigue in response to the treatments commonly employed to cure and control cancer will be presented and symptom correlates of cancer-related fatigue, as suggested by these models, will be discussed. Rather than present an exhaustive picture of the multiple factors that have been identified in previous empirical work and reviews, this chapter will appraise symptoms that have been consistently identified as holding some degree of significance. As other chapters in this book will critique the relationship between fatigue and anorexia/weight loss (Chapter 4) and fatigue and mood state (Chapter 10) such studies will not be revisited here.

Treatment-related fatigue

Surgery

Surgery can be used for prevention, diagnosis, definitive treatment, rehabilitation, or palliation and most patients with cancer will undergo surgery of some kind at least once. It remains the treatment of choice for many tumours, and it is not unusual for patients to undergo several surgical procedures for diagnosis and initial treatment of cancer. Whilst fatigue is a consistent finding in individuals recovering from all types of surgery (Christensen *et al.* 1985) and is generally assumed to have multiple causes, in-depth investigations in large samples of patients with cancer have not been conducted. Much of what we know (or extrapolate) is derived from studies with general surgical populations, in particular those undergoing elective abdominal surgery, and hence the specific pattern and profile of fatigue after cancer surgery is not clear. Surgical procedures performed for reasons unrelated to malignancy are associated with fatigue in the immediate postoperative period, and it persists for over a month (Petersson *et al.* 1990). The anaesthetic and surgical literature generally assumes that postoperative fatigue has a physical basis. One view intensely investigated is that it results from changes in muscle physiology, but attempts to identify changes which relate to fatigue have been contradictory (Christensen and Kehlet 1984; Christensen *et al.* 1987; Zeiderman *et al.* 1990). There is an association of fatigue with various cardiorespiratory parameters, including pulse rate (during orthostatic stress), oxygen consumption, and heart rate (following exercise on a bicycle ergometer) (Rose and King 1978; Christensen *et al.* 1982, 1989; Zeiderman *et al.* 1990).

The lack of consistent findings has resulted in the more recent suggestion that there may be an alternative physiological basis, arising from the view that fatigue is part of a general stress response to surgery and that, specifically, it might be related to the hormonal response to surgery. Pick *et al.* (1994) tested the link between fatigue and the catecholamine and emotional response to surgery. They determined, in a group of patients having coronary artery bypass surgery, that postoperative fatigue had both physiological and psychological correlates. Whilst results did little to illuminate the basis of fatigue early in the postoperative period, the study did reveal a link between perioperative noradrenaline levels and fatigue 1 month postoperatively. This study serves to emphasize the fact that different factors might play a role in the development and maintenance of fatigue, depending on the time that has elapsed since surgery was performed. There have also been attempts to predict the intensity of postoperative fatigue based on preoperative factors (Schroeder and Hill 1993). In this study the best predictor of postoperative fatigue was preoperative fatigue, with lesser but none the less significant correlations observed with diagnosis (especially cancer); preoperative weight, particularly total body protein; weight loss; grip strength; and age. The authors concluded that those presenting for surgery were more likely to suffer fatigue in the postoperative period if they were elderly, had a diagnosis of cancer, and had depleted body protein reserves. A more productive approach in searching for factors associated with surgical fatigue might entail viewing it as an aspect of perioperative emotional distress. Thus, complaints of fatigue postoperatively may reflect a tendency to complain of fatigue or negative mood preoperatively, rather than be attributable to surgical trauma.

Levels of fatigue in those undergoing diagnostic breast biopsy and subsequent surgery have been studied by Stanton and Snider (1993). Scores 24 h (Time 1) prebiopsy were similar in both groups, but women who received a diagnosis of cancer postbiopsy were more fatigued than those in whom the biopsy proved benign (Time 2). This assessment was undertaken 24 h prior to surgery in those with cancer and after a similar amount of time had elapsed in the benign group. Distress provoked as a result of a cancer diagnosis appeared related to fatigue. Three weeks after surgery (Time 3), women with breast cancer were significantly more fatigued than the women with benign disease who did not undergo surgery. The fact that cancer patients' fatigue remained elevated postsurgery might have resulted directly from the demands of diagnostic and surgical procedures. Cimprich (1992) has studied the attentional component of fatigue in women following surgery for breast cancer. More recently she has reported that age and more extensive surgery increase the likelihood of loss of attention, due, in part, to a greater risk of attentional fatigue (Cimprich 1998). Whilst her work has made an important contribution to the study of the discrete dimensions of fatigue in patients with cancer, the use of breast cancer as a model of postoperative fatigue in patients with cancer is limited for a number of reasons. These are that it does not reflect many of the physical aspects associated with major surgery, it tends to be technically standardized and performed in those who are predominately female, of a certain age range, and are in relatively good health. The propensity of other surgical populations to experience fatigue in either the pre- or postoperative period remains under-investigated. An exception to this is the study by Forsberg *et al.* (1996), who asked patients with colon, rectal, and stomach cancer to complete a battery of instruments both before surgery and 6 weeks postoperatively. Similar levels of fatigue were identified as always or often present before and after surgery (43% versus 49%), and there was very little difference in the pattern of symptoms identified on a checklist before and after surgery. Following surgery for cancer of the colon, the presence of fatigue prior to discharge has been confirmed by Galloway and Graydon (1996).

It can be seen that research is incomplete in describing the amount, qualities, and resolution of surgically associated fatigue in those with cancer. The possible cumulative effects of multiple surgical procedures on both the severity and duration of postoperative fatigue remain unstudied. The increasing use of other therapies in the pre- and postoperative phase adds to the complexity when identifying both cause(s) and course. Finally, the changing qualitative nature of fatigue in the postoperative period has not been studied in any depth. Future studies should pay attention to issues of measurement, in particular capturing the different dimensions of fatigue, charting its course over time, and examining associations with physical and mental health, both pre- and postoperatively.

Radiotherapy

Radiotherapy forms an essential component of many treatment protocols. It is used as a primary treatment, as an adjunct to other strategies such as surgery and/or chemotherapy, and has an important role to play in terms of palliation. It is very versatile in that it may be administered either through external radiation (teletherapy), interstitial implants, intracavitary treatment, and as systemic therapy (brachytherapy).

The association between radiotherapy and fatigue was first documented, empirically, in the seminal study of Haylock and Hart (1979). A steady stream of studies followed in the 1980s, which sought to examine both the incidence and course of this symptom, particularly during external beam therapy (Kubricht 1984; King *et al.* 1985; Kobashi-Schoot *et al.* 1985). Further work during the 1990s has extended our knowledge base (Blesch *et al.* 1991; Greenberg *et al.* 1992; Irvine *et al.* 1994, 1998; Hickock *et al.* 1996; Munro and Potter 1996; Mock *et al.* 1997; Hann *et al.* 1998; Smets *et al.* 1998*a*,*b*,*c*; Miaskowski and Lee 1999). A summary of key prospective studies is presented in Table 2.1. From such a synthesis it is possible to draw conclusions about certain aspects related to onset, frequency, and duration. Fatigue commonly occurs from the first day of treatment and then intensifies over the course of therapy. It reaches a plateau between the second and fourth week and then remains at that level. However, without sufficient studies which incorporate a pretreatment baseline, and a lack of consistency in the time points selected for data collection, it is not yet possible to outline a definitive pattern. It affects more people for more of the time as treatment progresses. In particular, it appears to adopt an intermittent pattern during the early part of treatment which then converts to a continuous phenomenon at the later stage of treatment. Patients often report the sensation of fatigue is heightened in the late afternoon. There is conflicting evidence as to whether fatigue lessens during the break in treatment at the weekend. On ceasing treatment the sensation of fatigue gradually diminishes and, in many individuals, does not persist beyond the first 3 months.

The evidence for variance in the incidence of fatigue, according to site of irradiation, is at present sparse and over-reliant on the study by King *et al.* (1985). Whilst other investigators have included samples with differing diagnoses and diverse sites of irradiation, up to the present subgroups (even in the largest study to date by Smets *et al.* (1998*b*,*c*) with a total sample of 250 have not proved large enough to state with any confidence whether differences exist based on these factors. The relationship of fatigue to disease and treatment-related factors such as aim of treatment, stage of disease at diagnosis and data collection, time elapsed since previous treatment, number of fractions, cumulative radiation dose, and scheduling remains to be rigorously investigated. But current evidence suggests that the experience of fatigue in those being treated with radiotherapy does appear to be treatment-related, as reflected by differences in prevalence rates between groups with differing radiation fields, by a gradual increase in fatigue over the course of treatment, and by a reduction in fatigue scores over the weekend, when treatment is temporarily suspended (King *et al.* 1985; Greenberg *et al.* 1992; Irvine *et al.* 1994; Smets *et al.* 1998*b*).

The incidence, severity, and pattern of fatigue in patients receiving therapy other than that delivered by an external beam remains relatively unknown. Exceptions to this include the work of Nail (1993), describing women's symptom experience during intracavitary radiotherapy for gynaecological cancer, and Fieler (1997), who studied a sample of patients receiving high-dose brachytherapy for either gynaecological or bronchial cancer. In both studies there were similarities in terms of side-effects experienced, as compared with studies of those receiving external radiation, and fatigue was

Table 2.1 Summary of prospective studies documenting external beam radiotherapy-related fatigue

Study reference	Sample	Time points for data collection	Measure of fatigue	Course	Correlates
Haylock and Hart (1979)	N = 30. Mixed diagnosis. Varying number of fractions.	No pretreatment baseline. Started on first day and then every day for duration of therapy. At the same time each day	Pearson Byars Fatigue Feeling Checklist	Consistent drop in fatigue scores on Sundays. Fatigue increased over course and was greatest in those with longer regimes	Positive: time since surgery. Negative: weight
King et al. (1985)	N = 96. Mixed diagnoses. Mixed radiation site (chest, head and neck, male and female pelvis). Varied fractionation protocols	No pretreatment baseline. Weekly during treatment and monthly for 3 months after treatment ended	Investigator-developed Symptom Profile Interview	Number reporting fatigue increased as treatment progressed and dropped during months after treatment finished. Intermittent during first few weeks, continuous as treatment progressed, and intermittent after treatment ended. Worse in the afternoon	Not studied but highest in lung cancer group receiving radiotherapy to chest
Kobashi-Schoot et al. (1985)	N = 95. Mixed diagnoses (lymphoma, uterus, breast, bladder). Varied fractionation protocols	No pretreatment baseline. Six times over a period of 3 weeks on Mondays and Fridays	Fatigue Symptom Checklist and investigator-developed visual analogue scales	Malaise increased in magnitude during treatment. Some groups suffered less malaise during weekend	Negative: age

Table 2.1 (Continued) Summary of prospective studies documenting external beam radiotherapy-related fatigue

Study reference	Sample	Time points for data collection	Measure of fatigue	Course	Correlates
Greenberg et al. (1992)	N = 15. Early stage breast cancer. 28 fractions plus 7–10 fraction electron boost	No pretreatment baseline. Fatigue rated daily during treatment and at 3rd and20th week post-treatment	Profile of Mood States. Pearson Byars Fatigue Feeling Checklist. Investigator-developed visual analogue scales	Fatigue did not increase in a linear manner with cumulative dose over time. Dropped from 1st to 2nd week, rise in 3rd week. Reached plateau in 4th week, maintained to end of treatment. Within 3 weeks of treatment had diminished. Patients were not less tired at weekends	Negative: correlation with selected biological markers
Munro and Potter (1996)	Total N = 110. N = 72: postop. radiotherapy; early stage breast cancer. N = 24: radical radiotherapy; head and neck cancer. N = 14: more than 5 fractions; localized lung cancer	Assessment schedule varied for each group but all patients had baseline before planning, at day 5–7, day 12–14, and day 19–21	Investigator-developed computerized linear analogue self-assessment type scale focused on symptom distress	At start of treatment 55% selected tiredness as a symptom, by end of treatment it was 71%. It increased steadily and significantly during treatment. In patients with breast cancer no significant difference between first follow-up visit and pretreatment baseline	Not studied

Study	Sample	Time points	Instrument	Results	Correlates
Irvine et al. (1998)	N = 76. Early stage breast cancer	Six points in time: before treatment, 1 week after start, 2 weeks after start, during last week, and at 3 and 6 months after completing	Pearson Byars Fatigue Feeling Checklist	Increased over course of treatment, highest at last week of treatment, and returned to pretreatment levels by 3 months after treatment. Significant increase at day 7 and 14. Plateaued from 14 days to last week of treatment and then significant decrease to pretreatment levels at 3 and 6 months. Pattern of symptom and psychological distress did not mirror that of fatigue	Negative: age, stage of disease, time since surgery, weight, length of time since diagnosis, and radiation dose. Positive: symptom distress, psychological distress, and self-reported fatigue strategies
Smets et al. (1998b,c)	N = 250. Mixed diagnoses. Varying number of fractions	2 weeks before start of treatment, 2 weeks after completion of treatment, and 2 weekly intervals during treatment	Multidimensional Fatigue Inventory	Gradual increase in fatigue over course of radiotherapy, decrease after completion. Fatigue scores obtained after treatment were only slightly, although significantly, higher than pretreatment scores	Association with post-treatment fatigue. Positive: diagnosis, physical distress, pain, quality of sleep, hours of sleep, functional disability, psychological distress, and depression

common across all groups. The pattern, however, was different. For example, in the study by Fieler (1997) a more stable pattern of symptoms (including fatigue) was evident, with incidence being high at the start of treatment and continuing to stay high, even 3 months later. Where patients received external radiation the pattern of onset was often acute, peaking during the last half of treatment, and gradually declining post-treatment.

Knowledge in this area does now have the benefit of a cohort of studies that have employed a prospective, longitudinal design. However, what accounts for fatigue in people undergoing radiation therapy remains unclear. Many fail to use robust measurement strategies, continuing to select one-off study-specific instruments or tools that were developed, in the first instance, for populations other than patients with cancer. Future studies will contribute little if they fail to establish a baseline prior to treatment commencing, lack a data collection strategy which takes into account what we already know about the pattern of fatigue, and persist in adopting measurement tools which make comparisons between studies difficult. The inclusion of a comparative group of age-matched healthy individuals would add the possibility of collecting normative data. Studies such as that designed by Irvine *et al.* (1998) should be replicated (albeit with more robust tools with which to measure fatigue) in order to determine the frequency, duration, and severity of fatigue with groups other than those with breast cancer. In addition, studies that seek to describe the physical, mental, and behavioural manifestations of fatigue and whether it varies across the days of the week or the time of day should be undertaken. If this does not occur clinicians will be forced to rely on studies with substantial limitations and which, due to their age, do not reflect current radiation oncology practice.

Chemotherapy

Documentation of the association between chemotherapy and fatigue has been under way since the early 1980s and gathered momentum in the 1990s. Investigations have been conducted with patients with breast cancer, lymphoma, lung cancer, ovarian cancer, and other solid tumour types, although by far the greatest number of data have been collected with those in the first group, namely breast cancer. It is now acknowledged as the most frequent and distressing side-effect of chemotherapy. Compelling descriptions of the impact of fatigue on patients' quality of life and ability to perform self-care are available (Fernsler 1986; Rhodes *et al.* 1988; Nail *et al.* 1991; Ferrell *et al.* 1996; Pearce and Richardson 1996; Hilfinger Messias 1997; Ream and Richardson 1997; Richardson and Ream 1997). Evidence suggesting an association between the administration of chemotherapy and feelings of fatigue has been collected during studies conducted to document the range of side-effects associated with this treatment modality. These include, for example, studies conducted by Meyerowitz *et al.* (1979), Cassileth *et al.* (1985), Love *et al.* (1989), Tierney *et al.* (1991), Greene *et al.* (1994), Sitzia and Dikken (1997), and Sitzia *et al.* (1997).

The severity of chemotherapy-induced fatigue, and the distress associated with it, vary among studies, apparently because measurement of fatigue, site of disease, drug regimes, and duration of treatment differ (Irvine *et al.* 1991; Smets *et al.* 1993; Richardson 1995*b*; Stone *et al.* 1998). Lack of congruence between expected and experienced side-effects is reported as a major cause of distress (Cassileth *et al.* 1985; Love *et al.* 1989; Griffin *et al.* 1996).

There are still only a relatively small number of investigations that have been designed to collect in-depth information about the factors linked with fatigue in this population and the ensuing pattern over a course of therapy. These are summarized in Table 2.2. Subjects report rapid onset of fatigue following administration of pulsed therapy, as early as 24–48 h after treatment (Greene *et al.* 1994) and lowest levels often occur immediately before the next treatment (Richardson *et al.* 1998). Due to inconsistencies in disease-related factors, such as chemotherapy regime, stage, and nature of disease, and both the timing and nature of measurement, it remains difficult to say with any certainty what the nature of the overall pattern of this symptom is, both between and within different groups of patients. There is evidence that fatigue varies in intensity over the course of treatment (Pickard-Holley 1991), within each cycle (Pickard-Holley 1991; Irvine *et al.* 1994; Richardson *et al.* 1998) and within each day (Berger 1998; Richardson *et al.* 1998). The length of each cycle is one factor predicted to influence the experience of fatigue (Richardson *et al.* 1998), although this has not been supported in the study by Berger (1998), as are timing and the manner in which drugs are administered. As the complexity of regimes increases, for example the combination of pulsed drugs with continuous therapy, the chance of patients experiencing fatigue is likely to multiply. With traditional pulsed regimes there is an opportunity for fatigue to decline post-treatment; however, it is possible that continuous therapy is associated with increased background levels of fatigue, with a cyclical pattern superimposed on top of this. The influence of different administration regimes on the pattern of fatigue remains under-researched. Studies in which patients are asked to document their experiences over a single treatment cycle fail to provide information about changes in fatigue that may already have occurred following the start of chemotherapy or that occur over repeated cycles. Since the experience of fatigue may vary by both disease site and stage (Glaus 1998), research designs that include heterogeneous samples are now of limited usefulness. Such studies will fail to provide detailed information about the nature of fatigue to be expected with specific regimes and for specific conditions.

The overwhelming lack of normative or comparison group data is a further negative feature of previous research. As Jacobsen *et al.* (1999) point out, in the absence of such data it is difficult to know the degree to which levels of fatigue reported by chemotherapy patients differ from levels that are commonly experienced by healthy individuals of the same age and gender. Previously small and relatively uncontrolled studies have produced conflicting results (Pickard-Holley 1991; Irvine *et al.* 1994). More recently, however, evidence points to the fact that women receiving adjuvant chemotherapy

Table 2.2 Summary of studies documenting chemotherapy-related fatigue

Study reference	Sample	Time points for data collection	Measure of fatigue	Course	Correlates
Jamar (1989)	$N = 16$. Stage I–IV ovarian cancer. Chemotherapy regime not stated	No pretreatment baseline. Retrospective and cross-sectional, not at uniform point in treatment	Profile of Mood States—Short Form (POMS-SF) and Pearson Byars Fatigue Feeling Checklist interview	Worse in first week following therapy and lessened prior to next injection	Positive: symptom distress, nausea, living arrangements, assistance with home responsibilities, and total score on POMS-SF. Negative: haematocrit
Pickard-Holley (1991)	$N = 12$: stage IIb–IIIC ovarian cancer; chemotherapy: cyclophosphamide and cisplatin. $N = 12$: healthy women	No pretreatment baseline. Prospective, on days 1, 7, 14, and 21, not at uniform point in treatment	Rhoten Fatigue Scale	Fatigue peaked at day 7 and then slowly declined during remainder of 28-day cycle	Positive: CA125. No relationship between fatigue and cycle of treatment
Irvine et al. (1994)	$N = 47$: breast, lung, cervical, or endometrial cancer; chemotherapy regime not stated. $N = 54$: radiotherapy. $N = 53$: healthy people	No pretreatment baseline. Prospective, comparative. Fatigue rated at two time points, Time 1, before received therapy, and Time 2, 10–14 days after therapy, not at uniform point in treatment	Pearson Byars Fatigue and Feeling Checklist	Increase in fatigue over two time points was observed	Positive: symptom distress, mood disturbance, weight loss, alteration in functional activities. No relationship with disease or treatment related variables
Berger (1998)	$N = 72$. Stage I or II breast cancer. Adjuvant chemotherapy: doxorubicin/	Prospective, descriptive, repeated measures during first 3 cycles, 48 h after	Piper Fatigue Scale and wrist actigraphs	Fatigue levels 48 h after each 3 cycles were not significantly different over time.	Negative: with activity levels except at MP2. Fatigue scores

Study	Sample	Design	Measures	Findings	Conclusions
	cyclophosphamide or cyclophosphamide, methotrexate, and fluorouracil or cyclophosphamide, doxorubicin, and fluorouracil	each new treatment (T1–T3) and at each cycle mid point (MP1–MP3)		Fatigue intensity was significantly lower at MP1–MP3 than at T1–T3. Activity levels mirror-image pattern of fatigue	higher in doxorubicin-based protocols
Richardson et al. (1998)	N = 109 Varied site of cancer (stated). Chemotherapy: varied regimes (stated)	No pretreatment baseline. Prospective, comparative repeated daily measures of fatigue over a cycle of treatment. Not at uniform point in treatment	Investigator-developed visual analogue scales	Levels of fatigue are high in first few days after bolus injection, drop slightly, and then rise at nadir, only to subside again. Varied throughout the day, more frequently occurring in afternoon and early evening	Differences in fatigue scores according to site of cancer, type of chemotherapy regime, and method of drug administration
Jacobsen et al. (1999)	N = 54: breast cancer; adjuvant chemotherapy regime not stated. N = 54: no history of breast cancer	Prospective, descriptive, repeated measure. Pretreatment baseline (home 1) and in week before next treatment at 2nd and 3rd cycle (home 2 and home 3) and immediately before first four cycles (clinic 1–4)	Profile of Mood States Fatigue Scale and Fatigue Symptom Inventory for home 1–3 measures. Memorial Symptom Assessment Scale at clinic 1–4.	Fatigue increased in prevalence, severity, and disruptiveness after start of treatment. No evidence that fatigue worsens over course of subsequent infusions	More severe fatigue was associated with poorer performance status, and presence of fatigue-related symptoms. Increases in fatigue after chemotherapy started was associated with development of chemotherapy side-effects

for breast cancer experience significantly worse fatigue than an age-matched comparison group of women with no cancer history (Berger 1998; Jacobsen *et al.* 1999). These careful pieces of research with women receiving adjuvant therapy for a diagnosis of breast cancer should be replicated in other groups of patients who commonly receive chemotherapy in curative, adjuvant, and palliative circumstances. It has been speculated whether the fatigue associated with chemotherapy, as is the case with radiotherapy, is cumulative. Jacobsen *et al.*'s (1999) and Berger's (1998) studies refute this, as both found no evidence that following the start of adjuvant chemotherapy fatigue worsened over the course of subsequent treatment cycles. However, this effect has not been studied beyond the end of the third cycle of therapy and data collection should now be extended beyond this period.

Over the last 10 years, the use of autologous and allogeneic bone marrow and stem cell transplants following dose-intensified chemotherapy have established themselves as important treatment approaches for both haematological and solid organ malignancies. Few studies have explicitly examined the course, characteristics, and correlates of fatigue in relation to this form of therapy. There is, however, a growing interest in the experience of side-effects as a result of transplantation, and the impact of these on quality of life. An exception to this is the work of Hann and her team (Hann *et al.* 1997, 1999), this in turn improved methodologically on two previous studies that focused, in part, on the fatigue experienced by patients during and after transplant (Andrykowski *et al.* 1995; McQuellon *et al.* 1996). Hann and colleagues have focused on autologous stem cell transplantation and documented that women undergoing this form of treatment experience fatigue that is worse than that normally experienced by a comparative group of healthy women, and that it interferes with daily functioning and quality of life.

Other therapies

Surgery, chemotherapy, and radiotherapy play a principal role in the management of cancer. However, hormone therapy and, with growing frequency, biological response modifiers, are employed in either a primary role or, as is more common, as part of a programme of treatment.

Fatigue is a side-effect of all biological response modifiers and is frequently accompanied by a flu-like syndrome, which includes myalgia, chills, fever, headache, and malaise (Dean *et al.* 1995). Despite recognition that fatigue is often described by patients receiving this group of therapies as overwhelming and intolerable, and, at times, acts as a dose-limiting toxicity, there are only a handful of studies that take fatigue as their explicit focus (Davis 1984; Rieger 1987; Robinson and Posner 1992; Dean *et al.* 1995). Hence our understanding of the pattern, intensity, duration, correlates, and resolution of biological response modifier-related fatigue is very limited. At the close of the 1980s Piper *et al.* (1989) synthesized what was currently known about patterns of fatigue with this treatment modality, but this was, in the main, based on clinical observation and unpublished data. That review concluded that the pattern and duration of fatigue are influenced by the type of clinical agent, dose, schedule, and route of administration (Piper *et al.* 1989). Since then little progress has been made in this area, apart from the publication of the work by Dean *et al.* (1995).

Hormone therapy plays a central role in the treatment of a number of common cancers, for example breast and prostate. Considering that this form of therapy is increasingly being given as an adjuvant and preventative agent, it is desirable that they are well tolerated and convenient. It is startling that little is known about the experiences of daily life and life quality in the men and women who receive these therapies. However, there is growing recognition that clinicians tend to underestimate the impact of side-effects of hormone therapy (Denton 1996). Research highlights that there are discrepancies between the perceptions patients and clinicians hold in terms of the level of distress caused by side-effects, and the impact such distress has on increasing the likelihood that patients will seek a change in therapy (Leonard *et al.* 1996). Lethargy and lack of energy feature as one of the most troublesome symptoms in this respect (Leonard *et al.* 1996). The Working Group on Living with Advanced Breast Cancer Hormone Treatment (Denton 1996) highlighted that side-effects of hormonal treatment are not generally well assessed. In response to this the Checklist for Patients on Endocrine Therapy (C-PET) was developed (Hopwood 1996). Through the process of development and pilot testing of the C-PET 'low energy' was confirmed, alongside hot flushes/sweats and weight gain, as one of the most frequently experienced symptoms.

Relationship of cancer-related fatigue with side-effects and symptoms of disease and treatment

There is fairly consistent evidence from studies of varying methodological quality that fatigue is related to many of the symptoms that accompany the experience of cancer and its treatment (Smets *et al.* 1993; Winningham *et al.* 1994; Nail and Winnigham 1995; Richardson 1995*a*). Symptoms linked with fatigue in the patient with cancer include pain, nausea, dyspnoea, and sleep disturbances. Table 2.3 lists these symptoms and a selection of the correlation coefficients reported in the literature. This highlights that the extent of the evidence is far from plentiful. Correlations between fatigue and other symptoms have only been assessed in a limited number of studies and the strength of these is inconsistent. This is not surprising as there is little similarity in the operational definitions adopted when measuring these symptoms, or in the context in which they are being assessed. However, based on the existing evidence, a degree of convergence is demonstrated. Because it is not wise to infer causation from data such as these, it is unclear whether such symptoms predispose the individual to fatigue, are consequences of it, or are simply concomitant symptoms.

Our understanding of what accounts for fatigue in patients with cancer has been supplemented by the opinions of patients themselves (see Chapters 5 and 6). These have been documented in a number of studies of both a qualitative and quantitative,

Table 2.3 Selected symptoms and reported correlations with fatigue

Symptom	Correlation coefficient	Authors
Pain	0.41	Miaskowski and Lee (1999)
	0.36	Smets et al. (1998b)
	0.24	Morant (1996)
	0.31	Richardson (1995b)
	0.48	Blesch et al. (1991)
Nausea	0.31	Richardson (1995b)
	0.39	Irvine et al. (1994)
	0.58	Jamar (1989)
Dyspnoea	0.41	Irvine et al. (1994)
Sleep disturbance	0.54	Miaskowski and Lee (1999)
	0.41	Smets et al. (1998b)
	0.40	Morant (1996)
	0.43	Richardson (1995b)
	0.31	Irvine et al. (1994)

and prospective and retrospective nature (Piper 1989; Pearce and Richardson 1996; Richardson and Ream 1996; Ream and Richardson 1997). In these studies patients consistently identify symptoms such as nausea, pain, and breathlessness as provoking increased feelings of fatigue, and, as a converse to this, that the relief of such symptoms often alleviates fatigue.

When designing future studies, researchers interested in uncovering the true picture of the relationship between fatigue and other symptoms associated with cancer need to acknowledge the dynamic nature of symptom expression and the manner in which symptoms are subject to change over time. Energy should be devoted to tracking symptoms across time and their relative position to each other in terms of quality, duration, distress, and intensity, as well as their subsequent influence on functional, cognitive, and physical performance. Dodd (1999) has recently raised the issue that it is likely that new methodologies/techniques will be needed in order to track symptoms across time, and we would add to this that a greater degree of rigour should be applied when selecting the timing of symptom assessments. Studies which have been carefully constructed to evaluate the pattern of symptoms which occur in discrete clusters now need to progress so that, for example, it is possible to discern which of the symptoms occurs first, and which followed. Miaskowski and Lee's (1999) study has made an important contribution in this respect.

Implications for practice and research

Although research indicates that it is common, data derived to date on the experience of fatigue are insufficient for understanding its trajectory in relation to disease severity or treatment factors. Researchers and clinicians alike now acknowledge the problems inherent in isolating causes of fatigue among patients with cancer who are the recipients of multiple forms of treatment. However, up to the present, few studies have examined patients' experiences of fatigue over the course of common treatment pathways. Little effort has been expended to assess the natural history of fatigue (i.e. starting with pre-treatment baselines and progressing through the acute period of therapy, the phases of intermediate and long-term recovery, and rehabilitation). Most studies have captured a snapshot of fatigue at a particular point in treatment or two or three assessments during a relatively short period of time. Although challenging to design, and costly to implement, prospective studies that include healthy people are essential to establish disease-free baselines and capture aspects of fatigue unique to the cancer experience. Most research describes the characteristics of fatigue associated with treatment, but there remains a significant problem when attempting to separate out both the quantity and qualities related to the cancer itself, and that portion that can be ascribed to treatment. Few studies have established baseline measures for fatigue that include a description of changes attributable to treatment. The recent study by Cimprich (1999) demonstrated that there is a discernible pattern of symptom distress even before treatment commences. Subjects in this study reported fatigue in the pretreatment period that cannot be attributed to the effects of treatment. Cimprich speculated that this might be due, in part, to the cognitive/attentional demands placed on patients during this particular time.

It remains difficult to determine whether cancer-related fatigue should be viewed as emanating from pathological mechanisms, or as concomitant with other disease-related symptoms which provoke discomfort. However, careful sifting of major contributing factors is needed, whilst paying particular regard to the various contexts in which they are likely to occur. Competing explanations of fatigue need to be carefully accounted for. Causal interpretation of results needs to be undertaken with a degree of caution, as studies that utilize cross-sectional designs lacking a control or comparative group are in the majority. Because fatigue is so closely linked with symptoms such as pain and dyspnoea, to name but a couple of factors, studies that incorporate multiple measures are likely to be more instructive in furthering our understanding of fatigue (see Box 2.1).

The interaction of fatigue with other symptoms is rarely evaluated. The importance of pursuing such lines of enquiry is crystallized in the theory of Lenz and colleagues: the 'middle range theory of unpleasant symptoms'. It is claimed that this theory now represents an accurate representation of the complexity and interactive nature of the symptom experience (Lenz *et al.* 1997). It acknowledges the cumulative burden that symptoms are likely to impose and suggests a relationship between the number of symptoms and increase in fatigue intensity. Tracking the onset, course, and resolution of different sets of symptoms, and the circumstances surrounding them, will help confirm some of these relationships. For example, work by Hickock *et al.* (1996) demonstrates

Box 2.1 Future areas for research

- ◆ Collaboration between basic scientists and clinical researchers might further understanding about the various physiological and psychological factors postulated to be related to fatigue.
- ◆ Pattern, intensity, duration, and resolution of fatigue should be studied in relation to each of the treatment modalities commonly employed in the treatment of cancer.
- ◆ Pretreatment baseline assessments, comparative samples, and psychometrically robust measurement instruments should be incorporated into future studies.
- ◆ Onset, course, and resolution of different sets of symptoms, including fatigue, and the circumstances surrounding them, should be tracked.

that whereas the frequency of pain is stable over the course of radiotherapy, the frequency of fatigue continues to increase, and many patients continue to experience fatigue while not reporting significant pain. The relationship between fatigue and other symptoms is complex; the presence of fatigue may lower the threshold of pain or increase its perceived intensity.

A significant amount of research has been undertaken examining either fatigue as a single symptom or alongside its associated symptoms. Whilst this approach has advanced our understanding to a certain degree, it has not always proved beneficial. Dodd (1999) has recently asserted that the next generation of symptom research should focus on frequently occurring groups of symptoms, what she refers to as 'symptom clusters'. If we are to take a leap forward in furthering our understanding of both cancer-related fatigue and other frequently experienced symptoms of cancer and its treatment, researchers will need to direct their energies at finding answers to the following sorts of questions (Dodd 1999):

- ◆ In a cluster of symptoms, which symptoms usually drive, or are antecedent to, the other symptoms?
- ◆ Will the use of single-symptom assessment instruments or single-item scales be sufficient to assess individual symptoms within a cluster?
- ◆ Is there a direct linear relationship among the symptoms in the cluster and their severity?

Conclusion

Whilst practice remains compromised by our lack of understanding about fatigue in people with a diagnosis of cancer, clinicians must now use the knowledge that has been generated through research to shape their clinical practice. Evidence suggests that they frequently encounter patients who are suffering from cancer-related fatigue. As has been documented in previous sections of this chapter, patients receiving chemotherapy, radio-therapy, surgery, hormone therapy, biological therapy, and bone marrow transplantation have reported it. Whilst not reviewed here, it has also been reported in those facing a diagnosis of cancer (Weisman 1976; Cimprich 1999), those recovering from cancer (Fobair *et al.* 1986; Devlen *et al.* 1987; Berglund *et al.* 1991; Smets *et al.* 1998*c*), and those at the advanced stage of their illness (Donnelly *et al.* 1995; Krishnasamy 1997). It is important, therefore, that all patients with cancer are assessed for fatigue, whether they are receiving treatment or not. Patients will benefit from ongoing assessment throughout the course of their illness. Patients often describe cancer-related fatigue as both quantita-tively and qualitatively different from the fatigue they experienced before having cancer, and this suggests that they may benefit from receiving explanations about possible causes, factors likely to worsen or lessen its intensity, and how it is likely to affect them.

Relieving fatigue in patients with cancer requires an appreciation of the various fac-tors that can contribute to it. It is important to emphasize that correlation does not indicate causation. However, the evidence from the studies summarized above indicates that it is wise to assess the patient who is experiencing fatigue for the presence of symp-tom distress. Specific symptoms that have been correlated with fatigue include pain, nausea, vomiting, lack of appetite, sleep disturbance, and breathlessness. Intervention in clinical practice is, by the very nature of the problems experienced by the client group in question, multifocused. This is currently based more on experience and intuition than evidence, and is compounded by the fact that there is little empirical support to suggest that a reduction in other symptoms will lead to a reduction in fatigue. However, because they have been related in a number of studies, interventions targeted at holistic symp-tom management may be effective at preventing and ameliorating fatigue. Programmes of management for fatigue that address several hypothesized causes are more likely to achieve success than a single isolated strategy.

The ideas discussed in this chapter are summarized in Box 2.2.

Box 2.2 Summary points

- A degree of evidence exists linking fatigue with the different treatment modali-ties used in the management of cancer.
- Evidence is less prevalent in relation to surgery, hormone therapy, and biological response modifiers.
- Factors linked with fatigue in relation to each treatment modality are insuffi-ciently described.
- Fatigue has been associated with many of the common symptoms experienced by those with cancer, including pain, nausea, breathlessness, and sleep disturbances.
- It remains unclear whether such symptoms predispose individuals to fatigue, are consequences of it, or are simply concomitant.

References

Andrykowski, M., Bruehl, S., Brady, M., and Henslee-Downey, P. (1995) Physical and psychosocial status of adults one year after bone marrow transplantation: a prospective study. *Bone Marrow Transplant*, **15**, 837–44.

Berger, A. (1998) Patterns of fatigue and activity and rest during adjuvant breast cancer chemotherapy. *Oncology Nursing Forum*, **25**(1), 51–62.

Berglund, G., Bolund, C., Fornanader, T., Rutqvist, L., and Sjoden, P.-O. (1991) Late effects of adjuvant chemotherapy and postoperative radiotherapy on quality of life among breast cancer patients. *European Journal Of Cancer*, **27**(9), 1075–81.

Blesch, K., Paice, J., Wickham, R., Harte, N., Schnoor, D., Purl, S., et al. (1991) Correlates of fatigue in people with lung and breast cancer. *Oncology Nursing Forum*, **18**(1), 81–7.

Cassileth, B., Lusk, E., Bodenheimer, B., Farber, J., Jochimsen, P., and Morrin-Taylor, B. (1985) Chemotherapeutic toxicity—the relationship between patients' pre-treatment expectations and the post-treatment results. *American Journal Of Clinical Oncology*, **8**, 419–25.

Christensen, T. and Kehlet, H. (1984) Postoperative fatigue and changes in nutritional status. *British Journal of Surgery*, **71**, 473–6.

Christensen, T., Bendix, T., and Kehlet, H. (1982) Fatigue and cardiorespiratory function following abdominal surgery. *British Journal of Surgery*, **69**(2), 417–19.

Christensen, T., Hougard, F., and Kehlet, H. (1985) Influence of pre- and intraoperative factors in the occurrence of postoperative fatigue. *British Journal of Surgery*, **72**(1), 63–5.

Christensen, T., Kehlet, H., Vetserberg, K., and Vinnars, E. (1987) Fatigue and muscle amino acids during surgical convalescence. *Acta Chirurgica Scandinavica*, **153**, 567–70.

Christensen, T., Stage, J., Galbo, H., Christensen, N., and Kehlet, H. (1989) Fatigue and cardiac and endocrine metabolic response to exercise after abdominal surgery. *Surgery*, **105**(1), 46–50.

Cimprich, B. (1992) Attentional fatigue following breast cancer surgery. *Research in Nursing and Health*, **15**(3), 199–207.

Cimprich, B. (1998) Age and extent of surgery affect attention in women treated for breast cancer. *Research in Nursing and Health*, **21**, 229–38.

Cimprich, B. (1999) Pretreatment symptom distress in women newly diagnosed with breast cancer. *Cancer Nursing*, **22**(3), 185–95.

Davis, C. (1984) Interferon induced fatigue. *Oncology Nursing Forum*, **11**(Supplement), 67 (abstract 72).

Dean, G., Spears, L., Ferrell, B., Quan, W., Groshon, S., and Mitchell, M. (1995) Fatigue in patients with cancer receiving interferon alpha. *Cancer Practice*, **3**(3), 164–72.

Denton, S. (1996) Exploring the impact of treatment, communications, perceptions, reality. *European Journal of Cancer Care*, **5**(Supplement 3), 3–4.

Devlen, J., Maguire, P., Phillips, P., Crowther, D., and Chambers, H. (1987) Psychological problems asssociated with diagnosis and treatment of lymphomas. I. Retrospective. II. Prospective. *British Medical Journal*, **295**, 953–7.

Dodd, M. (1999) A future perspective of symptom management research. *International Cancer Nursing News*, **11**(3), 8.

Donnelly, S., Walsh, D., and Rybicki, L. (1995) The symptoms of advanced cancer, identification of clinical and research priorities by assessment of prevalence and severity. *Journal of Palliative Care*, **11**, 27–32.

Fernsler, J. (1986) A comparison of patient and nurse perceptions of patients' self-care deficits ssociated with cancer chemotherapy. *Cancer Nursing*, **9**(2), 50–7.

Ferrell, B., Grant, M., Dean, G., Funk, B., and Ly, J. (1996) 'Bone tired', the experience of fatigue and its impact on quality of life. *Oncology Nursing Forum*, **23**(10), 1539–47.

Fieler, V. (1997) Side effects and quality of life in patients receiving high-dose rate brachytherapy. *Oncology Nursing Forum*, **24**(3), 545–53.

Fobair, P., Hoppe, R., Bloom, J., Cox, R., Varghese, A., and Spiegel, D. (1986) Psychosocial problems among survivors of Hodgkin's disease. *Journal of Clinical Oncology*, **4**(5), 805–14.

Forsberg, C., Bjorvell, H., and Cedermark, B. (1996) Well-being and its relation to coping ability in patients with colorectal and gastric cancer before and after surgery. *Scandinavian Journal of Caring Science*, **10**, 35–44.

Galloway, S. and Graydon, J. (1996) Uncertainty, symptom distress, and information needs after surgery for cancer of the colon. *Cancer Nursing*, **19**, 112–17.

Glaus, A. (1998) *Fatigue in Patients With Cancer*. Springer, Berlin.

Greenberg, D., Sawicka, J., Eisenthal, S., and Ross, D. (1992) Fatigue syndrome due to localised radio-therapy. *Journal of Pain and Symptom Management*, **7**(1), 38–45.

Greene, D., Nail, L., Fieler, V., Dudgeon, D., and Jones, L. (1994) A comparison of patient-reported side effects among three chemotherapy regimes for breast cancer. *Cancer Practice*, **2**(1), 57–62.

Griffin, A., Butow, P., Coates, A., Childs, A., Ellis, P., and Dunn, S. (1996) On the receiving end V, patient perceptions of the side effects of cancer chemotherapy in 1993. *Annals of Oncology*, **7**, 189–95.

Hann, D., Jacobsen, P., Martin, S., Kronish, L., Azzarello, L., and Fields, K. (1997) Fatigue in women treated with bone marrow transplantation for breast cancer, a comparison with women with no history of cancer. *Supportive Care in Cancer*, **5**, 44–52.

Hann, D., Jacobsen, P., Martin, S., Azzarello, L., and Greenberg, H. (1998) Fatigue and quality of life following radiotherapy for breast cancer; a comparative study. *Journal of Clinical Psychology in Medical Settings*, **5**(1), 19–33.

Hann, D., Garovoy, N., Finkelstein, B., Jacobsen, P., Azzarello, L., and Fields, K. (1999) Fatigue and quality of life in breast cancer patients undergoing autologous stem cell transplantation, a longitudinal study. *Journal of Pain and Symptom Management*, **17**(5), 311–19.

Haylock, P. and Hart, L. (1979) Fatigue in patients receiving localised radiation. *Cancer Nursing*, **2**(6), 461–7.

Hickock, J., Morrow, G., McDonald, S., and Bellg, A. (1996) Frequency and correlates of fatigue in lung cancer patients receiving radiation therapy, implications for management. *Journal of Pain and Symptom Management*, **11**(6), 370–7.

Hilfinger Messias, D., Yeager, K., Dibble, S., and Dodd, M. (1997) Patients' perspectives of fatigue whilst undergoing chemotherapy. *Oncology Nursing Forum*, **24**(1), 43–8.

Hopwood, P. (1996) A Checklist For Patients On Endocrine Therapy (C-PET) *European Journal of Cancer Care*, **5**(Supplement 3), 7–8.

Irvine, D., Vincent, L., Bubela, N., Thompson, L., and Graydon, J. (1991) A critical appraisal of the research literature investigating fatigue in the individual with cancer. *Cancer Nursing*, **14**(4), 188–99.

Irvine, D., Vincent, L., Graydon, J., Bubela, N., and Thompson, L. (1994) The prevalence and correlates of fatigue in patients receiving treatment with chemotherapy and radiotherapy. *Cancer Nursing*, **17**(5), 367–78.

Irvine, D., Vincent, L., Graydon, J., and Bubela, N. (1998) Fatigue in women with breast cancer receiving radiation therapy. *Cancer Nursing*, **21**(2), 127–35.

Jacobsen, P., Hann, D., Azzarello, L., Horton, J., Balducci, L., and Lyman, G. (1999) Fatigue in women receiving adjuvant chemotherapy for breast cancer: characteristics, course and correlates. *Journal of Pain and Symptom Management*, **18**, 233–42.

Jamar, S. (1989) Fatigue in women receiving chemotherapy for ovarian cancer. In: *Key Aspects of Comfort: Management of Pain, Fatigue and Nausea*, (ed. S. Funk, E. Tornquist, M. Champagne, L. Archer Copp, and R. Wiese). Springer, New York, pp. 224–8.

King, K., Nail, L., Kreamer, K., Strohl, R., and Johnson, J. (1985) Patients' descriptions of the experience of receiving radiation therapy. *Oncology Nursing Forum*, 12(4), 55–61.

Kobashi-Schoot, J., Hanewald, G., Van Dam, F., and Bruning, P. (1985) Assessment of malaise in cancer patients treated with radiotherapy. *Cancer Nursing*, 8(6), 306–13.

Krishnasamy, M. (1997) Exploring the nature and impact of fatigue in advanced cancer. *International Journal of Palliative Nursing*, 3(3), 126–31.

Kubricht, D. (1984) Therapeutic self-care demands expressed by out-patients receiving external radiation therapy. *Cancer Nursing*, 7(1), 43–52.

Lenz, E., Pugh, L., Milligan, R., Gift, A., and Suppe, F. (1997) The middle-range theory of unpleasant symptoms: an update. *Advances in Nursing Science*, 19(3), 14–27.

Leonard, R., Lee, L., and Harrison, M. (1996) Impact of side effects associated with endocrine treatments for advanced breast cancer: clinicians' and patients' perceptions. *The Breast*, 5, 259–64.

Love, R., Leventhal, H., Easterling, D., and Nerenz, D. (1989) Side effects and emotional distress during cancer chemotherapy. *Cancer*, 63(3), 604–12.

McQuellon, R., Craven, B., Russell, G., Hoffman, S., Cruz, J., Perry, J. *et al.* (1996) Quality of life in breast cancer patients before and after autologous bone marrow transplantation. *Bone Marrow Transplantation*, 18, 579–84.

Meyerowitz, B., Sparks, F., and Spears, I. (1979) Adjuvant chemotherapy for breast carcinoma: psychosocial implications. *Cancer*, 43, 1613–18.

Miaskowski, C. and Lee, K. (1999) Pain, fatigue and sleep disturbances in oncology outpatients receiving radiation therapy for bone metastasis: a pilot study. *Journal of Pain and Symptom Management*, 17(5), 320–32.

Mock, V., Hassey Dow, K., Meares, C., Grimm, P., Dienemann, J., Haisfield-Wolfe, M., *et al.* (1997) Effects of exercise on fatigue, physical functioning, and emotional distress during radiation therapy for breast cancer. *Oncology Nursing Forum*, 24(6), 991–1000.

Morant, R. (1996) Asthenia: an important symptom in cancer patients. *Cancer Treatment Reviews*, 22(Supplement A), 117–22.

Munro, A. and Potter, S. (1996) A quantitative approach to the distress caused by symptoms in patients treated with radical radiotherapy. *British Journal of Cancer*, 74, 640–7.

Nail, L. (1993) Coping with intracavitary radiation treatment for gynecologic cancer. *Cancer Practice*, 1(3), 218–24.

Nail, L. and Winnigham, M. (1995) Fatigue and weakness in cancer patients: the symptom experience. *Seminars in Oncology Nursing*, 11(4), 272–8.

Nail, L., Jones, L., Greene, D., Schipper, D., and Jensen, R. (1991) Use and perceived efficacy of self-care activities in patients receiving chemotherapy. *Oncology Nursing Forum*, 18(5), 883–7.

Pearce, S. and Richardson, A. (1996) Fatigue in cancer: a phenomenological perspective. *European Journal of Cancer Care*, 5(2), 111–15.

Petersson, B., Wernerman, J., Waller, S.-O., von der Decken, A., and Vinnars, E. (1990) Elective abdominal surgery depresses muscle protein synthesis and increases subjective fatigue: effects lasting more than 30 days. *British Journal of Surgery*, 77, 796–800.

Pick, B., Molloy, A., Hinds, C., Pearce, S., and Salmon, P. (1994) Post-operative fatigue following coronary artery bypass surgery: relationship to emotional state and to the catecholamine response to surgery. *Journal of Psychomatic Research*, 38(6), 599–607.

Pickard-Holley, S. (1991) Fatigue in cancer patients—a descriptive study. *Cancer Nursing,* **14**(1), 13–19.

Piper, B. (1989) Fatigue: current bases for practice. In: *Key Aspects of Comfort: Management of Pain, Fatigue and Nausea,* (ed. S. Funk, E. Tornquist, M. Champagne, L. Archer Copp, and R. Wiese). Springer, New York, pp. 187–98.

Piper, B., Rieger, P., Brophy, L., Haeuber, D., Hood, D., and Lyver, A. (1989) Recent advances in the management of biotherapy-related side effects: fatigue. *Oncology Nursing Forum,* **16**(6, Supplement), 27–34.

Ream, E. and Richardson, A. (1997) Fatigue in patients with cancer and chronic obstructive airways disease: a phenomenological enquiry. *International Journal of Nursing Studies,* **34**(1), 44–53.

Rhodes, V., Watson, P., and Hanson, B. (1988) Patients' descriptions of the influence of tiredness and weakness on self-care abilities. *Cancer Nursing,* **11**(3), 186–94.

Richardson, A. (1995*a*) Fatigue in cancer patients: a review of the literature. *European Journal of Cancer Care,* **4**(1), 20–32.

Richardson, A. (1995*b*) Patterns of fatigue in patients receiving chemotherapy. PhD Thesis. Department of Nursing Studies, King's College London.

Richardson, A. and Ream, E. (1996) The experience of fatigue and other symptoms in patients receiving chemotherapy. *European Journal of Cancer Care,* **5**(Supplement 2), 24–30.

Richardson, A. and Ream, E. (1997) Self-care behaviours initiated by chemotherapy patients in response to fatigue. *International Journal of Nursing Studies,* **34**(1), 35–43.

Richardson, A., Ream, E., and Wilson-Barnett, J. (1998) Fatigue in patients receiving chemotherapy: patterns of change. *Cancer Nursing,* **21**(1), 17–30. [Erratum. *Cancer Nursing,* **21**(3), 195.]

Rieger, P. (1987) Interferon-induced fatigue: a study of fatigue measurement. *Sigma Theta Tau International 29th Biennial Convention: Book of Proceedings,* November 10 A163. Sigma Theta Tau International, San Francisco.

Robinson, K. and Posner, J. (1992) Patterns of self-care needs and interventions related to biological response modifier therapy: fatigue as a model. *Seminars in Oncology Nursing (Supplement 1),* **8**(4), 17–22.

Rose, E. and King, T. (1978) Understanding post-operative fatigue. *Surgery, Gynaecology and Obstetrics,* **147**, 97–101.

Schroeder, D. and Hill, G. (1993) Predicting postoperative fatigue; importance of preoperative factors. *World Journal of Surgery,* **17**(2), 226–31.

Sitzia, J. and Dikken, C. (1997) Survey of the incidence and severity of side effects reported by patients receiving six cycles of FEC chemotherapy. *Journal of Cancer Nursing,* **1**(2), 61–73.

Sitzia, J., North, C., Stanley, J., and Winterberg, N. (1997) Side effects of CHOP in the treatment of non-Hodgkin's lymphoma. *Cancer Nursing,* **20**(6), 430–9.

Smets, E., Garssen, B., Schuster-Uitterhoeve, A., and de Haes, J. (1993) Fatigue in cancer patients. *British Journal of Cancer,* **68**(2), 220–4.

Smets, E., Visser, M., Garssen, B., Frijda, N., Ooosterveld, P., and de Haes, J. (1998*a*) Understanding the level of fatigue in cancer patients undergoing radiotherapy. *Journal of Psychosomatic Research,* **45**(3), 277–93.

Smets, E., Visser, M., Willems-Groot, A., Garssen, B., Oldenburger, F., van Tienhoven, G. *et al.* (1998*b*) Fatigue and radiotherapy: (A) experience in patients undergoing treatment. *British Journal of Cancer,* **78**(7), 899–906.

Smets, E., Visser, M., Willems-Groot, A., Garssen, B., Schuster-Uitterhoeve, A., and de Haes, J. (1998*c*) Fatigue and radiotherapy: (B) experience in patients 9 months following treatment. *British Journal of Cancer,* **78**(7), 907–12.

Stanton, A. and Snider, P. (1993) Coping with a breast cancer diagnosis: a prospective study. *Health Psychology*, **12**(1), 16–23.

Stone, P., Richards, M., and Hardy, J. (1998) Fatigue in patients with cancer. *European Journal of Cancer*, **34**(11), 1670–6.

Tierney, A., Leonard, R., Taylor, J., and Closs, J. (1991) Side effects experienced by women receiving chemotherapy for breast cancer. *British Medical Journal*, **302**, 272.

Weisman, A. (1976) Early diagnosis of vulnerability in cancer patients. *American Journal of Medical Sciences*, **271**(2), 187–96.

Winningham, M., Nail, L., Barton Burke, M., Brophy, L., Cimprich, B., Jones, L., *et al.* (1994). Fatigue and the cancer experience: the state of the knowledge. *Oncology Nursing Forum*, **21**(1), 23–36.

Zeiderman, M., Welchew, E., and Clark, R. (1990) Changes in cardiorespiratory and muscle function associated with the development of postoperative fatigue. *British Journal of Surgery*, **77**(5), 576–80.

Chapter 3

Mechanisms and models of fatigue associated with cancer and its treatment: evidence from preclinical and clinical studies

Paul Andrews, Gary Morrow, Jane Hickok, Joseph Roscoe, and Paddy Stone

Introduction

Defining non-exercise-induced fatigue in humans and identifying its correlates in other animals is one of the most difficult aspects of studying this widespread clinical problem. In humans an operational definition is 'a subjective state of overwhelming, sustained exhaustion and decreased capacity for physical and mental work that is not relieved by rest' (Piper *et al.* 1989; Piper 1992). Additionally, in contrast to exercise-induced fatigue, that which accompanies cancer and its treatment has a sustained duration of weeks, months, or even years. It is important to appreciate that this definition has both subjective (that is, self-reported) and objective (i.e. measurements that can be made independent of the subject) elements. Any explanation of the pathophysiology of this symptom must account for both dimensions. Other definitions such as that produced by the National Comprehensive Cancer Network (NCCN) Fatigue Guidelines Committee (Mock *et al.* 2000) also refer to both elements: 'Cancer related fatigue is an unusual, persistent, subjective sense of tiredness related to cancer or cancer treatment that interferes with usual functioning'.

Whatever the precise definition, it is clear that a symptom described as 'fatigue' is commonly reported by patients with cancer, and by people undergoing cancer treatment. It is present in more than 70% of patients in most published research studies (Jamar 1989; Hickok *et al.* 1996; Stone *et al.* 1998; Bower *et al.* 2000; Ahlberg *et al.* 2003), and is more common in cancer patients than in the general population and other medical populations (see Chapter 1).

Fatigue may be present even before treatment for cancer begins. It can increase during the course of cancer treatment with either radiation therapy or chemotherapy, and persist at a higher-than baseline rate, sometimes for years, after cancer treatment is finished (see Chapter 2) (Fobair *et al.* 1986; Nail and King 1987; Blesch *et al.* 1991; Irvine *et al.* 1991; Abrahamsen *et al.* 1998; Kaasa *et al.* 1998; Loge *et al.* 1999).

In patients with cancer, fatigue has a strong and direct negative impact on all aspects of their quality of life (QOL), particularly physical well-being. Fatigue during chemotherapy has also been associated with a cluster of other symptoms including pain, difficulty sleeping, and perceived muscle weakness, as well as with common adverse effects of treatment such as nausea and vomiting (see Chapter 2) (Foley 1985; Hickok *et al.* 1996; Abrahamsen *et al.* 1998). In addition to having a significant influence on QOL during chemotherapy, fatigue often lingers. For example, women with breast cancer who have been disease free for months or even years after completion of a course of adjuvant chemotherapy may still have their lives disrupted. Significant fatigue is reported by as many as 68% of women as long as 10 years following cessation of chemotherapy (Knobf 1986; Berglund *et al.* 1991; Beisecker *et al.* 1997; Broeckel *et al.* 1998). It does not appear to be related to the intensity of therapy or elapsed time following completion of primary treatment (Andrykowski *et al.* 1996, 1998). Studies on the late effects of chemotherapy for breast cancer have indicated that women often experience fatigue and rate fatigue, and related symptoms such as decreased stamina, insomnia, and other sleep problems, as among the most distressing of all symptoms (Knobf 1986; Berglund *et al.* 1991). The fatigue experienced interferes with QOL (Meyerowitz *et al.* 1983; Padilla and Grant 1985) and the ability to carry out daily tasks and activities (Piper 1988; Bloom *et al.* 1990).

Fatigue is still viewed by clinical staff, caregivers, and patients as an inevitable consequence of cancer and cancer treatment (Stone *et al.* 2000*a*), and has therefore been considered as something which could not particularly be treated by pharmacological interventions. This situation parallels the view held of chemotherapy-induced nausea and vomiting 20 years ago, but in the case of the latter, the situation changed dramatically due to the discovery of 5-hydroxytryptamine$_3$ receptor antagonists (5-HT$_3$) concomitant with an increased knowledge of the pathophysiology of chemotherapy-induced emesis (Morrow *et al.* 2001).

The current focus of research is description and aggregation of the symptoms of fatigue rather than prediction and integration of potential mechanisms (leading to the creation of testable hypotheses). A critical feature lacking to date in this field of research has been the basic science required to form a coherent framework that might guide the integration of observations. This chapter provides a comprehensive synthesis of current understanding and attempts to provide a basis upon which to build relevant but testable hypotheses.

A quote from Beard (1880) relating to subjective states gives an appropriate context for this chapter: 'neurasthenia [nervous exhaustion] has been the central Africa of medicine—an unexplored territory into which few may enter and those few have been compelled to bring back reports that have been neither credited or comprehended'.

Is fatigue a biologically appropriate response to cancer and therapy?

This teleological question may appear an irrelevant question to ask of a clinical symptom, but it addresses whether non-exercise-induced fatigue may have a 'useful' (or at the least a non-disadvantageous) function to an animal; otherwise why would we have the capacity to generate or express this state? To illustrate the importance of this question consider the nausea and vomiting associated with cancer chemo- and radio-therapy. These symptoms are now thought to be due to inappropriate activation of the emetic system that evolved to detect and respond to toxins accidentally ingested with the food (Andrews 1990). Nausea is viewed as a warning response (comparable to pain), and one that probably more importantly generates a learned aversion, such that the animal links the unpleasant sensation of nausea with the causal stimulus (that is, a specific food). Vomiting serves to void the contaminated gastric and upper intestinal contents in bulk, but in itself is not considered to be aversive.

In the absence of overt physical exertion, fatigue also appears to be an inappropriate response. However, in parallel with the previous studies into the mechanisms of nausea and vomiting, an examination of the ways in which an animal responds to infection suggests that it may be appropriate. Thus, the symptoms commonly associated with febrile infectious diseases such as lethargy, increased sleep, reduced plasma iron, changes in plasma lipids, depression, anorexia, and reduced grooming are all components of an organized response to defend the body against the pathogen (Weinberg 1984; Kluger 1991; Ewald 1994; Long 1996). This response is called 'illness behaviour' or 'sickness syndrome' and all components of the response play some role in combating the infection (Hart 1988). For example, the reduction in plasma iron retards bacterial growth (Long 1996). This cluster of behavioural responses is aimed at reducing energy consumption. The associated sensations can be argued to drive the animal to seek a safe haven where it can rest or sleep, further aiding recovery, or die if the defensive responses are over-whelmed. Many aspects of the body's response to cancer and chemotherapy suggest activation of the same response system. In this context it therefore becomes appropriate to consider the hypothalamic–pituitary–adrenal axis that has been implicated in responses to infection and chronic stress as well as in chronic fatigue syndrome (Chrousos and Gold 1991). Evidence for an involvement of this and other systems in cancer- and chemotherapy-induced fatigue is reviewed in detail below, forming the basis on which detailed research into the pathophysiology of this symptom can begin to be discussed further.

To summarize (see Fig. 3.1) the body responds to noxious challenges with four broad types of response:

(1) 'cleansing' to remove the stimulus from the body including vomiting, increased intestinal mucus secretion, increased lower gut secretion, and diarrhoea;

(2) immunological/antibacterial to directly attack the invading organism;

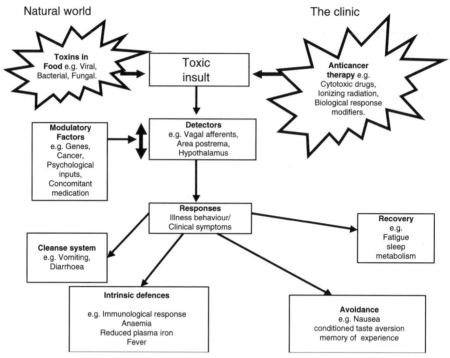

Fig. 3.1 A summary of some of the strategies employed by the body to defend itself against toxic insults but which also appear to be evoked by therapies used to treat cancer. See text for references.

(3) recovery and energy conservation measures such as fatigue and sleep, particularly increased slow wave sleep;

(4) avoidance of the problem by induction of learned aversions.

Each component of this defensive/protective system can be activated to a greater or lesser extent by cancer and its treatment. Particular note should be taken that the behavioural (that is, externally measurable) and allied (that is, subjective) sensations occur to help the animal cope with, and recover from, the insult. Provided the animal acquiesces to these internal signals the chances of recovery are optimized. In humans, although the same signals may operate, they are probably subject to a greater degree of cerebral (guilt at being ill) and external (inability to care for a spouse or child) modulation. This could lead to a serious dissonance between physiological attempts to recover ('sickness behaviour') and the patient's desire to be well. Thus, attempts to undertake or even a desire to undertake normal tasks in a physiologically 'weakened' state would lead to a mismatch between ability and expectation, and hence to reporting of fatigue.

Challenges in studying the mechanism(s) of fatigue

Studies in humans

The multidimensional nature of fatigue and the complexity of previously proposed (and largely descriptive) models of fatigue have all made it a difficult area for study. A critical aspect of cancer-induced fatigue is the consistent observation that it is not relieved by rest (Piper *et al.* 1989). This key observation distinguishes it from exercise-induced fatigue, which is readily relieved by rest, and suggests that even if the expression of the symptoms are similar the underlying causal mechanism differs. This implies that exercise-induced fatigue is not a useful model for understanding the aetiology and mechanisms of cancer-related fatigue.

There are a number of practical reasons why the study of fatigue is difficult. For example, fatigue is a common reason given by cancer patients for refusing to enter experimental protocols as their ability to retain information, deal with the increased demands of research participation (e.g. additional visits to hospital), or the consequences of additional interventions, discourage them from participating. Thus the potential pool of people available to participate is reduced (Kaempfer 1982; Holland 1989). Some researchers also think that fatigue, possibly resulting from its detrimental effect on concentration or ability to direct attention, may adversely affect patients' ability to comprehend and retain important information about the disease and its treatment. This may affect the ability of patients to adhere to treatment regimens (Kaempfer 1982; Cimprich 1992, 1995; Nail and Winningham 1995).

Objective measures of fatigue could complement the subjective assessments of fatigue obtained from questionnaires (Piper *et al.* 1989; Richardson 1998) (for a detailed consideration of problems associated with both subjective and objective assessment of fatigue see Chapter 9). An index of muscle activity can be obtained by the use of dynamometers (Fig. 3.2) (Dawson *et al.* 1998; Stone *et al.* 1999). Their portability makes them potentially useful in a clinical setting, but they suffer from the disadvantage that they monitor activity of a muscle group in performing a simple task (usually a manual one) which is then used as an index of overall ability to perform a motor task. Whilst this may be true, it is important that force generation is also investigated in postural muscles, particularly the legs. Also, repetitive tasks should be studied (Stone *et al.* 1999), as it may be the ability to sustain a task which may be impaired rather than the ability to perform it once (e.g. ascending one step as opposed to a flight of stairs). There may be natural variations in grip strength such as those reported to occur during the menstrual cycle (Sarwar *et al.* 1996). Of greater significance is that even if a reduction in a motor task such as a manual power grip is demonstrated in a single study, without further research evidence this does little to help identify mechanisms. The reason for this is that the reduction could be in the ability of the muscle itself to contract (see below), a problem with neuromuscular transmission (comparable to myasthenia gravis), or with the central motor drive.

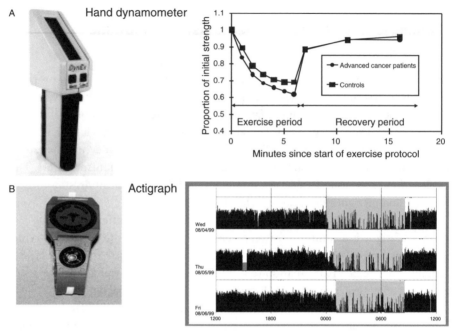

Fig. 3.2 An example of two techniques which have been used in patients with cancer to measure physical components of fatigue. Panel A shows a dynamometer used to measure hand grip strength and an example of the type of result obtained in patients with advanced cancer (Stone *et al.* 1999). Panel B shows the actigraph which is worn on the wrist and an example of the activity (vertical lines) pattern recorded each day for 3 days in a patient with cancer. The shaded area indicates the time the patient was 'in bed' or 'down' periods. Note that these periods are interrupted by bouts of activity indicating that the circadian rhythm is irregular. Reproduced with permission from Springer-Verlag. From Roscoe *et al.* (2002). Temporal interrelationships among fatigue, circadian rhythm and depression in breast cancer patients undergoing chemotherapy treatment. *Supportive Care in Cancer*, **10**, 329-36. © Springer-Verlag 2002. Permission also sought from the author.

An additional problem with asking patients to undertake voluntary motor tasks is that of motivation to complete the task, particularly when depression, that is known to reduce motivation, may coexist. The problem of motivation is encapsulated in the following, attributed to Leonardo da Vinci: he recalled seeing 'a mule which was almost unable to move through fatigue from a long journey under a heavy load, which on seeing a mare, multiplied its force so much and acquired such a velocity that it overtook the course of the mare which fled from it, and which was obliged to obey the desires of the mule'.

A more global measure of patient activity should give a better insight into their reported fatigue. Patient motion can be recorded using a Mini-Motionlogger actigraph (Ambulatory Monitoring, Inc., Ardsley, NY) (Patterson *et al.* 1993; Teicher 1995), an accelerometer and microprocessor with 32 kbyte of dedicated memory approximately the size of a wrist-watch, which is generally worn on the wrist, although it could be worn on the ankle (Fig. 3.2). The instrument computes activity based on wrist accelerations measured over preselected time periods. Motion logger actigraphs provide very sensitive measures of activity with high validity, intersubject reliability, reproducibility between instruments, and results that are independent of wrist placement (Patterson *et al.* 1993; Teicher 1995). We have shown that actigraph data confirm information obtained using standard paper and pencil questionnaires of depression completed by patients (Hickok *et al.* 1998, Roscoe *et al.* 2002). The actigraph has the advantage over the dynamometer in that it does not require the patient to be trained or motivated to undertake a task. Additionally it monitors activity over a period of time and not just at single points. Combining actigraph measurements with repeated blood sampling may provide important insights into the underlying pathophysiology (see below). Use of the actigraph is prompted not only by the face validity of the measure (fatigued patients universally report marked reductions in activity), but also by the fact that the original case definition of chronic fatigue syndrome (CFS), mandated a 50% reduction in physical activity (Holmes *et al.* 1998).

Studies in animals

The fundamental stumbling block of studying fatigue in laboratory animals is the same as studying nausea, that is, it is a subjective, self-reported symptom. Thus we have to measure correlates of, or surrogates for, the symptom. Nevertheless there is the advantage of being able to monitor a large number of variables in the same animal, as well as undertake and perform more pharmacological and surgical interventions to investigate aetiological mechanisms than is possible in humans. Whilst a 'sickness syndrome' has been described in animals following administration of pathogens, similar detailed studies have not been undertaken to examine the effects of cancer and chemotherapy agents alone and together.

Rats have been used to investigate the mechanism of 'sickness behaviours' including fatigue associated with cholestatic liver disease (Swain and Maric 1995). These studies showed that in rats with biliary duct resection there was reduction in exploratory behaviour and defective release of corticotrophin-releasing hormone (CRH) and a mechanistic link between the two is supported by additional studies showing that the intracerebroventricular injection of CRH stimulates locomotor activity in rats. Rats with cholestasis have an increased sensitivity to the locomotor effects of CRH (Burak *et al.* 2002) Such studies provide insights into the link between the hypothalamic–pituitary axis (HPA) and behaviour, and are of particular relevance in view of the growing number of patient studies showing modified HPA function in patients with CFS.

In addition to monitoring activity, food intake, and taking serial blood samples it is possible to study well-accepted equivalents of anxiety, depression, and motivation in animals. Animal studies provide a means of directly investigating hypotheses that may be generated from careful observations of patients.

What is the origin of the sensation of fatigue?

Much of what we know of fatigue mechanisms originates not surprisingly from studies of exercise-induced fatigue. Whilst such studies are relevant and provide important clues as to the types of study that may be undertaken in patients with cancer, they must also be viewed in light of the clear differences that exist between exercise-induced and cancer/therapy-induced fatigue. It is perhaps unfortunate that the word 'fatigue', which is so linked to exercise, is also used as the descriptor for the symptom reported by cancer patients, as this may lead to a biased view of mechanisms involved.

Exercise studies have identified two broad possible origins of fatigue: central and peripheral. These are encapsulated in the question 'is the problem with the driver or the machine?'(Edwards 1981). This draws the distinction between fatigue resulting from the inability of the peripheral neuromuscular apparatus itself to perform a task ('the machine') and that resulting from a reduced central drive ('the driver') (see Chapter 14).

The origin of the sense of muscular fatigue is clearly complex and it has been proposed to have at least three components:

- a greater sense of effort required to accomplish a task;
- weakness;
- sensations present in the fatigued muscle that are present even if it is not being used.

In recent years attention has shifted from the muscle to the central mechanisms. Studies of patients with CFS using transcranial magnetic stimulation to activate corticospinal motor pathways has provided some evidence for cortical changes (Brouwer and Packer 1994; Samii *et al.* 1996). However, recent studies, one of which examined intracortical inhibition in the motor cortex, failed to show a difference between CFS patients and matched controls (Davey *et al.* 2001; Zaman *et al.* 2001). An increase in simple reaction times is a consistent finding in CFS patients (see for example Prasher *et al.* (1990) and Davey *et al.* (2001)) suggesting a delay in the central processing of information or changes in signal transmission. Overall, we believe that the weight of current evidence for cancer fatigue and other types of chronic fatigue syndrome favours a central site, but further studies of the peripheral neuromuscular apparatus are required before a peripheral component can be excluded.

Whether the origin of the fatigue is in the muscle or in the central nervous system we still have to consider how the sensation is generated. Fatigue is a subjective, self-reported sensation, although it may be possible to objectively measure a physical manifestation of the sensation by monitoring activity patterns (actigraph) and measuring muscle strength (dynamometer). As with nausea, however accurate our descriptions of the sensation or its associated phenomena we still have to attempt to identify how the sensation is generated and where it is perceived. Fatigue is further complicated because it is intimately linked with the allied sensation of weakness. In essence there are two main ways in which the symptoms could be generated:

(1) by signalling from afferents in the muscles or closely related structures (for example, tendons, joints);

(2) by activation of pathways within the central nervous system, particularly the cerebral cortex.

The weight of evidence from psychophysical studies of the origin of the sense of effort (the sensation felt when holding a heavy object for a prolonged period when the object appears to increase in mass and the effort required to hold it increases), shows that the subject's perception is based more upon the effort required to generate a force rather than upon the magnitude of the force exerted (Enoka and Stuart 1992). The mechanism is central and is proposed to be due to a 'corollary discharge' (internal actions of motor commands) from the motor cortex (the output to the muscles) to the primary somatosensory cortex (McCloskey 1978). In patients with CFS, evidence has been presented for cortical motor abnormalities (Lloyd *et al.* 1991; Brouwer and Packer 1994; Samii *et al.* 1996), but this is not a universal finding (Davey *et al.* 2001; Zaman *et al.* 2001). It must be emphasized that the relationship between the sense of effort and reported sensations of fatigue in disease have yet to be fully explored and such central mechanisms do not exclude contributions from muscle afferents. Non-invasive psychophysical techniques are well established for the study of the sense of effort, and could be readily undertaken in cancer patients to elucidate fatigue mechanisms (McCloskey *et al.* 1974). In the sections discussing neuropharmacology of fatigue below, it is these central mechanisms that it is proposed are being affected to generate inappropriate sensations of the effort required to undertake a task.

Is it the cancer or its treatment?

One of major unresolved issues is the extent to which fatigue is caused by the tumour and its effects (for example cachexia (Plata-Salaman 1996)), the treatments used (for example chemotherapy, radiotherapy, or surgery), or an interaction between the two. Fatigue is a common presenting symptom of many different types of cancer (see Chapters 1 and 2) with little apparent difference in the incidence (except perhaps for haematological malignancies associated with severe anaemia), suggesting some commonality of mechanism associated with substances produced by, or in response to, the tumour (for example cytokines). In a study of 499 patients with cancer, Glaus (1998) found that reported fatigue was related to tumour type, with individuals with gynaecological cancers reporting more fatigue than patients with testicular cancer, who in turn reported more fatigue than patients with breast cancer. Fatigue was also influenced by stage of disease, with patients with metastatic disease reporting more fatigue than patients with localized disease, and those with localized disease reporting more than individuals in remission.

In a retrospective study of 50 consecutive patients (men and women) receiving radiotherapy for lung cancer, 39 individuals (78%) reported fatigue during the course of treatment, with the proportion of patients with fatigue increasing linearly over the course of therapy (Hickok *et al.* 1996). Fatigue frequency did not vary significantly by demographic variables such as age, gender, race, work, or marital status of the patients, or by disease or treatment characteristics, such as disease stage, radiation dose, and previous chemotherapy. A study of 183 men with prostate cancer (Stages 1, 2, or 3), receiving external beam radiation therapy extended these findings (Morrow *et al* 2001). Results presented in Table 3.1 show 75% feeling fatigued during treatment, and in 50% the fatigue was described as moderate or severe. This table also shows that approximately one-third had sleeping difficulties.

Taken together, these studies indicate that some patients with cancer have a degree of fatigue prior to treatment but that the incidence and severity of the fatigue is increased during radiotherapy. Studies of treatments have focused on radiotherapy and chemotherapy, and, as far as we are aware, the possible impact of surgery as an independent variable has not been examined. Many patients will have surgery at some point in their treatment and studies in patients undergoing elective surgery for diseases other than cancer have revealed fatigue as a sequela to surgery (Christensen *et al.* 1989; Zeiderman *et al.* 1990) (see also Chapter 2).

For obvious reasons it is not possible to study the effect of therapy in subjects who do not have a tumour in order to evaluate the relative contributions of cancer and its treatment to overall fatigue. Data collected from the victims of accidental nuclear fallout exposure show that they experience fatigue and that the incidence falls within the range of that found for radiotherapy patients (Anno *et al.* 1989). Although sparse and uncontrolled, these observations demonstrate that radiation is capable of inducing fatigue, and that the presence of a tumour is not an essential cofactor. However, it is not known whether the fatigue induced by radiotherapy in cancer patients has the same characteristics and mechanism(s) as that induced by nuclear fallout exposure.

To summarize, the sparse evidence available indicates that cancer, cytotoxic therapy, and surgery are all independently capable of inducing fatigue, although its characteristics and underlying mechanism(s) may differ. Some patients with cancer report fatigue at diagnosis, and this increases in incidence and severity with treatment.

Table 3.1 Frequency and severity of adverse effects in 183 men receiving external beam radiation treatment for prostate cancer

Adverse effect	Frequency	Intensity (moderate or severe)
Fatigue	N = 121 (74%)	N = 60 (50%)
Urinary problems	N = 118 (72%)	N = 72 (61%)
Diarrhoea	N = 105 (64%)	N = 49 (47%)
Difficulty sleeping	N = 52 (32%)	N = 25 (48%)

Mechanisms and models of cancer-related fatigue

In looking at fatigue from a broad mechanistic perspective two categories can be identified:

1. 'Known': by this we mean fatigue associated with conditions or diseases where a plausible mechanism can readily be identified based upon the known underlying pathophysiology. In this category would be included fatigue associated with exercise, myasthenia gravis, multiple sclerosis, cardiac disease, chronic lung disease, severe anaemia, hypothyroidism, polio, and steroid myopathy.

2. 'Unknown': in this category are conditions or diseases where the origin of the fatigue is obscure (although this is changing rapidly), such as cancer, chemotherapy, radiotherapy, viral, and bacterial infections, postsurgery fatigue, and CFS. It is possible that these types of fatigue have at least some mechanistic features in common.

The emerging body of cancer-related fatigue knowledge can be combined with findings from other related fields (particularly exercise and CFS) to generate several models for the aetiology of cancer-related fatigue. None of the models is complete, but each is presented as a plausible and testable model to suggest (and hopefully stimulate) further research on the aetiology of cancer-related fatigue. For each we state the basic hypothesis, the key evidence upon which it is based, and suggest approaches to testing.

The muscle metabolism hypothesis

Hypothesis

Cancer and/or its treatment, may lead to a defect in the mechanism for regeneration of adenosine triphosphate (ATP) in skeletal muscle, compromising the ability to perform mechanical work and resulting in symptoms of fatigue (Fig. 3.3).

Evidence

Muscle fatigue can be defined as 'any exercise-induced reduction in the ability to exert muscle force or power, regardless of whether or not the task can be sustained' (Gandevia *et al.* 1995). The fundamental mechanism of force generation in skeletal muscle is the interaction between actin filaments and myosin cross-bridges. Any situation that compromises this interaction will lead to a reduction in force, that is, fatigue. Substances in the muscle, including calcium (Ca^{2+}), potassium (K^+), hydrogen (H^+), adenosine diphosphate (ADP), and ATP are all able to directly or indirectly influence the actin–myosin interaction, and hence force generation. It is therefore possible that cancer or its treatment could produce fatigue by modulating any of these factors.

Adenosine triphosphate is a major source of energy, splitting high-energy phosphate bonds for a range of cellular processes, including those responsible for the generation of mechanical work (contraction) in skeletal muscle. Thus, it is self-evident that depletion of ATP would

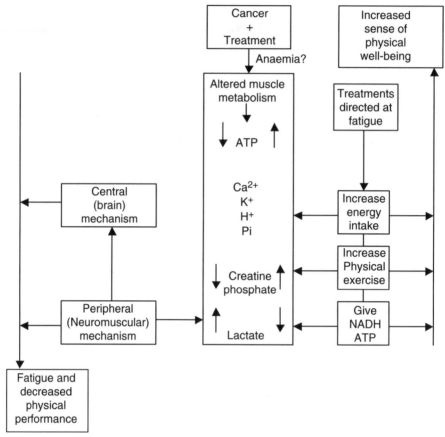

Fig. 3.3 Summary diagram of the possible involvement of changes in skeletal muscle metabolism induced by cancer and its treatment on the genesis of fatigue. See text for references.

compromise the ability to do mechanical work. Normally, ATP can be quickly replenished, with most cellular ATP being formed in mitochondria by oxidative phosphorylation.

Research has demonstrated a relationship between fatigue and physical performance ability in cancer patients (Dimeo *et al.* 1997; Akechi *et al.* 1999). Altered muscle metabolism, for example, due to decreased synthesis of various proteins or accumulation of certain metabolites, may contribute to cancer-related fatigue (Cella *et al.* 1998). ATP concentrations may be relatively low in certain areas of tumours themselves (Karczmar *et al.* 1989, 1991; Feller *et al.* 1994; Tamulevicius and Streffer 1995). Compromised blood supply to tumours can result in oxygen-depleted areas associated with deprivation of nutrients and energy, and a hostile metabolic microenvironment (that is, severe tissue acidosis) (Vaupel *et al.* 1989). Preclinical *in vitro* experiments have shown that treatment modalities often used successfully against cancer, such as radiation, are associated with alterations in cellular energy functions including decreased ATP in tumour cells (Karczmar *et al.* 1991) and peripheral lymphocytes (Robins *et al.* 1991). Incubation of malignant cell lines with cytostatic drugs has resulted in marked decreases in intracellular ATP levels, the degree of decrease varying with the strength of cytostatic drug (Kuzmits *et al.* 1986).

Patients diagnosed with CFS have been the focus of some studies of muscle fatigue, which do not consistently show that the problem resides in the periphery, that is, the muscle or its innervation (Wessely *et al.* 1998). In one study, increased $2'$-$5'$A synthetase, and RNAase L activity, led to depleted cellular ATP which was thought to be 'a pivotal lesion responsible for severe fatigue, cognitive difficulties, or other disturbances' (Forsyth *et al.* 1999). However, other investigators have found impaired synthesis of ATP and defective muscle energy metabolism, along with impaired voluntary activation of skeletal muscle during sustained intense exercise, in a proportion of patients with CFS (Lane *et al.* 1998). The latter finding is suggestive of the presence of a central component of fatigue (Kent-Braun *et al.* 1993). In non-dialysed patients with chronic renal failure who often complain of muscle weakness and fatigue after minor physical activity and may suffer from myopathy related to uraemia, muscle biopsies showed significantly low ATP and creatine phosphate levels (Pastoris *et al.* 1997).

A recent study of patients with CFS did provide some evidence for a defect in ATP metabolism. This randomized, double-blind, crossover study compared the ability of NADH (the reduced form of the coenzyme nicotinamide adenine dinucleotide (NAD), a key coenzyme in the process of oxidative phosphorylation) (Guyton 1992; Pastoris *et al.* 1997) and placebo to ameliorate symptoms of CFS including fatigue, cognitive dysfunction, and sleep disturbance. In the study by Forsyth *et al.* (1999), 31% ($n = 8$) of patients showed at a minimum 10% improvement in their score on a questionnaire measuring fatigue, memory, ability to concentrate, sleep disturbance, and mood. They also reported decreased fatigue, decreased symptoms overall, and improved QOL while taking the study drug compared with 8% ($n = 2$), while taking placebo ($p < 0.05$).

Alteration in energy metabolism has been postulated as a factor likely to influence the fatigue associated with cancer chemotherapy. Reasons for this include the quality and degree of fatigue in patients with CFS, other diseases associated with this symptom and cancer, and a correspondence between appetite changes and the course of post-chemotherapy fatigue. Repletion of intracellular stores of ATP, for example by giving NADH, might be expected to ameliorate feelings of lack of energy and promote enhanced physical performance.

Testing

Any investigation of muscle fatigue in cancer patients should include measurements of both voluntary muscle contraction and that evoked by electrical stimulation of the nerve supplying the same muscles ('twitch interpolation') (Gandevia *et al.* 1995). This important technique allows a distinction to be made between central mechanisms (brain) of fatigue and those operating at the level of the neuromuscular system. Research tools such as assessment of physical activity using actigraphy and concomitant measurement of metabolic activity (for example, ATP, creatine phosphate, and lactate levels) in muscle tissue biopsy samples, or preferably *in situ,* using nuclear magnetic resonance (NMR) and related techniques, could be used to further evaluate this hypothesis. Further indirect support would come from therapeutic trials of agents enhancing the formation of ATP, such at NAD (Forsyth *et al.* 1999).

The vagal afferent hypothesis

Hypothesis

Cancer, and or its treatment, leads to release of a neuroactive agent(s) (for example, 5-HT, interleukin 1β (IL-1β)), which activate a population of vagal afferents, leading to a reflex decrease in somatic motor outflow and sustained plastic changes in selected regions of the brain, including the hypothalamus (Fig. 3.4).

Evidence

In addition to supplying a number of visceral organs (heart, stomach) with efferent parasympathetic fibres, the vagus nerve also has a high percentage (in the abdominal vagus 90%) of afferent fibres conveying information from the viscera to the brainstem. The abdominal vagal afferents have been shown to play a major role in the acute phase of emesis induced by cytotoxic drugs and radiation, which is mediated by the local

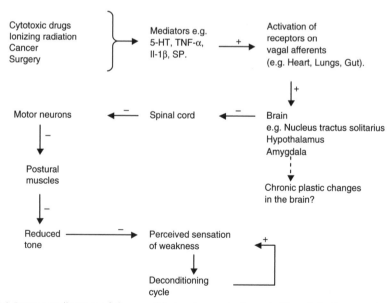

Fig. 3.4 Summary diagram of the possible involvement of vagal afferents in the genesis of reduced somatomotor tone induced by cancer and its treatment. See text for references.

release of 5-HT from gut mucosal enterochromaffin cells (Andrews and Davis 1995). Several pieces of evidence from animal studies suggest that some vagal afferents could be involved in the genesis of fatigue sensations by modulation of somatic muscle tone. The modulation of somatic muscle tone by vagal afferent activation was first reported in 1937 by Schweitzer and Wright. They showed that electrical stimulation of the central end of the vagus caused a reduction in the magnitude of the knee-jerk reflex. Further studies showed that activation of a population of visceral afferent receptors in the cardiopulmonary region (Ginzel *et al.* 1972), including vagal afferents supplying the lungs (juxtapulmonary capillary receptors (Paintal 1973), pulmonary C-fibres (Coleridge and Coleridge 1984)), caused reflex inhibition of somatic motor activity in decerebrate and anaesthetized cats. In a mesencephalic cat, activation of pulmonary receptors attenuated or abolished walking (Kalia 1973; Pickar *et al.* 1993). More recently, activation of vagal afferents by a 5-HT$_3$ receptor agonist has been shown to reduce steady-state exercise-induced EMG activity in conscious rats (Dicarlo *et al.* 1994), and intravenous injection of a thromboxane A2 receptor agonist has been shown to inhibit the knee-jerk reflex in anaesthetized cats (Pickar 1998).

Other relevant studies in the rat have shown that activation of abdominal vagal afferents reduced reflex activation of skeletal muscles (Kawaski *et al.* 1983), and in studies of dogs it was shown that shielding the abdomen prevented performance decrement caused by gamma radiation (Malkhovski *et al.* 1990).

The physiological function of the reflex, pulmonary, afferent suppression of somatic muscle activation was proposed to limit exercise by detecting the pulmonary congestion resulting from exercise (Paintal 1973, 1995). This hypothesis is not accepted universally. However, section of the vagal fibres to the right lung of a patient with right pulmonary obstruction relieved the associated dyspnoea and normalized the ventilatory response to exercise (Davies *et al.* 1987). The function of the abdominal vagal afferent suppression of somatic muscle activity has not been identified. One possible explanation may be its relation to the teleological requirement of an animal to rest and recover following ingestion of a noxious material (see above). It must be noted that the evidence for these vagosomatic inhibitory reflexes in humans is scant, and a recent study was unable to demonstrate a suppression of somatic muscle activity by pulmonary C-fibre activation, but the explanation may reside in technical rather than physiological considerations (Gandevia *et al.* 1998; Widdicombe 1998). Further studies of this reflex are required in humans. Although there are numerous differences in the physiological response to exercise in humans and animals, on teleological grounds it appears likely that a reflex from the lungs to the somatic muscles will be identified in humans when appropriate experimental conditions are identified.

If a vagosomatic inhibitory reflex is identified in humans, then it could play a role in the genesis of lethargy, weakness, and fatigue associated with cancer and its treatment. Studies in animals have shown that vagal afferent C-fibres can be stimulated by 5-HT (Blackshaw and Grundy 1993*a,b*), substance P, cytokines (for example IL-1β

(Ek *et al.* 1998)), and prostaglandins (Niijima 1996). These and other substances may be secreted as a result of the tumour and/or the anti-cancer treatment in appropriate locations (for example, lungs, gut mucosa, liver), where vagal afferents terminate, potentially evoking a reflex decrease in skeletal muscle tone. This decrease in tone would be perceived as a generalized weakness, particularly when standing, an inability to complete a motor task, or as a feeling that more effort (that is, central drive) was needed to complete the task than was usually required or anticipated. However, it is likely that other pathways might also be driven by inappropriate vagal afferent firing. Thus, studies predominantly in rats have suggested an additional role for abdominal vagal afferents relevant to the genesis of 'sickness syndrome', and involving signalling of information about peripheral pathogenic information to the brain. Such behaviour can be argued to be the teleological 'equivalent' of the symptoms evoked by anti-cancer treatment (see above). For example, in rats following intraperitoneal injection of either bacterial lipopolysaccharide or IL-1β, a 'sickness syndrome' is induced (Konsman *et al.* 2002). The initial phase consists of hyperalgesia/allodynia, increased activity and fever, and the later phase of hypoalgesia, decreased activity, increased sleep, and either fever or hypothermia. Abdominal vagotomy attenuates or abolishes the hyperalgesia, increased sleep, reduced activity, and fever (Hansen and Kreuger 1997; Opp and Toth 1998; Kapas *et al.* 1998). Activation of the vagal afferents by IL-1 influences brainstem, hypothalamic, and limbic nuclei and these actions are particularly important in the genesis of behavioural depression (Konsman *et al.* 2002).

To summarize, there are considerable data from animals to show that vagal afferents have the ability to generate many features of the 'sickness syndrome', which could therefore be regarded as a model of the vagal nerve mechanisms suggested to initiate a chronic fatigue syndrome. This non-specific host response to the invasion of a pathogenic organism, and the proinflammatory mediators released, has many features in common with the symptoms observed in patients with cancer or being treated. It is not unreasonable to suggest that vagal afferent activation contributes to the genesis of symptoms, including fatigue, in humans. However, it is not clear how such a mechanism would sustain symptoms of fatigue over years, indicating that a secondary and sustained degree of neuronal plasticity must be evoked separately, or as a consequence of the inappropriate vagal nerve activity. Evidence suggesting the latter is provided by the ability of intraperitoneal injection of IL-1β in rats to increase induction of IL-1β mRNA in rat brainstem, hippocampus, and hypothalamus. This induction was either reduced or abolished by abdominal vagotomy (Hansen *et al.* 1998). The authors proposed that 'the induction of brain cytokines is a critical step in the pathway by which vagal mediated signals result in centrally controlled symptoms of the acute phase response'. The importance of this for fatigue is twofold: firstly, it is hypothesized below that central cytokines (e.g. IL-1, IL-6) and 5-HT are involved in the pathogenesis of fatigue. Secondly, one of the areas in which brain cytokines are induced by vagal activation is the hypothalamus, which together with the pituitary gland has often been implicated in the genesis of fatigue (see below). Vagal afferent activation also influences 'higher' regions of the brain (e.g. the limbic system) which may also be involved in the pathogenesis of fatigue.

Thus, if correct, the vagal nerve hypothesis provides an ability to link each of the following hypotheses by providing both the substrate for the initiation of fatigue (or 'sickness behaviour'), and the vehicle and/or the stimulus for secondary, plastic changes in central nervous system functions.

Testing

Testing this hypothesis in humans would be problematic, as the clearest evidence would come from studies of patients receiving chemotherapy in which the effects of thoracic and abdominal vagal afferent blockade are investigated. Whilst blockade of the cervical vagi has been performed in volunteers using injection of local anaesthetic, and surgical abdominal vagotomy is still occasionally performed, neither approach is realistic here. Although vagal afferent modulation of somatic motor activity has been demonstrated convincingly in animals, the evidence for such modulation is weak in humans (see Gandevia *et al.* (1998) discussed above), and this clearly needs further investigation. An alternative approach in patients would be to pharmacologically modulate vagal afferent traffic either at a central or peripheral site. $5-HT_3$ and neuro-kinin 1 (NK1) receptor antagonists or cyclooxygenase (COX) inhibitors would be suit-able for such a study, but as 5-HT, substance P, and prostaglandins are not the only substances involved in afferent activation, a negative result would not be definitive. It may also be important to apply such treatment during periods in which symptoms of fatigue are induced, rather than at later stages in which secondary maintenance mechanisms may be operating. Thus, further testing of this hypothesis in humans probably awaits studies in animals to better characterize any temporal changes in peripheral and central vagal afferent and efferent nerve functions resulting from cancer and its treatment.

The serotonin dysregulation hypothesis

Hypothesis

Cancer and or its treatment causes an increase in brain serotonin (5-HT) levels in specific brain regions, and/or an upregulation of a population of 5-HT receptors leading to reduced somatomotor drive, modified HPA function, and a sensation of reduced capacity to perform physical work (Fig. 3.5).

Evidence

A growing body of evidence is accumulating from studies of exercise-induced fatigue and CFS to implicate a dysregulation of 5-HT in the mechanism(s) by which fatigue can be induced. These studies will be reviewed here because of the insights they give into cancer-related fatigue and the types of study that could be undertaken.

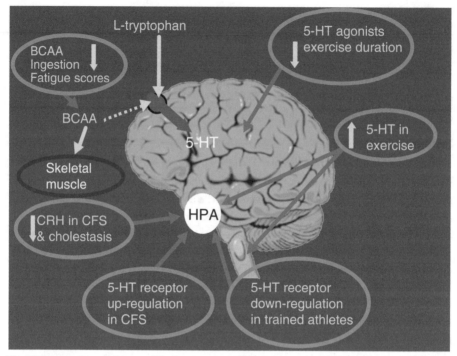

Fig. 3.5 Summary of the possible involvement of brain 5-hydroxytryptamine (5-HT) and the hypothalamic–pituitary axis (HPA) in the genesis of fatigue induced by exercise and associated with chronic fatigue syndrome (CFS). L-tryptophan (the precursor for 5-HT synthesis) and branched chain amino acids (BCAA) compete for the same transporter into the brain so that when muscles are exercising and using BCAA more L-tryptophan is able to enter the brain via the transporter. CRH = corticotrophin-releasing hormone. See text for references.

Exercise-induced fatigue

The amino acid tryptophan is the precursor for 5-HT synthesis and enters the brain via a carrier (transporter) system that can also be used by branch-chain amino acids (BCAA). During exercise, BCAA are transported into the active skeletal muscles and hence the levels free in the plasma decrease, leading to a decreased competition with tryptophan and hence an increase in the entry of tryptophan into the brain. This is argued to lead to an increase in the synthesis of 5-HT in the brain, although whether this is generalized or regionalized has not been determined. As central 5-HT was known to be involved in sleep, aggression, and mood (depression), it was hypothesized that an elevation in central 5-HT could mediate or contribute to the central component(s) of the fatigue occurring during and after heavy exercise (Newsholme and Blomstrand 1995). In human volunteers receiving single 5 mg oral doses of (-) tryptophan, subjects rated themselves as 'more slowed down' than on placebo, and mood self-rating scales revealed a significant increase in subjects' ratings of drowsiness, muzziness, and mental slowness (Greenwood *et al.* 1975).

Hypothalamic 5-HT receptor function is down-regulated in endurance-trained athletes (Jakeman *et al.* 1994). The 5-HT hypothesis has been studied directly in healthy volunteers by examining the effect of ingestion of BCAA on the fatigue scores during exercise. The perceived exertion and mental fatigue scores were reduced by ingestion of BCAA in subjects exercising on a bicycle ergometer at 70% of their $VO_{2\,max}$ (maximum volume of oxygen consumption) for 60 min (Blomstrand *et al.* 1997). However, there was no significant effect in subjects exercising maximally, an observation which may be consistent with evidence showing that consumption of BCAA increased performance in slower but not faster marathon runners (Newsholme and Blomstrand 1995). These results suggest that a study of the effects of BCAA may be warranted in patients with cancer-related fatigue once further evidence supporting an involvement is forthcoming (see below).

The possible role of central 5-HT has also been investigated using drugs to modify serotonergic transmission. In healthy volunteers the selective serotonin reuptake inhibitor (SSRI) paroxetine, given as a single 20 mg oral dose, was shown to reduce the time that exercise on a bicycle ergometer at 70% $VO_{2\,max}$ could be sustained (Wilson and Maughan 1992). A similar study used the 5-HT_{1A} receptor agonist buspirone in subjects exercising at 80% $VO_{2\,max}$, and showed a reduction in the time subjects could exercise, and an increase in the perceived exhaustion score (Marvin *et al.* 1997).

The results from the above studies are consistent in implicating an elevation in central 5-HT in the genesis of the 'central fatigue' associated with exercise, defined as 'a progressive exercise-induced reduction in voluntary activation of muscle' (Gandevia *et al.* 1995). The site(s) at which 5-HT is elevated in humans remains to be identified, but sustained exercise in rats demonstrated increased 5-HT levels in the hypothalamus and brainstem but not in four other areas studied (Blomstrand *et al.* 1989). Other studies in rats have also shown that administration of 5-HT produced a dose-related decrease in running (Bailey *et al.* 1992), and an improvement in performance by addition of an antagonist (Bailey *et al.* 1993). In cats, injection of 5-HT into the lateral ventricle of the brain produced 'lethargy' and 'diminished muscular tone' (Gaddum and Vogt 1956).

Chronic fatigue syndrome

5-HT has also been the focus of attention in patients with CFS, but this has been because a number of pituitary hormones have their secretion influenced by 5-HT. In patients with CFS (but not primary depression, potentially co-morbid with chronic fatigue, see below) the 5-HT_{1A} agonist buspirone and the 5-HT_2 agonist D-fenfluramine evoke an enhanced secretion of prolactin (Cleare *et al.* 1995; Bakheit *et al.* 1992; Sharpe *et al.* 1996, 1997). Overall these results suggest an up-regulation/hypersensitivity of a population of central 5-HT receptors in the hypothalamus and this contrasts with a down-regulation reported in endurance trained athletes (Jakeman *et al.* 1994).

These types of study could readily be undertaken in patients with cancer-related fatigue.

How could cancer and its therapy modify serotonin metabolism?

The above sections have identified ways in which changes in 5-HT and/or its receptors may alter in fatigue, but how could such changes be brought about by cancer and its therapy? The proinflammatory cytokines are well known to induce fatigue when administered (Blesch *et al.*1991; Borish *et al.* 1998; Holmes *et al.* 1988; Moldawer and Figlin 1988; Piper *et al.* 1989; Winningham *et al.*1994) and tumour necrosis factor (TNF) has been shown to prevent proteosome-dependent degradation of the regulator of G-protein signalling, RGS7 (Benzing *et al.* 1999). This has been proposed to produce changes in central nervous system (CNS) neurotransmission leading to behavioural changes associated with an inflammatory response (for example lethargy, fever, anorexia). Several pieces of evidence implicate the proinflammatory cytokines in the possible modulation of serotonergic transmission which itself plays a key role in the neuropharmacology of sleep:

1. The proinflammatory cytokine TNF is elevated in the circulation of patients with cancer and is further elevated by radiotherapy (Bianco *et al.* 1991; Hallahan *et al.* 1993), as is IL-1 (Greenberg *et al.* 1993). Central nervous system neurons increase synthesis of TNF-α in response to radiation (Hong *et al.* 1995).

2. TNF and IL-6 levels have been reported to be elevated in several studies of patients with CFS (Borish *et al.* 1998; Chao *et al.* 1990; Patarca *et al.* 1994).

3. TNF has been shown to increase neuronal release of 5-HT and to double the levels of the 5-HT transporter (Mossner *et al.* 1998), which is the main mechanism responsible for removal of 5-HT from the synaptic space. The net effects of these actions upon synaptic transmission, if they occurred in the same location, are impossible to predict.

4. TNF can increase the circulating level of L-tryptophan the precursor for 5-HT synthesis (Pauli *et al.* 1998).

It must be emphasized that the above observations are from a combination of clinical and preclinical studies and from them it is not possible to predict exactly what will happen to either synaptic 5-HT levels or 5-HT receptors. However, taken together with the studies of exercise and CFS they do provide a possible mechanistic link between cytokines, 5-HT, and fatigue that merits further investigation. If cytokines are involved then one major issue is how systemic cytokines could influence the CNS as they do not readily penetrate the brain. There are at least two possibilities, both of which could be involved in the genesis of fatigue:

(1) activation of peripheral afferents (for example the vagus) which project to the brain (see above);

(2) access to the brain via the circumventricular organs (for example the area postrema or anterior hypothalamus) where the blood–brain barrier is relatively permeable.

There is evidence that macrophage-like (phagocytic) cells in the circumventricular organs and the choroid plexus (e.g. in the region of the hypothalamus) produce IL-1 which can then diffuse into the brain to activate neurons and release other neuroactive agents (e.g. prostaglandin E_2) (Konsman *et al.* 2002).

Testing

The simplest way to investigate whether this hypothesis has any validity is to repeat the dietary modification studies using BCAA used in investigations of exercise-induced fatigue. Indications of modifications to the neuropharmacology of brain 5-HT could be gained from studies using selective antagonists, agonists, or uptake inhibitors to probe central systems known to be modulated by 5-HT (for example prolactin secretion). A study of the effects of 5-HT$_3$ receptor antagonists (for example granisetron, ondansetron) on fatigue would be of particular interest as such antagonists have been shown in case or open-label studies to improve performance status in two patients on high-dose interferon therapy (Drapkin *et al.* 1999), patients with profound fatigue associated with chronic liver disease (Jones 1999), and approximately one-third of patients in a small study of CFS (Spath *et al.* 2000). It will also be of value to study the acute and long-term changes in those animals with 'sickness behaviour', attempting to correlate changes in behavioural indices with vagal nerve function (see above), central changes in 5-HT turnover, as well as hypothalamic–pituitary function (see below).

The hypothalamic–pituitary axis dysfunction hypothesis

Hypothesis

Cancer and/or its treatment directly or indirectly cause a modification of hypothalamic–pituitary axis (HPA) function resulting in endocrine changes either causing or contributing to fatigue.

Evidence

Some of the evidence implicating a dysregulation of central 5-HT comes from the studies of hypothalamic–pituitary function discussed above (for example prolactin secretion) which could also be used to indicate a dysfunction of the hypothalamic–pituitary axis. However, additional evidence supporting a dysregulation of function comes from studies of patients with CFS.

A consistent finding in patients with CFS is the presence of mild hypocortisolism (Cleare *et al.* 2001) with the proposed cause being a 'defect' in hypothalamic neurons producing corticotrophin-releasing hormone (CRH). This observation is of particular interest, as patients with major depression are reported to have mild hypercortisolism and evidence of central upregulation of the HPA (Demitrack *et al.* 1991; Demitrack 1998; Komaroff and Buchwald 1998). Fatigue is one of the clinical symptoms of adrenocortical insufficiency (Nussey and Whitehead 2001). In addition glucocorticoids can repress genes for several interleukins (e.g. IL-1, IL-6) and TNF-α. It is possible

that if cancer and its therapy increase the secretion of these cytokines and this is combined with a suppression of cortical secretion, then the latter could conceivably facilitate
the secretion of the former.

The proposal of a defect in CRH secretion in patients with CFS is consistent with an
animal study of sickness syndrome induced by cholestatic disease, which showed
a reduction in CRH (Swain and Maric 1995).

Further evidence of a defect in the HPA comes from a study of patients with postviral
fatigue syndrome (Bakheit *et al.* 1993). The authors were unable to find the expected
correlation between plasma osmolarity and levels of plasma vasopressin (antidiuretic
hormone) synthesized by the supraoptic nuclei in the hypothalamus and secreted into
the blood in the posterior lobe of the pituitary.

Testing

Initial testing of this hypothesis would involve a detailed study of the hypothalamic–
pituitary–adrenal function in matched populations of control subjects, patients with
cancer, and the same patients during therapy. Although basal secretion of hormones
may be affected, it is essential that studies use provocative challenges of
differing intensity to investigate the ability of the system to respond, and also the sensitivity of the response and its feedback control. As the 5-HT$_2$ receptor agonist fenfluramine produces a dose-related increase in prolactin secretion after acute
administration, this would provide a suitable stimulus in which the sensitivity of
central 5-HT receptors could be investigated in humans (Quattrone *et al.* 1983).
Prolactin secretion from the anterior pituitary is under tonic inhibitory control by
hypothalamic dopaminergic neurons. Metoclopramide and domperidone are still in
use as antiemetics and both have dopamine receptor antagonist properties leading to
an increase in plasma prolactin levels after acute and subchronic administration
(Brouwers *et al.* 1980). This property could be utilized to make an opportunistic
assessment of hypothalamic dopaminergic neuronal activity in patients undergoing
chemotherapy in whom either metoclopramide or domperidone are being used as
antiemetics.

The availability of selective corticotrophin-releasing factor 1 (CRF1) and CRF2
receptor antagonists will enable direct testing in animal models of the role that CRH
may have in fatigue.

Conditions that may covary with fatigue

The hypotheses outlined above summarize the major aetiological associations supported by currently available data from both clinical and preclinical investigations.
There are other conditions that have been linked to fatigue. Among the other health-
related conditions that often occur along with cancer-induced fatigue are depression,
anaemia, and changes in circadian rhythm. They are found significantly less frequently
than fatigue among cancer patients—thus bringing into question their role as primary

aetiological contributors—but none the less may play some potential role in the development or expression of cancer related fatigue.

Depression

Depression frequently occurs together with fatigue in cancer patients. Five studies that used a structured clinical interview to classify depression by the Diagnostic and Statistical Manual of Mental Disorders (revised third edition) (DSM IIIR) criteria diagnosed depression in 40% to 82% of patients, with a mean percentage (weighted by the number of people per study) of 58% (Nerenz *et al.* 1982; Devlen *et al.* 1987; Peck and Boland 1977; Kubricht 1984; Mitchell and Glicksman 1977). However common in cancer patients, depression is not as prevalent as fatigue, suggesting that while there is some covariation fatigue is not equivalent to depression (see Chapter 10 for a detailed consideration of the relationship between fatigue and depression).

The covariance of fatigue with depression is of particular interest, as a history of depression is a predisposing factor for the development of chronic fatigue syndrome, again suggesting a degree of common aetiology (Wessely *et al.* 1998). However, a recent study of the selective serotonin re-uptake inhibitor (SSRI) paroxetine in cancer patients undergoing treatment showed that whilst scores of depression were reduced, there was no effect on fatigue scores (Morrow *et al.* 2003).

Disruption of circadian rhythms

Patients often report sleep disturbance as a very common feature of cancer treatment. Results presented in Table 3.1 showed sleep disturbance (one of the pre-eminent symptoms of circadian disruption) to be commonly reported by prostate patients during radiation treatment.

Berger (1998) and Mormont *et al.* (1996, 1998) used actigraphy to measure relative levels of activity in patients with breast cancer and colorectal cancer. Both found a negative relationship between fatigue and activity levels during the day and a positive relationship between fatigue and restless sleep at night. Mormont *et al.* (1996, 1998) also found a strong reduction in activity levels of patients with colorectal cancer during the day and an increase in activity levels during the night as compared with a matched group of controls. In addition, the difference between daytime and night-time activity levels in cancer patients was less than in the matched group of controls. Furthermore, Mormont *et al.* (1996, 1998) found the circadian alternation of activity and rest to be altered in the group of colorectal cancer patients but not in the control group and concluded that cancer patients may have a disruption in their activity circadian rhythm cycle.

Further results from a study outlined below (Roscoe *et al.* 2002) indicate that disruption of circadian rhythms may be associated with both fatigue and depression and that the association between fatigue and circadian disruption is independent of depression. Results shown in Table 3.2 are intercorrelations among fatigue, depression, and

Table 3.2 Partial correlations of study measures from patient's second on-study treatment, controlling for baseline performance status.[a] (From Roscoe *et al.* 2002)

Measure	1	2	3	4	5	6	7	8
1. Circadian rhythm[b]	—							
2. Mean activity[c]	65**	—						
3. Per cent sleep[d]	− 0.52**	− 0.82**	—					
4. FSCL	− 0.26*	− 0.21	0.27*	—				
5. MAF	− 0.27*	− 0.23*	0.30**	0.63**	—			
6. CESD	− 0.32**	− 0.30**	0.40**	0.63**	0.66**	—		
7. HDI	− 0.25*	− 0.25*	0.31**	0.66**	0.68**	0.75**	—	
8. POMS	− 0.37**	− 0.26*	0.36**	0.78**	0.75**	0.83**	0.74**	—

Abbreviations: FSCL, Fatigue Symptom Checklist; MAF, Multidimensional Assessment of Fatigue; CES-D, Center for Epidemiological Studies Depression Scale; HDI, Hamilton Depression Inventory; POMS, Profile of Mood States.

$N = 76–78$; * $p < 0.05$; ** $p < 0.01$.

[a] Measured on the Karnofsky Performance Scale.

[b] Actigraph measurement of autocorrelation.

[c] Actigraph measurement of daytime activity level.

[d] Actigraph measurement of daytime nap and rest periods.

circadian rhythm measured concomitantly 1 week after the second or later treatment in 76 patients receiving chemotherapy for breast cancer.

Fatigue was assessed by the Fatigue Symptom Checklist (FSCL) and the Multidimensional Assessment of Fatigue (MAF); depression with the Center for Epidemiological Studies Depression Scale (CES-D) and the depression–dejection subscale of the Profile of Mood States (POMS-D). Circadian rhythm was assessed over 72 h period with a Mini-Motionlogger actigraph. Daily patterns of sleep and activity were compared across the 3 day period (Fig. 3.5) by autocorrelation analyses to calculate a circadian rhythm score for each patient. Higher circadian rhythm scores (i.e. a more consistent day-to-day pattern of rest and activity) were significantly related to lower fatigue reports on all measures (all $r > 0.30$, all $p < 0.01$), and also to depression ($r = 0.28$, $p = 0.02$). The relationship between fatigue and circadian rhythm remained significant or marginally significant for all measures even after controlling for depression (all partial correlation $r > 0.20$, all $p < 0.1$).

Anaemia

Anaemia is sometimes equated with fatigue in cancer patients, but whilst anaemia may be caused by chemotherapy, it occurs at a significantly lower rate than fatigue.

While exact incidence figures are not available, transfusions (presumably for anaemia) have been noted in up to 18% of patients receiving chemotherapy (Demetri *et al.* 1998). It may be more frequent in patients treated with cisplatin and less frequent in patients treated with radiation. As with depression and circadian rhythm disruption, anaemia may be a contributing factor in patients reporting fatigue. The fact that it occurs significantly less frequently than fatigue in patients treated with chemotherapy, and is quite infrequently found as a result of radiation therapy (even though fatigue is reported by perhaps a greater proportion of cancer patients receiving radiation than chemotherapy), argues for a relatively minor contribution to the general experience of fatigue (see also Chapter 12).

Whatever the relative contribution of anaemia to the genesis of fatigue, understanding more about anaemia is important as anaemia is treatable (blood transfusion or recombinant erythropoietin (EPO)), and because anaemia itself is relatively well characterized it may provide an important insight into one mechanism of fatigue in cancer patients.

Recent studies have identified an important role for cytokines in the genesis of anaemia associated with cancer and its treatment (Groopman and Itri 1999; Bron 2001). However, the relationships between the degree of anaemia and magnitude of fatigue are unclear. Bruera *et al.* (1989) were unable to find a relationship between fatigue and haemoglobin (Hb) level in patients with advanced breast cancer, although other studies have demonstrated weak correlations (Morant 1996). Using the FACT-An questionnaire to assess the impact of anaemia on QOL, Demetri *et al.* (1998) showed a significant correlation between an improvement in QOL and the change in Hb brought about by treatment with recombinant EPO; patients with the largest increases in Hb had the largest changes in overall QOL score. It is important to appreciate that this study looked at the change in, rather than the absolute level of, Hb and therefore the relationship between fatigue and Hb remains to be elucidated. This is of relevance to understanding the mechanism(s) by which cancer-related anaemia 'causes' fatigue, which itself is unclear. The usual mechanism implicated is hypoxia-related impairment of organ function (Mercuriali and Inghilleri 2001), but there appears to be a paucity of evidence supporting this in cancer patients. Furthermore, if this is the case, which is the critical organ(s) or system(s) (for example brain, skeletal muscle) affected? The absence of a clear relationship between fatigue and Hb may indicate that the functionality of the Hb itself is reduced in cancer patients (for example by therapy alone or in combination with cytokines) thereby reducing its ability to transport oxygen. Haemoglobin function could also be altered by cancer or therapy-induced changes to membrane transport characteristics of the erythrocyte (for example K^+, chloride (Cl^-), magnesium (Mg^{2+}) fluxes), and in this context it is of interest that the lifespan of erythrocytes is reduced in cancer-related anaemia (Bron 2001). In addition, in a small study of patients with CFS, red cell Mg^{2+} concentrations were lower than matched controls. Red cell magnesium concentrations were restored to normal by 6 weeks of magnesium sulphate injections and this was associated with improved energy levels (Cox *et al.* 1991).

Whilst attention has focused on the erythropoietic effects of recombinant EPO, other pharmacological effects should not be overlooked as:

(1) receptors for EPO have been found on neurons, glia, and brain capillary endothelial cells (Yamaji *et al.* 1996; Juul *et al.* 1998; Morishita *et al.* 1997);

(2) increased EPO receptor expression and EPO synthesis occurs in the CNS in response to hypoxia (Masuda *et al.* 1994; Bernaudin *et al.* 2000);

(3) administration of EPO protects against neuronal damage in stroke models (Sakanaka *et al.* 1998);

(4) EPO normalizes the autoregulation of cerebral blood flow after subarachnoid haemorrhage (Springborg *et al.* 2002).

Although anaemia is involved in the pathogenesis of cancer-related fatigue its importance should not be overestimated. For example, a study of the correlates of fatigue amongst 227 assorted cancer patients and 98 controls revealed that although there was a statistically significant association between fatigue severity and haematocrit the magnitude of the correlation was quite weak ($R = -0.22$, $p < 0.05$) (Stone *et al.* 2000*b*). Equally 'weak' correlations have been found between haematocrit and QOL (Crawford *et al.* 2002) and in another study of a mixed group of cancer patients it was reported that anaemia could explain only 8% of the variation of fatigue scores (Lind *et al.* 2002). In view of these observations we argue that anaemia should be regarded as a significant but modest contributor to fatigue in the majority of cancer patients.

The relationships between fatigue and other biochemical indices in the plasma have been less extensively studied in cancer patients than haemoglobin, but significant associations have been found between fatigue severity and serum sodium, urea, and testosterone (Stone *et al.* 1999). The size of the correlations is at least as large as that between fatigue and haemoglobin and the mechanism by which they could be involved in the pathogenesis of fatigue awaits further study (see Box 3.1).

Closing comment

In this often speculative review we have attempted to identify the specific mechanisms by which the fatigue associated with cancer and its treatment may be caused, but it is conceivable that other, as yet unidentified, mechanisms may be involved. It is apparent that much of the material reviewed is from studies of fatigue unrelated to cancer in humans (that is, exercise and CFS), or from animal studies of behaviour or pathways. This serves to highlight the relative lack of specific studies into the fatigue described by cancer patients as well as the urgent need to start integrating each of these areas of research into a set of common hypotheses. This area is, therefore, clearly a fertile one for research and this should be further prompted by the increasing concern expressed by patients, caregivers, and health-care professionals about the impact of this symptom on quality of life. Our discussions are summarized in Box 3.2.

Box 3.1 Future areas for research

1. The mechanisms and models of cancer-related fatigue represent a fertile and fundamental area for future research.

2. Further refinement of the emergent models of fatigue are needed to confirm or discomfirm their potential:

   ◆ Muscle metabolism hypothesis: future investigation of muscle fatigue in cancer patients should include measurement of voluntary muscle contraction as well as electrical stimulation of nerves supplying the same muscles in order to distinguish between central mechanisms of fatigue and those operating at the level of the neuromuscular system.

   ◆ Vagal afferent hypothesis: further studies in animals are needed to better characterize any changes in peripheral or central vagal afferent and efferent nerve functions resulting from cancer or its treatment.

   ◆ Serotonin dysregulation hypothesis: studies are needed to confirm or reject the potential of 5-HT_3 receptor antagonists to decrease fatigue and increase performance status in patients receiving treatment for cancer, for example patients receiving high-dose interferon therapy. Changes in serotonergic transmission also need to be investigated in cancer patients.

   ◆ Hypothalamic–pituitary axis hypothesis: a detailed study of the hypothalamic–pituitary axis function in matched populations of control subjects, patients with cancer, and the same patients during treatment is needed to further refine appreciation of this emergent model.

Box 3.2 Summary points

1. The origin and sensation of fatigue are multifactorial and poorly understood.

2. Several models for the aetiology of cancer-related fatigue have been generated but none is complete:

   ◆ muscle metabolism hypothesis
   ◆ vagal afferent hypothesis
   ◆ serotonin dysregulation hypothesis
   ◆ hypothalamic–pituitary axis hypothesis.

3. The development of or experience of cancer-related fatigue may be influenced by several conditions that may covary with fatigue, such as depression, circadian sleep disruption, or anaemia.

Acknowledgement

We wish to acknowledge Dr Peter Blower and Dr Gareth Sanger for provocative discussions.

References

Abrahamsen, A.F., Loge, J.H., Hannisdal, E., Holte, H., and Kvaloy, S. (1998) Socio-medical situation for long-term survivors of Hodgkin's disease: a survey of 459 patients treated at one institution. *European Journal of Cancer*, **34**, 1865–70.

Ahlberg, K., Ekman, T., Gaston-Johasson, F., and Mock, V. (2003) Assessment and management of cancer related fatigue in adults. *The Lancet*, **362**, 640–50.

Akechi, T., Kugaya, A., Okamura, H., Yamawaki, S., and Uchitomi, Y. (1999) Fatigue and its associated factors in ambulatory cancer patients: a preliminary study. *Journal of Pain and Symptom Management*, **17**, 42–8.

Andrews, P.L.R. (1990) Vomiting : a gastrointestinal tract defensive reflex. In: *Pathophysiology of the Gut and Airways—an Introduction*, (ed. P.Andrews and J. Widdicombe). Portland Press, London, pp. 97–114.

Andrews, P.L.R. and Davis, C.J. (1995) The physiology of emesis induced by anti-cancer therapy. In: *Serotonin and the Scientific Basis of Anti-emetic Therapy*, (ed. D.J.M. Reynolds, P.L.R. Andrews, and C.J. Davis), pp. 25–49. Oxford: Oxford Clinical Communications.

Andrykowski, M.A., Curran, S.L., Studts, J.L., Cunningham, L., Carpenter, J.S., McGrath, P.C. *et al.* (1996) Psychosocial adjustment and quality of life in women with breast cancer and benign breast problems: a controlled comparison. *Journal of Clinical Epidemiology*, **49**, 827–34.

Andrykowski, M.A., Curran, S.L., and Lightner, R. (1998) Off-treatment fatigue in breast cancer survivors: a controlled comparison. *Journal of Behavioral Medicine*, **21**, 1–18.

Anno, G.H., Baum, S.J., Withers, H.R., and Young, R.W (1989) Symptomatology of acute radiation effects in humans after exposure to doses of 0.5–30 Gy. *Health Physics*, **56**, 821–38.

Bailey, S.P., Davis, J.M., and Ahlborn, E.N. (1992) Effect of increased brain serotonergic activity on endurance performance in the rat. *Acta Physiologica Scandinavica*, **145**, 75–6.

Bailey, S.P., Davis J.M., and Ahlborn, E.N. (1993) Neuroendocrine and substrate responses to altered brain 5-HT activity during prolonged exercise to fatigue. *Journal of Applied Physiology*, **74**, 3006–12.

Bakheit, A., Behan, P., Dinan, T., Gray, C., and O'Keane, V. (1992) Possible upregulation of hypothalamic 5-hydroxytryptamine receptors in patients with postviral fatigue syndrome. *British Medical Journal*, **304**,1010–12.

Bakheit, A.M.O., Behan, P.O., and Watson, W.S. (1993) Abnormal arginine-vasopressin secretion and water metabolism in patients with postviral fatigue syndrome. *Acta Neurolgica Scandinavica*, **87**, 234–8.

Beard, G.M. (1880) A practical treatise on nervous exhaustion (neurasthenia): its symptoms, nature, sequences, treatment. William Wood, New York.

Beisecker, A., Cook, M.R., Ashworth, J., Hayes, J., Brecheisen, M., Helmig, L. *et al.* (1997) Side effects of adjuvant chemotherapy: perceptions of node-negative breast cancer patients. *Psycho-Oncology*, **6**, 85–93.

Benzing, T., Brandes, R., Sellin, L., Schermer, B., Lecker, S., Walz, G. *et al.* (1999) Upregulation of RGS7 may contribute to tumour necrosis factor-induced changes in central nervous function. *Nature Medicine*, **5**, 913–18.

Berger, A.M. (1998) Patterns of fatigue and activity and rest during adjuvant breast cancer chemotherapy. *Oncology Nursing Forum*, **25**, 51–62.

Berglund, G., Bolund, C., Fornander, T., Rutqvist, L.E., and Sjoden, P.O. (1991) Late effects of adjuvant chemotherapy and postoperative radiotherapy on quality of life among breast cancer patients. *European Journal of Cancer*, **27**, 1075–81.

Bernaudin, M., Bellail, A., Marti, H.H., Yvon, A., Vivien, D., Duchatelle, I. *et al.* (2000) Neurons and astrocytes express EPOmRNA: oxygen-sensing mechanisms that involve the redox-state of the brain. *Glia*, **30**, 271–8.

Bianco, J.A., Appelbaum, F.R., Nemunaitis, J., Almgren, J., Andrews, F., Kettner, P. *et al.* (1991) Phase I–II trial of pentoxifylline for the prevention of transplant-related toxicities following bone marrow transplantation. *Blood*, **78**, 1205–11.

Blackshaw, L.A. and Grundy, D. (1993a) Effects of 5-hydroxytryptamine on discharge of vagal mucosal afferent fibres from the upper gastrointestinal tract of the ferret. *Journal of the Autonomic Nervous System*, **45**, 41–50.

Blackshaw, L.A. and Grundy, D. (1993b) Effects of 5-hydroxytryptamine (5-HT) on discharge of vagal mechanoreceptors and motility in the upper gastrointestinal tract of the ferret. *Journal of the Autonomic Nervous System*, **45**, 51–9.

Blesch, K.S., Paice, J.A., Wickham, R., Harte, N., Schnoor, D.K., Purl, S. *et al.* (1991) Correlates of fatigue in people with breast or lung cancer. *Oncology Nursing Forum*, **18**, 81–7.

Blomstrand, E., Perrett, D., Parry-Billings, M., and Newsholme E.A. (1989) Effect of sustained exercise on plasma amino acid concentrations and on 5-hydroxytryptamine metabolism in six different brain regions in the rat. *Acta Physiologica Scandinavica*, **136**, 473–81.

Blomstrand, E., Hassmen, P., Ekblom, B., and Newsholme, E.A. (1997) Influence of ingesting a solution of branched-chain amino acids on perceived exertion during exercise. *Acta Physiologica Scandinavica*, **159**, 41–9.

Bloom, J.R., Gorsky, R.D., and Fobair, P. (1990) Physical performance at work and at leisure: validation of a measure of biological energy in survivors of Hodgkin's disease. *Journal of Psycho-Social Oncology*, **8**, 49–63.

Borish, L., Schmaling, K., DiClementi, J.D., Streib, J., Negri, J., and Jones, J.F. (1998) Chronic fatigue syndrome: identification of distinct subgroups on the basis of allergy and psychologic variables. *Journal of Allergy and Clinical Immunology*, **102**, 222–30.

Bower, J.E., Ganz, P.A., Desmond, K.A., Rowland, J.H., Meyerowitz, B.E., and Belin, T.R. (2000) Fatigue in breast cancer survivors: occurrence, correlates, and impact on quality of life. *Journal of Clinical Oncology*, **18**, 743–53.

Broeckel, J.A., Jacobsen, P.B., Horton, J., Balducci, L., and Lyman, G.H. (1998) Characteristics and correlates of fatigue after adjuvant chemotherapy for breast cancer. *Journal of Clinical Oncology*, **16**:1689–96.

Brouwer, B. and Packer, T. (1994) Corticospinal excitability in patients diagnosed with chronic fatigue syndrome. *Muscle and Nerve*, **17**, 1210–12.

Bron, D. (2001) Biological basis of cancer-related anaemia. In: *Fatigue and Cancer. European School of Oncology Scientific Updates*, 5. (ed. M. Marty and S. Pecorelli). Elsevier, Amsterdam, pp. 45–50.

Brouwers, J.R.B.J., Assies, J., Wiersinga, W.M., Hizing, G., and Tytgat, G.N. (1980) Plasma prolactin levels after acute and subchronic oral administration of domperidone and of metoclopramide. *Clinical Endocrinology*, **12**, 435–40.

Bruera E., Brenneis, C., Michaud, M., Rafter, J., Magnan, A., Tennant, A. *et al.* (1989) Association between asthenia and nutritional status, lean body mass, anemia, psychological status, and tumour mass in patients with advanced breast cancer. *Journal of Pain Symptom Management*, **4**, 59–63.

Buchwald, D., Umali, P., Umali, J., Kith, P., Pearlman, T., and Komaroff, A.L. (1995) Chronic fatigue and the chronic fatigue syndrome: prevalence in a Pacific Northwest health care system. *Annals of Internal Medicine*, **123**, 81–8.

Burak, K.W., Le, T., and Swain, M.G. (2002) Increased sensitivity to the locomotor-activating effects of corticotropin -releasing hormone in cholestatic rats. *Gastroenterology*, **122**, 681–8.

Cathebras, P.J., Robbins, J.M., Kirmayer, L.J., and Hayton, B.C. (1992) Fatigue in primary care: prevalence, psychiatric comorbidity, illness behavior, and outcome. *Journal of General Internal Medicine*, **7**, 276–86.

Cella, D., Peterman, A., Passik, S., Jacobsen, P.B., and Breitbart, W. (1998) Progress toward guidelines for the management of fatigue. *Oncology*, **12**, 369–77.

Chao, C.C., Gallagher, M., Phair, J., and Peterson, P.K. (1990) Serum neopterin and interleukin-6 levels in chronic fatigue syndrome. *Journal of Infectious Diseases*, **162**, 1412–13.

Christensen, T, Stage, J.G., Galbo, H., Christensen, N.J., and Kehlet, H. (1989) Fatigue and cardiac and endocrine metabolic response to exercise after abdominal surgery. *Surgery*, **105**, 46–50.

Chrousos, G.P. and Gold, P.W. (1991) Evidence for impaired activation of the hypothalamic–pituitary–adrenal axis in patients with chronic fatigue syndrome. *Journal of Clinical Endocrinology and Metabolism*, **73**, 1224–34.

Cimprich, B. (1992) Attentional fatigue following breast cancer surgery. *Research in Nursing and Health*, **15**, 199–207.

Cimprich, B. (1995) Symptom management: loss of concentration. *Seminars in Oncology Nursing*, **11**, 279–88.

Cleare, A.J., Bearn, J., Allain, T., McGregor, A., Wessely, S., Murray, R.M. *et al.* (1995) Contrasting neuroendocrine responses in depression and chronic fatigue syndrome. *Journal of Affective Disorders*, **34**, 283–9.

Cleare, A.J., Blair, D., Chambers, S., and Wessely, S. (2001) Urinary free cortisol in chronic fatigue syndrome. *American Journal of Psychiatry*, **158**, 641–3.

Coleridge, J.C.G. and Coleridge, H.M. (1984) Afferent vagal C-fibre innervation of the lungs and airways and its functional significance. *Reviews in Physiology, Biochemistry and Pharmacology*, **99**, 1–110.

Cox, I.M., Campbell, M.J., and Dowson, D. (1991) Red blood cell magnesium and chronic fatigue syndrome. *The Lancet*, **337**, 757–60.

Crawford, J., Cella, D., Cleeland, C.S., Cremieux, P.Y., Demetri, G.D., Sarokhan, B.J. *et al.* (2002) Relationship between changes in haemoglobin level and quality of life during chemotherapy in anemic cancer patients receiving epoetin alfa therapy. *Cancer*, **95**, 888–95.

Davey, N.J., Puri, B.K., Nowicky, A.V., Main, J., and Zaman, R. (2001) Voluntary motor function in patients with chronic fatigue syndrome. *Journal of Psychosomatic Research*, **50**, 17–20.

Davies, S.F., McQuaid, K.R., Iber, C., McArthur, C.D., Path, M.J., Beebe, D.S. *et al.* (1987) Extreme dyspnea from unilateral pulmonary venous obstruction. Demonstration of a vagal mechanism and relief by right vagotomy. *American Review of Respiratory Diseases*, **136**, 184–8.

Dawson, N.M. Felle, P., and O'Donovan, D.K. (1998) A new manual power grip. *Acta Anatomica*, **163**, 224–8.

Demetri, G.D., Kris, M., Wade, J., Degos, L., and Cella, D. (1998) Quality-of-life benefit in chemotherapy patients treated with epoetin alfa is independent of disease response or tumor type: results from a prospective community oncology study. *Journal of Clinical Oncology*, **16**, 3412–25.

Demitrack, M.A. (1998) Neuroendocrine aspects of chronic fatigue syndrome: a commentary. *American Journal of Medicine*, **105**, 11S–14S.

Demitrack, M.A., Dale, J.K., Straus, S.E., Laue, L., Listwak, S.J., Kruesi, M.J.P. *et al.* (1991) Evidence for impaired activation of the hypothalamic–pituitary–adrenal axis in patients with chronic fatigue syndrome. *Journal of Clinical Endocrinology and Metabolism*, **73**, 1224–34.

Devlen, J., Maguire, P., Phillips, P., and Crowther, D. (1987) Psychological problems associated with diagnosis and treatment of lymphomas. II: prospective study. *British Medical Journal*, **295**, 955–7.

Dicarlo, S.E., Collins, H.I., and Chen, C.-Y. (1994) Vagal afferents reflexly inhibit exercise in conscious rats. *Medicine and Science in Sports and Exercise*, **26**, 459–62.

Dimeo, F., Stieglitz. R., Novelli-Fischer, U., Fetscher, S., Mertelsmann, R., and Keul, J. (1997) Correlation between physical performance and fatigue in cancer patients. *Annals of Oncology*, **8**, 1251–5.

Drapkin, R., Barolo, J.L., and Blower, P.R. (1999) Effect of granisetron on performance status during high-dose interferon therapy. *Oncology*, **57**, 303–5.

Edwards, R.H.T. (1981) Human muscle function and fatigue. In: *Human Muscle Fatigue: Physiological Mechanisms*, Ciba Foundation Symposium No 82 (ed. R. Porter and J. Whelan). Pitman Medical, London, pp. 1–18.

Ek, M., Kurosawa, M., Lundeberg, T., and Ericsson, A. (1998) Activation of vagal afferents after intravenous injection of interleukin-1-B: role of endogenous prostaglandins. *Journal of Neuroscience*, **18**, 9471–9.

Enoka, R.M. and Stuart, G. (1992) Neurobiology of muscle fatigue. *Journal of Applied Physiology*, **72**, 1631–48.

Ewald, P.W. (1994) *Evolution of Infectious Diseases.* Oxford: Oxford University Press.

Feller, N., Versantvoort, C.H., Boven, E., Lankelma, J., Pinedo, H.M., and Broxterman, H.J. (1994) ATP dependence and activity of drug transporters *in vivo*, and in intact tumor cells. *Proceedings of the Annual Meeting of the American Association for Cancer Research*, **35**, A2076.

Fobair, P., Hoppe, R.T., Bloom, J., Cox, R., Varghese, A., and Spiegel, D. (1986) Psychosocial problems among survivors of Hodgkin's disease. *Journal of Clinical Oncology*, **4**, 805–14.

Foley, K.M. (1985) The treatment of cancer pain. *New England Journal of Medicine*, **313**, 84–95.

Forsyth, L.M., Preuss, H.G., MacDowell, A.L., Chiazze, L., Birkmayer, G.D., and Bellanti, J.A. (1999) Therapeutic effects of oral NADH on the symptoms of patients with chronic fatigue syndrome. *Annals of Allergy, Asthma and Immunology*, **82**, 185–91.

Gaddum, J.H. and Vogt, M. (1956) Some central actions of 5-hydroxytryptamine and various antagonists. *British Journal of Pharmacology*, **11**, 175–9.

Gandevia, S.C., Allen, G.M., and McKenzie, D.K. (1995) Central fatigue. Critical issues, quantification and practical implications. In: *Fatigue. Neural and Muscular Mechanisms*, (ed. S.C. Gandevia, R.M. Enoka, A.J. McComas, D.G. Stuart, and C.K. Thomas). Plenum Press, New York, pp. 281–94.

Gandevia, S.C., Butler, J.E., Taylor, J.L., and Crawford, M.R. (1998) Absence of viscerosomatic inhibition with injections of lobeline designed to activate human pulmonary C fibres. *Journal of Physiology*, **511**, 289–300.

Ginzel, K.H., Eldred, E., and Estavillo, J.A. (1972) Depression of alpha-motoneuron activity by excitation of visceral afferents in the cardiopulmonary region. *International Journal of Neuroscience*, **4**, 203–14.

Glaus, A. (1998) The relationship between fatigue and type and stage of cancer. In: *Fatigue in Patients with Cancer; Analysis and Assessment*, Recent Results in Cancer Research, Vol. 145. Springer, New York, pp. 105–150.

Greenberg, D.B., Sawicka, J., Eisenthal, S., and Ross, D. (1992) Fatigue syndrome due to localized radiation. *Journal of Pain and Symptom Management*, **7**, 38–45.

Greenberg, D.B., Gray, J.L., Mannix, C.M., Eisenthal, S., and Carey, M. (1993) Treatment-related fatigue and serum interleukin-1 levels in patients during external beam irradiation for prostate cancer. *Journal of Pain and Symptom Management*, **8**, 196–200.

Greenwood, M.H., Lader, M.H., Kantameneni, B.D., and Curzon, G. (1975) The acute effects of oral (-) tryptophan in human subjects. *British Journal of Clinical Pharmacology*, **2**, 165–172.

Groopman, J.E. and Itri, L.M. (1999) Chemotherapy-induced anaemia in adults: incidence and treatment. *Journal of the National Cancer Institute*, **91**, 1616–35.

Guyton, A.C. (1992) *Human Physiology and Mechanisms of Disease*. Philadelphia: W.B. Saunders.

Hallahan, D.E., Haimovitz-Friedman, A., Kufe, D.W., Fuks, Z., and Weichselbaum, R.R. (1993) The role of cytokines in radiation oncology. In: *Important Advances in Oncology, 1993*, (ed. V.T. DeVita, S. Hellman, and S.A. Rosenberg). Lippincott, Philadelphia, pp. 71–80.

Hansen, M.K. and Krueger, J.M. (1997) Subdiphragmatic vagotomy blocks the sleep- and fever-promoting effects of interleukin-1-B. *American Journal of Physiology*, **273**, 1246–53.

Hansen, M.K., Taishi, P., Chen, Z., and Krueger, J.M. (1998) Vagotomy blocks the induction of interleukin-1b (IL-1b) mRNA in the brain of rats in response to systemic IL-1b. *Journal of Neuroscience*, **18**, 2247–53.

Hart, B.L. (1998) Biological basis of the behavior of sick animals. *Neuroscience and Biobehavioural Reviews*, **12**, 123–37.

Hickok, J.T., Morrow, G.R., McDonald, S., and Bellg, A.J. (1996) Frequency and correlates of fatigue in lung cancer patients receiving radiation therapy: implications for management. *Journal of Pain and Symptom Management*, **11**, 370–7.

Hickok, J.T., Roscoe, J.A., Morrow, G.R., and Bushunow, P. (1998) Wrist actigraphy as a measure of fatigue. *Proceedings of the American Society of Clinical Oncology*, **17**, 60a.

Holmes, G.P., Kaplan, J.E., Gantz, N.M., Komaroff, A.L., Schonberger, L.B., Straus, S.E. *et al.* (1988) Chronic fatigue syndrome: a working case definition. *Annals of Internal Medicine*, **108**, 387–9.

Hong, J.H., Chiang, C.S., Campbell, I.L., Sun, J.R., Withers, H.R., and McBride, W.H. (1995) Induction of acute phase gene expression by brain irradiation. *International Journal of Radiation Oncology Biology Physics*, **33**, 619–26.

Irvine, D.M., Vincent, L., Bubela, N., Thompson, L., and Graydon, J. (1991) A critical appraisal of the research literature investigating fatigue in the individual with cancer. *Cancer Nursing*, **14**, 188–99.

Jakeman, P.M., Hawthorne, J.E., Maxwell, S.R.J., Kendall, M.J., and Holder G. (1994) Evidence for down regulation of hypothalamic 5-hydroxytryptamine receptor function in endurance-trained athletes. *Experimental Physiology*, **79**, 461–4.

Jamar, S.C. (1989) Fatigue in women receiving chemotherapy for ovarian cancer. In: *Key Aspects of Comfort: Management of Pain, Fatigue and Nausea* (ed. S.G. Funk, E.M. Tournquist, M.T. Champagne, L.A. Copp, and R.A. Weise). Springer, New York, pp. 224–8.

Jones, E.A. (1999) Relief from profound fatigue associated with chronic liver disease by long-term ondansetron therapy. *The Lancet*, **354**, 397.

Juul, S.E., Anderson, D.K., Li, Y., and Christensen, R.D. (1998) Erythropoietin and erythropoietin receptor in the developing human central nervous system. *Pediatric Research*, **43**, 40–9.

Kaasa, S., Knobel, H., and Loge, J.H. (1998) Hodgkin's disease: quality of life in future trials. *Annals of Oncology*, **9**, 137–45.

Kaempfer, S.H. (1982) Relaxation training reconsidered. *Oncology Nursing Forum*, **9**, 15–18.

Kalia, M. (1973) Effects of certain cerebral lesions on the J reflex. *Pflügers Archives*, **343**, 297–308.

Kapas, L., Hansen, M.K., Chang, H-Y, and Krueger, J.M. (1998). Vagotomy attenuates but does not prevent the somnogenic and febrile effects of lipopolysaccharide in rats. *American Journal of Physiology*, **274**, 406–11.

Karczmar, G.S., Meyerhoff, D.J., Speder, A., Valone, F., Wilkinson, M., Shine, N. *et al.* (1989) Response of tumors to therapy studied by 31p magnetic resonance spectroscopy. *Investigative Radiology*, **24**, 1020–3.

Karczmar, G.S., Meyerhoff, D.J., Boska, M.D., Hubesch, B., Poole, J., Matson, G.B. *et al.* (1991) P-31 spectroscopy study of response of superficial human tumors to therapy. *Radiology*, **179**, 149–53.

Kawaski, K., Kodama, M., and Matsushita, A. (1983) Caerulein, a cholecystokinin-related peptide, depresses somatic function via the vagal afferent system. *Life Science*, **33**, 1045–50.

Kent-Braun, J.A., Sharma, K.R., Weiner, M.W., Massie, B., and Miller, R.G. (1993) Central basis of muscle fatigue in chronic fatigue syndrome. *Neurology*, **43**, 125–31.

Kluger, M.J. (1991) Fever: role of pyrogens and cryogens. *Physiological Reviews*, **71**, 93–127.

Knobf, M.T. (1986) Physical and psychologic distress associated with adjuvant chemotherapy in women with breast cancer. *Journal of Clinical Oncology*, **4**, 678–84.

Komaroff, A.L. and Buchwald, D.S. (1998) Chronic fatigue syndrome: an update. *Annual Review of Medicine*, **49**, 1–13.

Konsman, J.P., Parnet, P., and Dantzer, R. (2002) Cytokine-induced sickness behaviour: mechanisms and implications. *Trends in Neurosciences*, **25**, 154–9.

Kubricht, D.W. (1984) Therapeutic self-care demands expressed by outpatients receiving external radiation therapy. *Cancer Nursing*, **7**, 43–52.

Kuzmits, R., Rumpold, H., Muller, M.M., and Schopf, G. (1986) The use of bioluminescence to evaluate the influence of chemotherapeutic drugs on ATP-levels of malignant cell lines. *Journal of Clinical Chemistry and Clinical Biochemistry*, **24**, 293–8.

Lane, R.J., Barrett, M.C., Taylor, D.J.,.Kemp, G.J., and Lodi, R. (1998) Heterogeneity in chronic fatigue syndrome: evidence from magnetic resonance spectroscopy of muscle. *Neuromuscular Disorders*, **8**, 204–9.

Lind, M., Vernon, C., Cruickshank, D., Wilkinson, P., Littlewood, T., Stuart, N.S.A. *et al.* (2002) The level of haemoglobin in anaemic cancer patients correlates positively with quality of life. *British Journal of Cancer*, **86**, 1243–9.

Lloyd, A.R., Gandevia, S.C., and Hales, J.P. (1991) Muscle performance, voluntary activation, twitch properties and perceived effort in normal subjects and patients with chronic fatigue syndrome. *Neurology*, **43**, 125–31.

Loge, J.H., Abrahamsen, A.F., Ekeberg, O., and Kaasa, S. (1999) Hodgkin's disease survivors more fatigued than the general population. *Journal of Clinical Oncology*, **17**, 253–61.

Long, N.C. (1996) Evolution of infectious disease: how evolutionary forces shape physiological responses to pathogens. *News in Physiological Sciences*, **11**, 83–90.

Malkhovski, V.N., Stemparzhetski, O.A., and Bokk, M.I. (1990) The mechanism of the neuromotor disorders in the period of the primary reaction to irradiation. *Radiobiologia*, **30**, 238–42.

Marvin, G., Sharma, A., Aston, W., Field, C., Kendall, M.J., and Jones, D.A. (1997) The effects of buspirone on perceived exertion and time to fatigue in man. *Experimental Physiology*, **82**, 1057–60.

Masuda, S., Okano, M., Yamagishi, K., Nagao., Ueda, M., and Sasaki, R. (1994) A novel site of erythropoietin production. Oxygen-dependent production in cultured rat astrocytes. *Journal of Biological Chemistry*, **269**, 19488–93.

McCloskey, D.I. (1978) Kinesthetic sensibility. *Physiological Reviews*, **58**, 763–820.

McCloskey, D.I., Ebeling, P., and Goodwin, G.M. (1974) Estimation of weights and tensions and apparent involvement of a 'sense of effort'. *Experimental Neurology*, **42**, 220–32.

Mercuriali, F. and Inghilleri, G. (2001) Treatment of anaemia in cancer patients: transfusion of rHuEPO. In: *Fatigue and Cancer. European School of Oncology Scientific Updates*, 5, (ed. M. Marty and S. Pecorelli). Elsevier, Amsterdam, pp. 185–200.

Meyerowitz, B.E., Watkins, I.K., and Sparks, F.C. (1983) Quality of life for breast cancer patients receiving adjuvant chemotherapy. *American Journal of Nursing*, **83**, 232–5.

Mitchell, G.W. and Glicksman, A.S. (1977) Cancer patients: knowledge and attitudes. *Cancer*, **40**, 61–6.

Mock, V., Atkinson, A., Barsevick, A., Cella, D., Cimprich, B., Cleeland, C. *et al.* (2000) National Comprehensive Cancer Network practice guidelines for cancer-related fatigue. *Oncology (Huntingt)*, **14**(11A), 151–61.

Moldawer, N.P. and Figlin, R.A. (1988) Tumor necrosis factor: current clinical status and implications for nursing management. *Seminars in Oncology Nursing*, **4**, 120–5.

Morant, R., Bacchus, L., Meyer, J., and Reisen, W.F. (1994) Tumoranämie und Entzündungsmarker [Tumor-induced anemia and markers of inflammation]. *Schweizerische Medizinische Wochenschrift Journal Suisse de Medecine*, **124**, 2267–71. (In German.)

Morant, R. (1996) Asthenia: an important symptom in cancer patients. *Cancer Treatment Reviews*, **22** Suppl. A, 117–22.

Morishita, E., Masuda, S., Nagao, M., Yasuda, Y., and Sasaki, R. (1997) Erythropoietin receptor is expressed in rt hippocampal and cerebral cortical neurons, and erythropoietin prevents *in vitro*, glutamate-induced neuronal death. *Neuroscience*, **76**, 105–16.

Mormont, M.C., De Prins, J., and Levi, F. (1996) Study of circadian rhythms of activity by actometry: preliminary results in 30 patients with metastatic colorectal cancer. *Pathologie Biologie (Paris)*, **44**, 165–71.

Mormont, M.C., Hecquet, B., Bogdan, A., Benavides, M., Touitou, Y., and Levi, F. (1998) Non-invasive estimation of the circadian rhythm in serum cortisol in patients with ovarian or colorectal cancer. *International Journal of Cancer*, **78**, 421–4.

Morrow, G.R., Hickok, J.T., Roscoe, J.A., Raubertas, R.F., Andrews, P.I., Flynn, P.J. *et al.* (2003) Differential effects of paroxetine on fatigue and depression: a randomised, double-blind trial from the University of Rochester cancer center community clinical oncology program. *Journal of Clinical Oncology*, **21**, 4635–41.

Mossner, R., Heils, A., Stober, G., Okladnova, O., Daniel, S., and Lesch, K.P. (1998) Enhancement of serotonin transporter function by tumor necrosis factor alpha but not by interleukin-6. *Neurochemistry International*, **33**, 251–4.

Nail, L.M. and King, K.B. (1987) Fatigue... a side effect of cancer treatments. *Seminars in Oncology*, **3**, 257–62.

Nail, L.M. and Winningham, M.L. (1995) Fatigue and weakness in cancer patients: the symptoms experience. *Seminars in Oncology Nursing*, **11**, 272–8.

Nerenz, D.R., Leventhal, H., and Love, R.R. (1982) Factors contributing to emotional distress during cancer chemotherapy. *Cancer*, **50**, 1020–7.

Newsholme, E.A. and Blomstrand, E. (1995) Tryptophan, 5-hydroxytryptamine and a possible explanation for central fatigue. In: *Fatigue*, (ed. S.C. Gandevia, R.M. Enoka, A.J. McComas, D.G. Stuart, and C.K. Thomas). Plenum, New York, pp. 315–20.

Niijima, A. (1996) The afferent discharges from sensors for interleukin-1-B in the hepatoportal system of the anaesthetized rat. *Journal of the Autonomic Nervous System*, **61**, 287–91.

Nussey, S.S. and Whitehead, S.A. (2001) Endocrinology—an integrated approach. BIOS Scientific Publishers Ltd., Oxford, p. 358.

Opp, M.R and Toth, L.A. (1998) Somnogenic and pyrogenic effects of interleukin-1beta and lipopolysaccharide in intact and vagotomized rats. *Life Science*, **62**, 923–36.

Padilla, G. and Grant, M. (1985) Quality of life as a cancer nursing outcome variable. *Advances in Nursing Science*, **8**, 45–9.

Paintal, A.S. (1973) Vagal sensory receptors and their reflex effects. *Physiological Reviews*, **53**, 159–227.

Paintal, A.S. (1995) Sensations from J receptors. *News in Physiological Sciences*, **10**, 238–43.

Pastoris, O., Aquilina, R., Foppa, P., Bovio, G., Segagni, S., Baiardi, P. *et al.* (1997) Altered muscle energy metabolism in post-absorptive patients with chronic renal failure. *Scandinavian Journal of Urology and Nephrology*, **31**, 281–7.

Patarca, R., Klimas, N.G., Lugtendorf, S., Antoni, M., and Fletcher, M.A. (1994) Dysregulated expression of tumor necrosis factor in chronic fatigue syndrome: interrelations with cellular sources and patterns of soluble immune mediator expression. *Clinics in Infectious Diseases*, **18**(Supplement 1), S147–S153.

Patterson, S.M., Krantz, D.S., Montgomery, L.C., Deuster, P.A., Hedges, S.M., and Nebel, L.E. (1993) Automated physical activity monitoring: validation and comparison with physiological and self-report measures. *Psychophysiology*, **30**, 296–305.

Pauli, S., Linthorst, A.C., and Reul, J.M. (1998) Tumour necrosis factor-alpha and interleukin-2 differentially affect hippocampal serotonergic neurotransmission, behavioural activity, body temperature and hypothalamic–pituitary–adrenocortical axis activity in the rat. *European Journal of Neuroscience*, **10**, 868–78.

Peck, A. and Boland, J. (1977) Emotional reactions to radiation treatment. *Cancer*, **40**, 180–4.

Pickar, J.G. (1998) The thromboxane A2 mimetic U-46619 inhibits somatomotor activity via vagal reflex from the lung. *American Journal of Physiology*, **275**, R706–R712.

Pickar, J.G., Hill, J.M., and Kaufman, M.P. (1993) Stimulation of vagal afferents inhibits locomotion in mesencephalic cats. *Journal of Applied Physiology*, **74**, 103–10.

Piper, B.F. (1998) Fatigue in cancer patients: current perspectives on measurement and management. *Fifth annual conference on cancer nursing. Monograph on Nursing Management of Common Problems: State of the Art*. American Cancer Society, New York.

Piper, B.F. (1992) Subjective fatigue in women receiving six cycles of adjuvant chemotherapy for breast cancer. Unpublished Doctoral Dissertation. University of California–San Francisco.

Piper, B.F., Lindsey, A.M., Dodd, M.J., Ferketich, S., Paul, S.M., and Weller, S. (1989) The development of an instrument to measure the subjective dimension of fatigue. In: *Key Aspects of Comfort: Management of Pain, Fatigue, and Nausea*, (ed. S.G. Funk, E.M. Tornquist, M.T. Champagne, L.A. Copp, and R.A. Wiess). Springer, New York, p. 199.

Plata-Salaman, C.R. (1996) Anorexia during acute and chronic disease. *Nutrition*, **12**, 69–78.

Prasher, D., Smith, A., and Findley, L. (1990) Sensory and cognitive event-related potentials in myalgic myoencephalitis. *Journal of Neurology, Neurosurgery and Psychiatry*, **53**, 247–53.

Quattrone, A., Tedeschi, G., Aguglia, U., Scopacasa, F., Direnzo, G.F., and Annunziato, L. (1983) Prolactin secretion in man: a useful tool to evaluate the activity of drugs on central 5-hydroxytryptaminergic neurones. Studies with fenfluramine. *British Journal of Clinical Pharmacology*, **16**, 471–5.

Richardson, A. (1998) Measuring fatigue in patients with cancer. *Supportive Care in Cancer*, **6**: 94–100.

Robins, H.L., Jonsson, G.G., Jacobson, E.L., Schmitt, C.L., Cohen, J.D., and Jacobson, M.K. (1991) Effect of hypothermia *in vitro* and *in vivo* on adenine and pyridine nucleotide pools in human peripheral lymphocytes. *Cancer*, **67**, 2096–102.

Roscoe, J.A., Morrow, G.R., Hickok, J.T., Bushunow, P., Matteson, S., Rakita, D. *et al.* (2002) Temporal interrelationships among fatigue, circadian rhythm and depression in breast cancer patients undergoing chemotherapy treatment. *Supportive Care in Cancer*, **10**, 329–36.

Sakanaka, M., Wen, T.C., Matsuda, S.S., Masuda, S., Morishita, E., Nagao, M. *et al.* (1998) *In vivo*, evidence that erythropoetin protects neurons from ischemic damage. *Proceedings of the National Academy of Sciences of the United States of America*, **95**, 4635–40.

Samii, A., Wassermann, E.M., Ikoma, K., Mercuri, B., Georger, M.S., O'Fallon, A. *et al.* (1996) Decreased post-exercise facilitation of motor evoked potentials in patients with chronic fatigue syndrome or depression. *Neurology*, **47**, 1410–14.

Sarwar, R., Niclos, B.B., and Rutherford, O.M. (1996) Changes in muscle strength, relaxation rate and fatiguability during the human menstrual cycle. *Journal of Physiology (London)*, **493**, 267–72.

Schweitzer, A. and Wright S. (1937) The anti-strychnine action of acetylcholine, prostigmine and related substances, and of central vagus stimulation. *Journal of Physiology*, **90**, 310–29.

Sharpe, M., Clements, A., Hawton, P., Young, A., Sargent, P., and Cowen, P. (1996) Increased prolactin response to buspirone in chronic fatigue syndrome. *Journal of Affective Disorders*, **41**, 71–6.

Sharpe, M., Hawton, K., Clements, A., and Cowen, P. (1997) Increased brain serotonin function in men with chronic fatigue syndrome. *British Medical Journal*, **315**, 164–5.

Spath, M., Welzel, D., and Farber, L. (2000) Treatment of chronic fatigue syndrome with 5-HT3 receptor antagonists-preliminary results. *Scandinavian Journal of Rheumatology*, **29** (Supplement 113), 72–7.

Springborg, J.B. Ma, X. D., Rochat, P., Knudsen, G.M., Amtrop, O., Paulson, O.B. *et al.* (2002) A single subcutaneous bolus of erythropoietin normalizes cerebral blood flow autoregulation after subarachnoid haemorrhage in rats. *British Journal of Pharmacology*, **135**, 823–9.

Stone, P. (1999) Fatigue in patients with cancer. MD Thesis. University of London.

Stone, P., Richards, M., and Hardy, J. (1998) Fatigue in patients with cancer. *European Journal of Cancer*, **34**, 1670–6.

Stone, P., Hardy, J., Broadley, K., Tookman, A.J., Kurowska, A., and Hern, R.A. (1999) Fatigue in advanced cancer: a prospective controlled cross-sectional study. *British Journal of Cancer*, **79**, 1479–86.

Stone, P., Richardson, A., Ream, E., Smith, A.G., Kerr, D.J., and Kearney, N. (2000*a*) Cancer-related fatigue: inevitable, unimportant, and untreatable? Results of a multi-centre patient survey. Cancer Fatigue Forum. *Annals of Oncology*, **11**, 971–5.

Stone, P., Richards, M., A'Hern, R., and Hardy, J. (2000*b*) A study to investigate the prevalence, severity and correlates of fatigue among patients with cancer in comparison with a control group of volunteers without cancer. *Annals of Oncology*, **11**, 561–7.

Swain, M.G. and Maric, M. (1995) Defective corticotropin-releasing hormone mediated neuroendocrine and behavioral responses in cholestatic rats: implications for cholestatic liver disease-related sickness behaviors. *Hepatology*, 1560–1564.

Tamulevicius, P. and Streffer, C. (1995) Metabolic imaging in tumours by means of bioluminescence. *British Journal of Cancer*, **72**, 1102–12.

Teicher, M.H. (1995) Actigraphy and motion analysis: new tools for psychiatry. *Harvard Review of Psychiatry*, **3**, 18–35.

Vaupel, P., Kallinowski, F., and Okunieff, P. (1989) Blood flow, oxygen and nutrient supply, and metabolic microenvironment of human tumors: a review. *Cancer Research*, **49**, 6449–65.

Weinberg, E.D. (1984) Iron withholding: a defense against infection and neoplasia. *Physiological Reviews*, **64**, 65–102.

Wessely, S., Chalder, T., Hirsch, S., Pawlikowska, T., Wallace, P., and Wright, D.J. (1995) Postinfectious fatigue: prospective cohort study in primary care. *The Lancet*, **345**, 1333–8.

Wessely, S., Hotopf, M., and Sharpe, M. (ed.) (1998) *Chronic Fatigue and its Syndromes.* Oxford University Press, Oxford, p. 428.

Widdicombe, J.G. (1998) The J reflex. *Journal of Physiology*, **511**, 2.

Wilson, W.M. and Maughan, R.J. (1992) Evidence for a possible role of 5-hydroxytryptamine in the genesis of fatigue in man: administration of paroxetine, a 5-HT re-uptake inhibitor, reduces the capacity to perform prolonged exercise. *Experimental Physiology*, **77**, 921–4.

Winningham, M.L., Nail, L.M., Burke, M.B., Brophy, L., Cimprich, B., Jones, L.S. *et al.* (1994) Fatigue and the cancer experience: the state of the knowledge. *Oncology Nursing Forum*, **21**, 23–36.

Yamaji, R., Okada, T., Moriya, M., Naito, M., Tsuruo, T., Miyatake, K. *et al.* (1996) Brain capillary endothelial cells express two forms of erythropoietin receptor mRNA. *European Journal of Biochemistry*, **239**, 494–500.

Zaman, R. Puri, B.K., Min, J., Nowicky, A.V., and Davey, N.J. (2001) Corticospinal inhibition appears normal in patients with chronic fatigue syndrome. *Experimental Physiology*, **86**(5), 547–50.

Zeiderman, M.R., Welchew, E.A., and Clark, R.G. (1990) Changes in cardiorespiratory and muscle function associated with the development of postoperative fatigue. *British Journal of Surgery*, **77**, 576–80.

Chapter 4

Cancer cachexia and anorexia and their role in cancer fatigue

Mónica Castro and Eduardo Bruera

Introduction

Cancer cachexia is one of the most devastating effects of cancer and an independent negative predictive factor for treatment outcome (Capra *et al.* 2001) and survival (De Wys *et al.* 1980; Vigano *et al.* 2000; Tilignac *et al.* 2002) in advanced cancer patients. It results in decreased quality of life (Seligman *et al.* 1998), decreased performance status (Barber *et al.* 1999*a*; Langer *et al.* 2001), altered body image (Hopwood *et al.* 2001), and other symptoms such as asthenia (MacDonald *et al.* 1995), chronic nausea (Bruera *et al.* 1987*b*), cognitive impairment (Lawlor *et al.* 2000), and dyspnoea (Coats 2002). This constellation of symptoms is sometimes present before cachexia becomes clinically apparent and can be a direct consequence of the process of weight loss. Fatigue is a major component of cancer cachexia (Coats 2002). However, cachexia is not a mandatory requirement for the development of severe fatigue. Fatigue can precede weight loss and changes in body composition, it can be present for years after the cure of cancer (Servaes *et al.* 2002; Morrow *et al.* 2002), and it may be absent in patients who present with severe malnutrition.

Cachexia and fatigue share a number of common links, mostly related to the development of a proinflammatory state. In addition, there are a number of factors that contribute to each of these syndromes in an independent way. This chapter discusses the pathophysiology, assessment, clinical presentation, and management of cachexia and outlines possible links with cancer-related fatigue (CRF). Suggestions for future research on the assessment and management of this poorly understood syndrome are also made.

Definitions and frequency of anorexia/cachexia and cancer-related fatigue

Anorexia

Anorexia is defined as an involuntary decline in food intake (Capra *et al.* 2001). It is one of the main features of the cachectic syndrome (Inui 1999) and is a major contributing factor to cachexia (Bruera *et al.*1990). However, anorexia is not always a part of the cachexia syndrome. In some animal models cachexia develops in complete absence of anorexia (Baracos 2000). Moreover, loss of muscle and adipose tissue in some patient populations may precede a fall in food intake (Tisdale 2002). It is one the most frequent symptoms in patients with advanced cancer (66%, range from 6–84%) (Walsh *et al.* 2000; Vainio and Auvinen 1996). This wide range reflects differences in frequency among patients according to histology and disease stage, as well as different modalities for assessing this symptom.

Cachexia

This is a complex, debilitating state of involuntary weight loss complicating the course of both malignancy (Barber *et al.* 1999*a*; Tisdale 2000; Scott *et al.* 2001; Staal-van den Brekel *et al.* 1995), and acute (Argiles *et al.* 2001*a*) and chronic inflammatory non-malignant conditions (Doehner and Anker 2002; Witte and Clark 2002). This results in loss of fat and lean body mass and is associated with high levels of mortality in these diseases (Argiles *et al.* 2001*a*). It is usually defined as weight loss of more than 5% of premorbid weight during the previous 2–6 months (Straisser and Bruera 2002). Cachexia is present in approximately 80% of cancer patients prior to death (Nelson 2000); this varies according to cancer site. For example, 80% of patients with upper gastrointestinal cancers and 60% of those with lung cancer have substantial weight loss at the time of diagnosis (Bruera 1997).

Cancer-related fatigue

Fatigue is a subjective sensation of weakness, lack of energy, and tiredness (Stone *et al.* 1998). Fatigue and the term asthenia are related terms; however, asthenia evokes even more clearly both the physical and mental components of fatigue sensation. The three components of fatigue perception (Barnes and Bruera 2002) are illustrated in Fig. 4.1. CRF has been reported in 70–100% of patients undergoing treatment (Morrow *et al.* 2002; Mock 2001) and it can persist for years after its completion (Morrow *et al.* 2002; Barnes and Bruera 2002). Up to 80% of all cancer patients experience fatigue (Smith and de Boer 2002). It is present in almost the same proportion of patients with cancer cachexia. Fatigue can precede weight loss, and this is probably, in a number of cancer patients, a direct consequence of treatment with chemotherapy (Servaes *et al.* 2002; Morrow *et al.* 2002; Richardson 1995; Ancoli-Israel *et al.* 2001), radiotherapy (Morrow *et al.* 2002; Richardson 1995; Visser and Smets 1998; Greenberg *et al.* 1993), and bio-therapy (Richardson 1995; Quesada *et al.* 1986; Kurzok 2001; Malik *et al.* 2001).

Mechanisms of cachexia/anorexia and their relationship with fatigue

Cancer-related cachexia/anorexia is a multifactorial syndrome caused by both the presence of a tumour and the host response to that stimulus. A number of proinflammatory

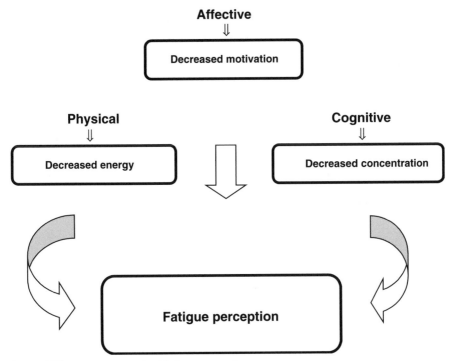

Fig. 4.1 Different components of fatigue perception.

cytokines, probably in connection with neuroendocrine mediators and second messengers, generate an inflammatory state and changes in the central nervous system. This results in a marked loss of fat and lean body mass, diminished muscle function, and a number of severe signs and symptoms, such as anorexia, chronic nausea, cognitive changes, and fatigue (see Fig. 4.2). In acute inflammatory conditions, such as severe and prolonged sepsis, and chronic non-malignant inflammatory processes, such as infection, rheumatological disease (Roubenoff *et al.* 1997), chronic obstructive pulmonary disease (COPD) (Di Francia *et al.* 1994), AIDS (Thea *et al.* 1996), and chronic heart failure (CHF) (Levine *et al.* 1990), cytokines also seem to be associated with weight loss (Kotler 2000).

Impaired food intake and gastrointestinal absorption can add a component of starvation to the previously described abnormalities. These are direct or indirect consequences of the presence of the tumour, treatment-related toxicity, and associated co-morbidities (e.g. infection, COPD, and CHF). Deconditioning, related to the primary tumour or associated co-morbidities, further contributes to cachexia because of the loss of muscle tissue resulting from decreased muscle activity (Straisser and Bruera 2002) (see Table 4.1).

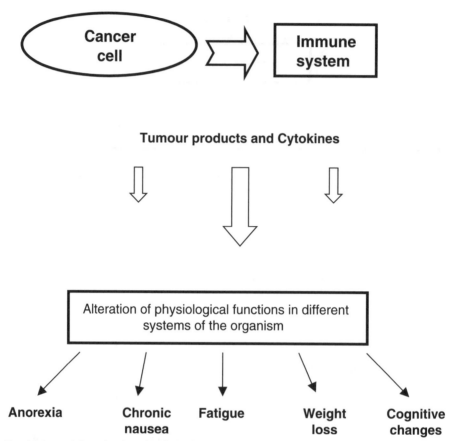

Fig. 4.2 Potential mechanisms implicated in the development of different clinical symptoms observed in advanced cancer patients.

Energy expenditure

Basal metabolism has been found to be low, normal, or increased in cancer patients as compared with healthy individuals (Tisdale 2002). Pancreatic and lung tumours are consistently associated with increased metabolic rates as compared with other cancers (Tisdale 2002; Staal-van den Brekel *et al.* 1995). A 12% increase in metabolic rate can contribute to a loss of 1–2 kg of body weight in a month (Lindmark *et al.* 1984). The mechanism for the increase in metabolic rate is complex and poorly understood. The uncoupling proteins 1, 2, and 3 have been linked with the control of energy metabolism. They are a family of mitochondrial membrane proteins that mediate protein leakage and decrease the coupling of respiration to ADP phosphorylation, leading to the generation of heat instead of ATP (Tisdale 2002). Uncoupling proteins can be

Table 4.1 Clinical conditions that contribute to cachexia in cancer

Impaired food intake	Mucositis (stomatitis, pharyngo-oesophagitis) related to chemotherapy, radiotherapy, and infections
	Xerostomia: secondary to radiotherapy and drug side-effects (tricyclics, opioids)
	Tumour presence (mechanical) induced dysphagia, bowel obstruction
	Chronic nausea and/or vomiting
	Decreased gastrointestinal motility: autonomic failure
	Cognitive impairment or delirium
	Others: severe pain, dyspnoea, depression, taste abnormalities
Decrease absorption of nutrients	Malabsorption: related to intestinal atrophy secondary to decreased food intake, mucositis, infections
	Treatment-related complications
	Exocrine pancreatic insufficiency
Associated co-morbidities	Acute and chronic infections
	Chronic heart failure
	Chronic lung disease
	Renal failure
Other causes of muscle loss	Deconditioning, hypogonadism, aging

induced by tumour products or cytokines (Tisdale 2002). For example, increased expression of mRNA levels of uncoupling proteins have been found in skeletal muscle of cachectic cancer-bearing animals and humans (Bing *et al.* 2000; Collins *et al.* 2002).

Metabolic abnormalities

Carbohydrates

The increase in glucose synthesis, insulin resistance, and activity of the Cori cycle (Mantovani *et al.* 2001) are characteristic features of cachexia. The Cori cycle is an energy-consuming process in which lactate produced by tumour cells and other tissues is converted to glucose in the liver (Langer *et al.* 2001).

Lipids

One of the most characteristic abnormalities in cancer cachexia is the loss of substantial amounts of adipose tissue. Lipolysis appears to be activated (Tisdale 2002; Argiles *et al.* 2001*a*; Inadera *et al.* 2002) and lipogenesis appears to be decreased, except in the liver (Argiles *et al.* 2001*a*). The activity of the enzyme lipoprotein lipase (LPL) is decreased in catabolic conditions, probably secondary to the action of cytokines (Argiles *et al.* 2001*a*). Tumour necrosis factor-alpha (TNF-α) opposes the differentiation and recruitment of new adipocytes (Zhang *et al.* 1996). It also decreases the expression of enzymes that contribute to lipogenesis (Zhang *et al.* 1996) and is capable of increasing the rate of lipolysis (Tisdale 2002).

In recent years some authors have emphasized the role of peroxisome proliferator-activated receptor gamma (PPAR-γ). This subtype transcription factor can exert control over adipogenesis by inducing adipocyte differentiation (Inadera *et al.* 2002).

Proteins

Whole body protein turnover is increased (Fearon and Moses 2002) with a resulting net negative nitrogen balance (Wray *et al.* 2002). Skeletal muscle represents approximately 45% of body weight, being the main source of total body nitrogen (Argiles *et al.* 2001*a*). In cancer cachexia, the liver shifts its protein synthesis pattern, resulting in an increased production of acute phase reactants (Mantovani *et al.* 2001) and a decrease in other substantial proteins such as albumin (Kotler 2000). This picture is observed in other stress conditions such as sepsis (Mantovani *et al.* 2001), trauma, and infection (Argiles *et al.* 2001*a*). In several types of cancer, changes in the acute phase response have been associated with disease progression (Fearon and Moses 2002). The maintenance of this situation over time results in muscle protein breakdown, weight loss, and asthenia (Argiles *et al.* 2001*a*). Cytokines are capable of reducing amino acid uptake, decreasing protein synthesis, and activating proteolysis in cancer patients (Argiles *et al.* 2001*a*).

All these changes are different from those observed in simple starvation (Langer *et al.* 2001) where the main physiological endpoint is the preservation of lean body mass. In cancer cachexia there is a loss of both adipose tissue and lean body mass. Starvation is characterized by an equal loss of skeletal and visceral protein (Tisdale 2002), while cancer cachexia results in a relatively larger loss of muscle mass with a relatively unchanged visceral protein compartment (Whitehouse *et al.* 2001).

Regulation of food intake: role of neuropeptides

Leptin is a protein encoded by the gene *LEP*, and is a member of cytokine receptor family (Aleman *et al.* 2002). It is produced by adipocytes and acts on specific receptors in the hypothalamus (Brown *et al.* 2001). Leptin levels regulate a network of orexigenic and anorexigenic neuropeptides and are correlated with body fat mass (Brown *et al.* 2001). Neuropeptide Y (NPY) and ghrelin (an orexigenic signal from the gut to the brain, mostly expressed in neuroendocrine cells of the gastric fundus) (Pinkney and Williams 2002), are the most potent feeding stimuli. They are released with falling levels of leptin, in conjunction with other orexigenic peptides (orexin, endorphin dynorphine, and melanin-concentrating hormone (MCH)) (Inui 1999). Corticosteroids and medroxyprogesterone acetate (MPA) stimulate the release of NPY (Tisdale 2002). Conversely an increase in leptin generates the release of potent anorexigenic substances, such as neurotensin, melanocortin, colecistokinine, corticotropin-releasing factor (CRF), and cocaine and amphetamine-related transcript (CART) (Inui 1999).

The hypothalamus seems to be the area with highest density of receptors for cytokines. It has been suggested that they might mimic hypothalamic negative feedback signalling from leptin (Fearon and Moses 2002). However, some authors found no correlation between plasma levels of cytokines and leptin (Aleman *et al.* 2002). Moreover in non-malignant diseases leading to cachexia, such as COPD (Takabatake *et al.* 1999) and chronic heart failure (CHF) (Filippatos *et al.* 2000), leptin levels were found to be normal or decreased and did not correlate with cytokine levels. On the other hand, a recent report of 76 patients with newly diagnosed non-surgically treated non-small cell lung cancer (prior to treatment) demonstrated a direct relationship between leptin levels and body fat mass. However, these levels were inversely correlated with proinflammatory cytokines and acute phase proteins (Aleman *et al.* 2002).

Cachexia is not a direct consequence of a dysregulation of leptin production (Aleman *et al.* 2002; Brown *et al.* 2001; Mantovani *et al.* 2000). It is unlikely that weight loss in cancer arises primarily from a reduction in food intake. Proof of this is that nutritional support alone cannot reverse the process of wasting, body composition changes differ from those found in anorexia, and loss of muscle and adipose tissue often precede a decrease in food intake and can occur without anorexia (Inadera *et al.* 2002).

Cytokines

TNF-α, interleukin-6 (IL-6), interleukin-1 (IL-1), and interferon-gamma (INF-γ) have been implicated in the development of cancer anorexia/cachexia syndrome (CACS) (Inui 1999; Mantovani *et al.* 2000, 2001). Cytokine plasma levels do not correlate with local production; high levels have been found in animal models and humans with cachexia (Mantovani *et al.* 2001) and there was no such elevation in patients with pronounced weight loss (Fearon and Moses 2002; Maltoni *et al.* 2001). Cancer cells are capable of producing cytokines constitutively (Dunlop and Campbell 2000). Production of cytokines by macrophages in tissues may be of much greater importance than circulating plasma levels (Falconer *et al.* 1994). CACS results from a complex network of cytokine interactions rather than one individual type (Mantovani *et al.* 2001).

Tumour-specific catabolic factors

Two tumour-specific products have been isolated from animal models and humans with cancer. Proteolysis-inducing factor (PIF), a sulphated glycoprotein associated with protein breakdown in animal models (Fearon and Moses 2002; Todorov *et al.* 1999), has been identified in the urine of humans and mice with cachexia (Cariuk *et al.* 1997). It seems to up-regulate the ubiquitin-proteosome proteolytic system (Lorite *et al.* 2001), which is involved in breakdown of muscle protein. It also seems to activate transcription factors (e.g. nuclear factor-κB (NF-κB)) and so the production of cytokines, such as IL-6, interleukin-8 (IL-8) and C-reactive protein (Tisdale 2002). In this way, PIF contributes to the cytokine cycle. The glycoprotein lipid mobilizing factor (LMF) was found in the urine of weight-losing cancer patients (Barber *et al.* 1999*a*; Fearon and Moses 2002);

this has been shown to cause catabolism of skeletal muscle and adipose tissue in mice (Dunlop and Campbell 2000).

Skeletal muscle homeostasis

Decreasing muscle mass and the loss of functional ability results in generalized weakness and decreased quality of life (QOL) (Diffee *et al.* 2002). Sarcopenia is not the only manifestation of skeletal muscle damage. Proinflammatory cytokines have been found to induce functional changes with a shift in myosin isoform expression. The result is an increase in type IIB chains ("fast" myosin isoforms) and decrease in "slow" myosin isoforms (type I) (Diffee *et al.* 2002), thereby inducing an increase in the velocity of muscle shortening and decrease in maximal force and power output.

The ATP-dependent ubiquitin-proteolytic pathway is the main mechanism for degradation of contractile protein in skeletal cell muscle (Mitch and Price 2001). This system is up-regulated in various catabolic processes including denervation atrophy, glucocorticoid treatment, metabolic acidosis, trauma, and infection (Baracos 2000). Recent data propose a skeletal muscle homeostasis system regulated indirectly by a number of cytokines through the NF-κB transcription factor. NF-κB could be activated by several cytokines, including TNF-α (Mitch and Price 2001), and seems to be an important molecular target in the modulation of inflammatory disease (Schwartz *et al.* 1999). NF-κB seems to balance two different effects (Tisdale 2000). Firstly, the inhibition of protein degradation by blocking a subunit of the proteosome system implicated in the degradation of polyubiquitinated muscle proteins. Glucocorticoids oppose this action (Tisdale 2000; Lorite *et al.* 2001), but eicosapentaenoic acid (EPA) stimulates this system, perhaps via its action on PIF and 15-hydroxyeico-satetraenoic acid (15-HETE).

Secondly, the decreased expression of the transcription factor MyoD. This factor is essential in the process of differentiation and replenishment of wasted muscle; mice lacking MyoD develop normally but have impaired ability to regenerate skeletal muscle after tissue injury (Guttridge *et al.* 2000). Thus, it seems that an imbalance between these two processes can be clinically extrapolated to muscle weakness or asthenia. Aggravating factors are deconditioning and co-morbidities associated with sarcopenia. (see Fig. 4.3).

The relationship between fatigue and cancer cachexia

Many of the postulated mechanisms for cachexia are applicable to fatigue, as is shown in Fig. 4.4. However, cachexia is not always accompanied by fatigue and fatigue can be present in diseases other than cancer.

Areas of overlap and discrepancy

Cytokines, as mentioned before, seem to be pivotal in the development and perpetuation of cancer cachexia (see Chapter 3). In addition, increased levels of cytokines have been observed in other clinical non-malignant conditions associated with fatigue. INF-γ

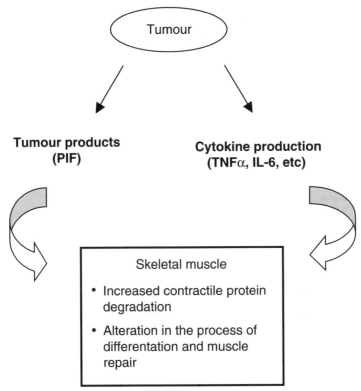

Fig. 4.3 Proposed role of cytokines and tumour products on skeletal muscle homeostasis (PIF = proteolysis-inducing factor).

is increased following dialysis (Gustein 2001) and transforming growth factor-beta (TGF-β), IL-1, and interleukin-2 (IL-2) in patients with chronic fatigue (Dunlop and Campbell 2000). Fatigue related to cancer treatment is another example of the development of this symptom outside the context of cancer cachexia. Increased IL-1 levels coincided with increased fatigue perception in the fourth week of external beam irradiation in a study of prostate cancer patients (Greenberg *et al.* 1993). It is also well known that fatigue is a major symptom of biotherapy (Richardson 1995; Quesada *et al.* 1986; Kurzok 2001; Malik *et al.* 2001). However, other studies found no relationship between fatigue and cytokine levels (Stone *et al.* 1998).

The muscles and the central nervous system (CNS) play a major role in the perception and expression of asthenia (Neuenschwander and Bruera 1998). Muscle function was tested in a study performed with non-cachectic, asthenic breast cancer patients (Bruera *et al.* 1987a). Compared with the control group, these patients showed decreased strength and relaxation speed, and increased muscle fatigue after sustained stimulation. Muscle energy sources are inadequate in cachectic patients and it has been postulated that there is a decrease in intracellular ATP levels in cells exposed to

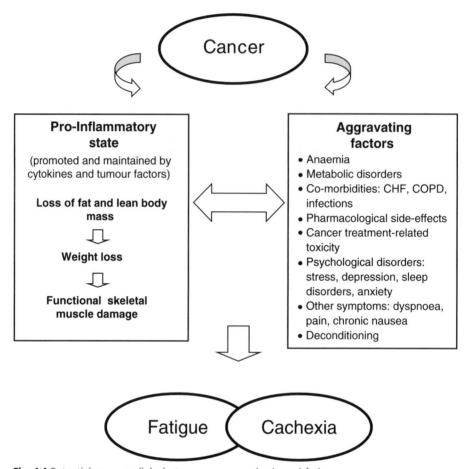

Fig. 4.4 Potential common links between cancer cachexia and fatigue.

cytostatic drugs (Morrow *et al.* 2002), owing to impaired oxidative phosphorylation (Morrow *et al.* 2002; Neuenschwander and Bruera 1996). This energy imbalance, associated with extensive loss of muscle mass and function, can be perceived as fatigue and, as such, may be another cause of CRF (Barnes and Bruera 2002).

Motor pathways and affective sensations are integrated in the CNS, involving the generation of physiological fatigue with or without cachexia. The peripheral autonomic nervous system also appears to play a role in general asthenia (Neuenschwander and Bruera 1996). Autonomic dysfunction is a frequent finding in cachectic patients. However, non-malignant disorders such as chronic fatigue syndrome have been associated with autonomic nervous system failure (Neuenschwander and Bruera 1998). Vagal afferents could be involved in fatigue perception by modulating somatic muscle tone (Morrow *et al.* 2002) (see Chapter 3).

Neuroendocrine dysfunction could be another contributing factor in the development of fatigue in cachectic patients. However, there is no conclusive data for an increase or decrease in hypothalamic–pituitary–adrenal (HPA) axis function. Hypogonadism in cancer patients has been associated with poor nutritional states and the use of opioids (Verhelst *et al.* 2000; Finch *et al.* 2000). Hormone ablative therapy for prostate cancer seems to increase the incidence of fatigue. Stone *et al.* (2000) found 66% of patients with prostate cancer had raised levels of fatigue after 3 months of treatment with luteinizing hormone (LH) analogues and cyproterone acetate. INF-α also generates acute and chronic hypothalamic–pituitary–gonadal axis inhibition with decreased levels of oestrogens, progesterone, testosterone, and decreased growth hormone activity (Gustein 2001).

Stress (Stone *et al.* 1998), mood-related factors, for example anxiety, depression, personality type (Hopwood *et al.* 2001; Magnusson *et al.* 1996), and sleep disorders (Ancoli-Israel *et al.* 2001) are present in patients with and without asthenia in the context of cancer cachexia. Cancer-related symptoms, such as pain and dyspnoea, may interact to produce fatigue (Richardson 1995) without the presence of cachexia. The use of opioid analgesics (which induce sedation) can also aggravate fatigue (Gustein 2001).

Clinical assessment

A systematic symptom assessment, alongside a complete clinical history, should be made initially in order to prioritize problems. Visual analogue scales and other verbal rating scales are useful tools for measuring symptom intensity and effects. In addition, performance status and the rate of weight loss are reliable tools in assessing the extent of the cachexia. For clinical research purposes, body compartment analysis through anthropometric measurements, and bioelectrical impedance analysis, as well as dual-photon absorptiometry (DEXA), are useful.

Screening for cachexia/anorexia

The following should be performed:

- Complete clinical oncological history: disease status, prognosis, and survival.
- Signs and symptoms: it is necessary to address correctly all the clinical details related to cachexia and possible aggravating factors. Table 4.2 lists signs and symptoms to consider in the global assessment.

Evaluation tools

Subjective global assessment

The Visual Analog Scale (VAS) permits a subjective assessment of a number of symptoms, including anorexia, fatigue (Vigano *et al.* 2000), and other associated symptoms such as dyspnoea and pain.

Table 4.2 Signs and symptoms in the global assessment of nutritional status

General	Anorexia, food aversion
	Fatigue, weakness
	Weight loss
	Decreased subcutaneous fat and muscle mass
Gastrointestinal	Nausea, vomiting
	Early satiety, dyspepsia
	Stomatitis, oesophagitis
	Xerostomia
	Abdominal pain, cramping, bloating
	Constipation, diarrhoea
	Fat malabsorption
Other associated complaints	Delirium
	Pain
	Depression
	Anxiety
	Dyspnoea

The Edmonton Symptom Assessment Scale (ESAS) consists of nine visual analogue scales for measuring symptom intensity (Vigano *et al.* 2000). This is a simple method to assess patients' cachexia and fatigue-related symptoms in clinical practice.

The following can be used for fatigue assessment: verbal rating scales (Wray *et al.* 2002), National Cancer Institute (NCI) toxicity criteria (NCI 1999), the Piper Fatigue Scale (Piper *et al.* 1998), the Profile of Moods States (POMS) (Norcross *et al.* 1984), and the Brief Fatigue Inventory (BFI) (Mendoza *et al.* 1999). Most of these scales are used in the context of clinical research (see Chapter 9).

Objective assessment

A number of methods can be used for the objective evaluation of cachexia:

◆ Daily functioning: performance status scales measure individual functional capacity. The two most widely used scales are the Karnofsky Performance Status (KPS) scale (Karnofsky and Burchenal 1949) and the Eastern Cooperative Oncology Group (ECOG) scale (Taylor *et al.* 1999) (see Chapter 13).

◆ Weight loss: weight loss is considered as one of the major objective signs in the evaluation of cachexia. Cachexia is suspected when weight loss is more than the 5% of premorbid weight within a 6 month period (in obese patients it is more than 10%) (Straisser and Bruera 2002). There is no analysis of body compartment differentiation.

◆ Body mass index (BMI) is the representation of an individual's weight per height as an index number (Nelson and Walsh 2002). There is no analysis of body compartment differentiation.

◆ Body compartment analysis:

1. Anthropometric measurements are measurements of body fat mass using body circumferences and skin-fold thickness in standardized anatomical sites— triceps skin fold, biceps skin fold, and subscapular and suprailiac skin folds. Their use is limited by interoperator variability (Langer *et al.* 2001), only body fat mass is directly assessed, subcutaneous adipose tissue is not the same in all sites, and the presence of oedema leads to overestimates of fat.

2. Bioelectrical impedance analysis (BIA) is based on the observation that different body tissues possess distinct conductive and resistive properties (Nelson and Walsh 2002). Total body impedance comprises the ratio of conductive to resistance components. A limitation of this analysis is that the actual conductive path through the body is unknown, so correlations between measured impedance and biological tissues are not absolute, and are based on statistical correlations. It is also affected by differences in tissue composition in the trunk (an important reservoir of fat), small-diameter limbs, alterations in electrolyte balance, and third-space fluid (Mantovani *et al.* 1998). Nevertheless if used correctly it is an excellent tool for measuring body composition.

◆ Other tools for objective assessment include:

1. Densitometry: body density is a calculated using body weight and volume. This permits the estimation of fat mass and fat-free mass because of density differences in a two-compartmental model.

2. Dual-photon absorptiometry (DEXA) is based on the fact that the ratio of absorbance of two different energy level photons, applied by X-ray, is linearly related to the percentage of fat and fat-free mass of the body (Straisser and Bruera 2002). It is performed on the supine subject at rest (Nelson and Walsh 2002).

3. Dynamometry: the grip strength in a non-dominant hand is used as index of muscle function for the follow-up of cachectic patients (Burman and Chamberlain 1996), mostly in the context of clinical research. It is a useful tool, especially for studying fatigue related to cachexia.

4. Total body potassium: estimation of potassium allows extrapolation of lean body mass because it is the major intracellular cation in lean tissue. The radioactive ^{40}K decay is used to detect the total amount of potassium present in the body. Measurement of the extracellular potassium (4% is the estimated proportion of extracellular potassium) is the major source of error with this method because it can be altered in wasting conditions. Potassium transport may also be altered in severe protein calorie malnutrition. It is not a feasible method for routine use in clinical practice, but it provides a highly accurate estimation of lean body mass (Koch 1998).

Laboratory tests: nutritional parameters

◆ Serum hepatic transport proteins (albumin, pre-albumin, transferrin): sensitivity can vary due different half-lives and pool sizes (Langer *et al.* 2001). Transferrin and albumin appear to be the best global indicators (Burman and Chamberlain 1996).

◆ Nitrogen balance (24 h urinary nitrogen excretion): this is a measure of catabolic protein loss and can estimate the need for protein when parenteral or enteral nutrition is used. It is also used in clinical trials.

◆ Total lymphocyte count: this is an estimation of immune function and delayed hypersensitive reaction, but has no relevance for this subject in this population (Burman and Chamberlain 1996).

◆ Creatinine to weight ratio: shown to be the most sensitive indicator of protein calorie malnutrition (Langer *et al.* 2001). Ninety-eight per cent of creatinine is located in skeletal muscle in the form of creatinine phosphate. Urinary creatinine excretion over 24 h can be affected if the patient has impaired renal function, a meat-free diet, etc.

◆ Haemoglobin levels and electrolyte disturbance are other possible contributing factors to the development of fatigue and decreased appetite.

◆ C-reactive protein (CRP) levels may be a useful tool for monitoring treatment, especially in the context of clinical research.

Management of cancer anorexia/cachexia syndrome with reference to cancer-related fatigue

The management of CACS is a real challenge. As our understanding of the pathophysiology of this syndrome is clarified, potential new treatments appear. A comprehensive and multidisciplinary management approach is required to control all the factors related to cachexia and fatigue in cancer patients. Physical, psychosocial, and spiritual issues need to be considered, alongside pharmacological interventions and nutritional support. Specific pharmacological interventions for fatigue are not discussed in this chapter (see Chapter 12). Instead the aim is to identify interventions for used in the management of cancer cachexia that may also relieve CRF in this population. The purpose of the treatment is to control specific symptoms, such as asthenia, anorexia, chronic nausea, and pain and so improve QOL, if not life expectancy.

Pharmacological treatment: established drugs

Progesterone derivatives

Weight gain and appetite stimulation are now recognized as secondary effects of treatment for hormone-sensitive cancers using progesterone derivatives (Gregory *et al.* 1985; Tchekmedyian *et al.* 1987). Randomized controlled trials have been conducted to evaluate the efficacy of megestrol acetate (MA) and medroxyprogesterone (MPA) (Downer *et al.* 1993) as appetite stimulants (Simons *et al.* 1996). In some studies weight gain seems to be related to a gain in fat mass (Lambert *et al.* 2002; Engelson *et al.* 1999; Loprinzi *et al.* 1993) and, to a lesser extent, fluid retention, whilst others found no weight gain but instead an improvement in QOL related to increased appetite (Beller *et al.* 1997). The data on improvements in QOL are equivocal (Simons *et al.* 1996; Jatoi *et al.* 2000; Rowland *et al.* 1996), although this may reflect the differing measures used to assess it.

The exact mechanism of action of these agents remains to be elucidated. It has been postulated that central appetite stimulation effect (probably mediated by NPY) (Engelson *et al.* 1999; McCarthy *et al.* 1994), reduction of serotonin and cytokine release (Mantovani *et al.* 1997, 1998), and a corticosteroid-like effect (Beller *et al.* 1997), suppressing baseline cortisol levels, suggest an impact on the HPA axis (Oster *et al.* 1994). MA inhibits secretion of LH and follicle-stimulating hormone (FSH) in males and females (Engelson *et al.* 1999) and reduces testosterone levels (Engelson *et al.* 1999; Venner *et al.* 1988). *In vitro* studies have identified that MA enhances the differentiation of pre-adipocyte mouse fibroblasts to adipocytes (Engelson *et al.* 1999) which suggests that MA increases not only cell size, but also cell number (Neuenschwander and Bruera 1998). Data are contradictory on the possible down-regulation of IL-6 levels by MA (Mantovani 2002; Jatoi *et al.* 2002). The effect of these drugs on lean body mass is controversial. In patients with AIDS administering MA 800 mg/day was associated with a gain in fat mass (not a shift in water content) but not in lean body mass (Oster *et al.* 1994). Thus it has been suggested that one of the possible antianabolic muscle effects of progestagens is decreased testosterone levels. MA seems to induce suppression of androgens, both testicular and adrenal, and impairs their intracellular metabolism (Venner *et al.* 1988). However, in a recent study on aging-related weight loss and sarcopenia, testosterone in conjunction with MA was unable to demonstrate enhanced gains in muscle mass. The combination of these with resistance exercise appears to bring about gains in muscle mass (Lambert *et al.* 2002). Well-conducted randomized controlled clinical trials have shown these drugs to be a reasonable option when anorexia and body image are major matters of concern. Evidence on this antianabolic effect requires further clarification in a cancer population.

MA has shown a dose-related effect on appetite (Jatoi *et al.* 2002), weight gain, and feelings of well-being (Mantovani *et al.* 1998) in a dose range of 160–1600 mg. However, the related side-effects also increase with dose (peripheral oedema, hypertension, Cushing syndrome, thromboembolic disease, and adrenal insufficiency with abrupt cessation) (Bruera *et al.* 1990; Straisser and Bruera 2002). The suggested starting dose is 160 mg/day (Loprinzi *et al.* 1993), and this is titrated according to the balance between clinical response and side-effects. MPA is used at a dose of 1000 mg/day orally (equivalent to MA 160 mg/day) (Mantovani *et al.* 2001).

Corticosteroids

In advanced cancer patients, dexamethasone (Moertel *et al.*1974) and methylprednisolone (Bruera *et al.* 1985) have been shown to relieve anorexia and increase sense of well-being (Bruera *et al.* 1985) and QOL (Robustelli Della Cuna *et al.* 1989) in randomized controlled trials. This improvement is probably the result of a euphoric effect (Moertel *et al.* 1974; Bruera *et al.* 1985). Alternative mechanisms of action include inhibition of prostaglandin synthesis (Bruera *et al.* 1985; Faisinger 1996) and the effects and cytokines. The use of corticosteroids is limited, due to the wide range of side-effects experienced in the long term (Needham *et al.* 1992) and with high-dose treatment. Proximal myopathy is one of the major concerns with prolonged use (Twycross 1992; Watanabe and Bruera 1994). Increased loss of function and number of muscle cells, probably through NF-κB action in the ubiquitin-proteolytic pathway, is one of the suggested pathophysiological mechanisms (Tisdale 2000). For this reason steroids are not a good treatment option for cachectic and fatigued ambulatory cancer patients. However, corticosteroids are effective in the management of symptoms, such as nausea (Watanabe and Bruera 1994; Bruera *et al.* 1996) and pain (Watanabe and Bruera 1994), and so they are useful for non-ambulatory symptomatic advanced cancer patients where there are no major contraindications. Symptom improvement is limited to a few weeks (Faisinger 1996; Watanabe and Bruera 1994), so short treatment courses are recommended (Faisinger 1996). Results can be assessed after 1 week of treatment and treatment should be stopped if there is no therapeutic response (Needham *et al.* 1992).

Other drugs

Anabolic drugs

Testosterone analogues have the advantage of greater anabolic effect and less androgenic activity than testosterone (Mantovani *et al.* 2001). In randomized controlled trials oxandrolone substantially increased lean body mass and strength in HIV patients with weight loss (Langer *et al.* 2001; Strawford *et al.* 1999). In this population it is recommended to enhance the effects of anabolic drugs with nutritional support and exercise (Langer *et al.* 2001).

Oral stanazolol (12 mg per day for 27 weeks) was administered to malnourished subjects with COPD; the findings of this study demonstrated an increase in lean body mass with no significant changes in endurance exercise capacity (Ferreira *et al.* 1998). There are few data to support its use in a cancer population. In a randomized, prospective trial of patients with lung cancer receiving chemotherapy with or without nandrolone 200 mg/day intramuscularly weekly for 1 month, no significant difference was seen between groups with respect to weight loss (Langer *et al.* 2001).

Growth hormone (GH), seems to have a positive effect on nitrogen balance and protein mass (Mantovani *et al.* 2001) through insulin growth factor-1 (IGF-1), which is produced by the liver. IGF-1 stimulates amino acid uptake and protein synthesis (Argiles *et al.* 2001*b*). However, concern that these agents may enhance tumour growth has precluded their use in this population. Recent basic data showed GH resistance in patients with newly diagnosed cancer and loss of lean mass (Crown *et al.* 2002).

Thalidomide

Thalidomide has been shown to be a modulator of the production of TNF-α and other cytokines (Peuckmann *et al.* 2000), probably via NF-κB transcription factor suppression (Majumdar *et al.* 2002; Richardson *et al.* 2002). In a preliminary study of 37 advanced cancer patients with cachexia, thalidomide was associated with a significant improvement in appetite, nausea, and sensation of well-being (Bruera *et al.* 1999), whilst HIV patients with tuberculosis, who were treated with thalidomide, showed a mean body weight gain (Klausner *et al.* 1996). However, its use in cancer patients remains to be established in future studies. It is possible that the recently synthesized thalidomide analogues, immunomodulatory derivatives (IMIDS) (Richardson *et al.* 2002), exhibit fewer adverse effects and so it is possible that they could be useful in this setting, either alone or in combination with other drugs.

Cannabinoids

The role of delta-9-tetrahydrocannabinol (THC) in the treatment of the wasting syndrome associated with cancer remains controversial. Preliminary data described this cannabinoid as an effective antidepressant and appetite stimulant for advanced cancer patients (Regelson *et al.* 1976). However, the design of most of the studies conducted in cancer patients preclude definitive conclusions being made (Bagshaw 2002). The endocannabinoid system seems to be linked with hypothalamic regulation of food intake. Administration of leptin in mice has been associated with reduced levels of both 2-arachidonylglycerol (2-AG) and anandamide (Berry and Mechoulam 2002). The endogenous endocannabinoid system seems to have a role in the modulation of feeding (Berry and Mechoulam 2002) and the oral reward of the process of feeding (Goutopoulos and Makriyannis 2002).

Endogenous endocannabinoids are derived from omega-6 essential polyunsaturated fatty acids (Berry and Mechoulam 2002). More research is needed to establish if dietary manipulation is capable of modifying endocannabinoid levels.

Prokinetics

Chronic nausea and early satiety are frequently present in advanced and cachectic cancer patients (Baines 1988). It is a multifactorial syndrome, mainly caused by autonomic failure (Bruera *et al.* 1987*b*, 1994; Komurku *et al.* 2000) and opioid therapy (Komurku *et al.* 2000). Gastroparesia is also believed to be a consequence of direct action of cytokines on the intrinsic nervous system in the gut. Indeed, the administration of cytokines is capable of inducing nausea (Dunlop and Campbell 2000). Metoclopramide (MCP), an antidopaminergic drug, has both an effective central antiemetic effect and gastric emptying properties (Loo *et al.* 1984). MCP 10 mg, orally or subcutaneously, every 4 h, in immediate release form, is the commonest mode of administration (Straisser and Bruera 2002). Controlled released MCP (administered every 12 h) is also effective in this setting (Bruera *et al.* 2000).

Drugs with poor or negative results in cancer cachexia

Pentoxyfilline (Goldberg *et al.* 1995), hydrazine sulfate (Loprinzi *et al.* 1994*a*, *b*) and cyproheptadine (Kardinal *et al.* 1990) were not found to be useful in placebo controlled trials.

Emerging drugs

In the recent years, basic research and pilot studies have demonstrated promising results with new compounds. The modulation of the proinflammatory effects exerted by cytokines and tumour products seems to be the rationale of some of the new emerging drugs and these will now be discussed.

Omega-3 polyunsaturated fatty acids

The omega-3 (ω-3) and omega-6 (ω-6) fatty acids are essential fatty acids, and they must be taken from the diet (Baracos 2001). Arachidonic acid (AA) is an ω-6 fatty acid and is a component of cell membranes and a precursor for prostaglandin synthesis (Rex *et al.* 2002). AA and one of its major metabolites, prostaglandin E2 (PgE2) (Rex *et al.* 2002), play important roles in complex signalling pathways that involve a series of second messengers.

Diets high in ω-6 content have been associated with increased cell proliferation (Rex *et al.* 2002). On the other hand, diets rich in ω-3, such as fish oil which contains 18% EPA (Tisdale 2002), are thought to reduce cell proliferation (Rex *et al.* 2002) by a reducing AA in plasma cell membranes. There is a subsequent decrease in production of PgE2 (Rex *et al.* 2002) and other potential mitogens, for example 13-hydroxyoctadecadienoic acid (13-HODE) (Sauer *et al.* 2000). Eicosanoid synthesis depends on the relative abundance of AA and EPA in the cell membrane (Baracos 2001).

Patients with advanced pancreatic cancer showed attenuation of weight loss with EPA alone (Wigmore *et al.* 1996) or in combination with nutritional supplementation (Baracos 2001; Barber *et al.* 1999*b*). In a phase I study, 22 patients were treated with EPA and docosahexaenoic acid (DHA), another ω-3; the dose-limiting toxicity was gastrointestinal, mainly diarrhoea (Burns *et al.* 1999).

PgE2 and 15-hydroxyeicosatetraenoic acid (15-HETE) are two metabolites of AA that have been found to activate protein catabolism in skeletal muscle *in vitro* (Baracos 2001). Cachectic mice, bearing the MAC 16 tumour, were treated with EPA and showed an attenuation of the up-regulated ATP-dependent proteolytic pathway. This correlated with an increase in myosin expression, confirming retention of contractile proteins (Whitehouse *et al.* 2001). EPA affects the expression of proteosome subunits, rather than acting as a direct inhibitor of this system (Whitehouse *et al.* 2001), and is correlated with the inhibition of PIF (Lorite *et al.* 1997). This probably occurs as a result of its ability to suppress 15-HETE production. Omega-3 fatty acids also seem to suppress expression of cyclooxygenase-2 and activation of NF-κB in tumours (Hardman 2002).

Non-steroidal anti-inflammatory drugs (NSAIDs)

Ibuprofen (a COX-1 inhibitor) has been found to improve survival in patients with cancer, and this correlated with an increase in body weight and a decrease in C-reactive protein (Wigmore *et al.* 1995; Lundholm *et al.* 1994). Similar results were found with other NSAIDs. Sodium salicylate, aspirin, and sulindac have been shown, amongst other effects, to decrease NF-κB activation through I-κBα phosphorylation (I-κB proteins regulate the subcellular localization of NF-κB) (Schwartz *et al.* 1999). COX-2 inhibitors are drugs with an improved safety profile and they have demonstrated suppression of tumour growth in animal models (Masferrer *et al.* 2000) and human cancer cells (Shureiqui *et al.* 2000). Over-expression of COX-2 is significantly correlated with invasiveness and mortality in some cancers (Koki and Masferrer 2002; Uefuji *et al.* 2000).

In an open uncontrolled pilot study, 15 patients with advanced lung adenocarcinoma and CACS received MA (500 mg twice a day), a COX-2 inhibitor (celecoxib 200 mg twice a day), and oral food supplementation (polymeric diet) for 6 weeks. After treatment 13 out of 15 patients had maintained or gained weight and levels of interleukin-10 (IL-10) were inversely correlated with weight change (all the patients had higher levels of IL-10 than the healthy control group). There were also significant improvements in nausea, early satiety, fatigue, performance status, and the rate of weight change. The authors conclude that this study encourages further work with multitargeted approaches (Cerchietti *et al.* 2004).

Cytokine modulation

Transcription factors, such as NF-κB and activation protein-1 (AP-1), are seen as the most important signal transducers for proinflammatory stimuli (von Haehling *et al.* 2002). Fumaric acid has an anti-inflammatory potency, and is capable of targeting the translocation of activated NF-κB (Loewe *et al.* 2002). However, complete inhibition of NF-κB in knock-out mice models leads to severe immunodeficiency (Ghosh *et al.* 1998). Glucocorticoid anti-inflammatory action has been linked with NF-κB inhibition (von Haehling *et al.* 2002). Injection of anti-TNF-α antibodies was not able to suppress the development of cachexia (Inadera *et al.* 2002). Thus it is essential to bear in mind that no single cytokine is responsible for the development and maintenance of cachexia. Also, the extent to which antibodies with limited tissue penetration can effectively extinguish paracrine-acting cytokines is unclear (Cahlin *et al.* 2000).

Proteosome inhibitors

Beta-2 agonists, like clenbuterol, can potentially suppress the ubiquitin-proteosome-dependent proteolytic system in animals (Costelli *et al.* 1995*a*). Beta-2 agonists can also suppress increased branched chain amino acid oxidation in skeletal muscle during cachexia in animal models (Costelli *et al.* 1995*b*).

Melatonin

In a controlled trial of 100 patients with metastatic cancer the administration of melatonin was associated with a significant decrease in weight loss (Lissoni *et al.* 1996). It is thought that this occurs as a result of a decrease in cytokine activity. In addition, melatonin appears to block tumour n-6 fatty acid uptake and 13-HODE formation (Sauer *et al.* 2000).

Peroxisome proliferator-activated receptor gamma ligands

Troglitazone is a peroxisome proliferator-activated receptor gamma (PPAR-γ) ligand that is associated with decreased levels of uncoupling protein 2 (UCP2) and 3 (UCP3) mRNA in mouse myotubes. The UCP expression is probably induced by cytokines and tumour product (Cabrero 2000).

Approaches to fatigue management

It is well known that many factors can contribute to fatigue in patients with cancer cachexia. It is necessary to identify any potential causes of fatigue, such as anaemia, metabolic disturbance, endocrine alteration, and sleep disturbance that can be effectively corrected. Non-pharmacological interventions, particularly exercise, are recommended in patients with good functional status, as well as educational and counselling measures (see Chapter 12).

With regard to the pharmacological approaches mentioned above for the management of cancer cachexia, there are controversies that need highlighting:

- ◆ Corticosteroids may show an improvement in fatigue over a short duration, as a consequence of a euphoric effect (Bruera *et al.* 1985; Robustelli Della Cuna *et al.* 1989). However, the prolonged use of corticosteroids produces loss of function and muscle mass (Tisdale 2000), which is counterproductive for relieving fatigue.

- ◆ More data are needed to achieve clearer conclusions about the potential benefit of progestational agents in the treatment of fatigued sarcopenic patients, possibly in conjunction with exercise and other drugs for managing cachexia (Lambert *et al.* 2002).

- ◆ With reference to the new agents identified for the management of cachexia, those that aim to decrease and control the production of cytokines and associated proinflammatory states (COX-1 inhibitors (Schwartz *et al.* 1999; Wigmore *et al.* 1995; Lundholm *et al.* 1994), COX-2 inhibitors (Cerchietti *et al.* 2004), melatonin (Lissoni *et al.* 1996), thalidomide (Majumdar *et al.* 2002; Richardson *et al.* 2002; Bruera *et al.* 1999) and PPAR-γ ligands (Tisdale 2002) may also be a reasonable option for improving fatigue, at least in those who also have cachexia.

Nutritional support

There is strong evidence that nutritional supplementation alone is not able to reverse the process of cachexia (Tisdale 1997). No improvements in survival, strength, QOL, or decreases in complication rates were observed when nutritional supplements were administered to patients undergoing treatment (chemotherapy and radiotherapy) (Straisser and Bruera 2002). Nevertheless, when starvation is a major contributor to the impairment of nutritional status in these patients, it may be possible to improve nutritional parameters with nutritional support (e.g. patients undergoing treatment for bowel obstruction) (Straisser and Bruera 2002). In selected patients, when their gastrointestinal tract is functional, enteral feeding is preferable to parenteral nutrition (Vignano and Bruera 1996).

Supplementation with specific nutrients that modulate protein synthesis and proteolysis have been studied in non-malignant inflammatory conditions. Glutamine seems to be a regulator of muscle proteolysis and synthesis (Tisdale 2002). It is the most abundant free amino acid in the body and becomes 'conditionally essential' during sepsis and other conditions of hypercatabolism (Wray *et al.* 2002). Both glutamine and arginine have immune stimulatory effects (Wray *et al.* 2002). Enteral provision of glutamine significantly decreased infectious complications in patients with severe multiple trauma (Wray *et al.* 2002). It has been suggested that arginine may enhance anabolism by stimulating GH and insulin release (Wray *et al.* 2002). A randomized study performed with 32 cachectic patients compared an isonitrogenous control mixture of non-essential amino acids with an experimental treatment of glutamine, arginine, and β-hydroxy-methylbutyrate. At week four the experimental group showed improvements in non-fatty mass (May *et al.* 2002).

Psychological and spiritual issues

Cancer cachexia is the most easily recognizable external sign of serious illness and is a major concern to patients and their families (Higginson and Winget 1996). Above all, cachexia is seen as a sign of impending death. Changes in body image impact on emotional well-being, one of the primary domains of health-related QOL (Fallowfield 2002). Fatigue appears to be an independent predictor factor of QOL. In fact, it was claimed as being the most distressing symptom experienced during cancer treatment (Richardson 1995).

Psychological disorders, such as anxiety (Sivesind and Baile 2001), adjustment disorders, and depression may play a part in this situation. Also cachexia may result in secondary depression (Higginson and Bruera 1996). Fatigue has been connected with depression, but this is not a constant relationship (Visser and Smets 1998) (see Chapter 10). The use of psychological and behavioural interventions in combination with pharmacological treatment could significantly improve QOL in fatigued and cachectic patients (see Chapter 12). A multidisciplinary approach in the treatment of this syndrome seems more reasonable than isolated approaches.

Future perspectives

CACS requires a multidisciplinary management approach. Changes in body image impact dramatically on emotional well-being, as well as a patient's QOL. Psychological and behavioural interventions must be an integral part of the management of this syndrome. As discussed in this chapter, CRF probably shares common pathophysiological pathways with cancer cachexia. In recent years knowledge of basic biology in this area has greatly increased. But it is necessary also to extrapolate this knowledge into clinical research in rational, controlled, randomized clinical studies (see Box 4.1).

Combined modalities of treatment appear to be an attractive option (see Box 4.2). Progestational derivatives associated with cytokine or eicosanoid metabolism modulators warrant further study. Aggressive nutritional support has not been proven to have major symptomatic effects in these patients. However, supplementation with anticatabolic amino acids, such as arginine and glutamine, in conjunction with other pharmacological approaches seems to be a rational tool in the early management of weight loss in cancer patients. Further clinical trials are needed to assess their impact in terms of improvement in nutritional parameters and QOL. Probably the stabilization or gain in weight in this population will not only be an achievement in the management of CACS but also in that of cachexia-related fatigue.

Box 4.1 Chapter summary

- CACS is a multifactorial syndrome caused by the presence of the tumour itself as well as the host response to that stimulus. It is one of the most devastating causes of poor QOL and death in cancer patients.

- The persistent activity of circulating mediators (cytokines, pro-inflammatory mediators) leads to alterations in physiological metabolic processes that characterize cancer cachexia.

- Fatigue is frequently present in the cancer cachexia population and it is possible that both share common links in their pathophysiology.

- It is necessary to identify any potential causes of fatigue, such as anaemia, metabolic disturbance, endocrine alterations, and sleep disturbance, so that they can be effectively corrected.

- There is still no optimal available treatment to relieve cachexia and fatigue in cancer; however, pharmacological plus non-pharmacological interventions (education, counselling, exercise (in good performance patients), and supplementation with specific nutrients) are recommended.

Box 4.2 Implications for research and practice

- The development of new bioimmunomodulators to treat cancer is a promising area for future research in the cachectic and fatigue cancer population.

- Multitarget therapies are a rational way of managing a multifactorial syndrome like cachexia and this may also contribute to relieving fatigue.

- More research on the intrinsic pathways implicated in the development of cachexia, such as the relationship between the immune, endocrine, and psychoneural systems, is needed.

- A rational use of the available tools, as well as the development of more accurate measures for the assessment of cachexia and fatigue, is also needed.

References

Aleman, M.R., Santolaria, F., Batista, N., de la Vega, M.J., Gonzalez-Reimers, E., Milena, A. *et al.* (2002) Leptin's role in advanced lung cancer. A mediator of the acute phase response or a marker of the status of nutrition? *Cytokine*, **19**, 21–6.

Ancoli-Israel, S., Moore, P.J., and Jones, V. (2001) The relationship between fatigue and sleep in cancer patients: a review. *European Journal of Cancer Care*, **10**, 245–55.

Argiles, J.M., Meijsing, S.H., Pallares-Trujillo, J., Guirao, X., and Lopez-Soriano, F.J. (2001*a*) Cancer cachexia: a therapeutic approach. *Medical Research Reviews*, **21**, 83–101.

Argiles, J.M., Busquets, S., and Lopez-Soriano, F.J. (2001*b*) Metabolic interrelationships between liver and skeletal muscle in pathological states. *Life Sciences*, **69**, 1345–61.

Bagshaw, S.M. (2002) Medical efficacy of cannabinoids and marijuana: a comprehensive review of the literature. *Journal of Palliative Care*, **18**, 111–22.

Baines, M. (1988) Nausea and vomiting in the patient with advanced cancer. *Journal of Pain and Symptom Management*, **3**, 81–5.

Baracos, V. (2001) Management of muscle wasting in cancer-associated cachexia. Understanding gained from experimental studies. *Cancer*, **92**, 1669–77.

Baracos, V.E. (2000) Regulation of skeletal-muscle-protein turnover in cancer-associated cachexia. *Nutrition*, **16**, 1015–18.

Barber, M.D., Ross, J.A., and Fearon, K.C.H. (1999*a*) Changes in nutritional, functional, and inflammatory markers in advanced pancreatic cancer. *Nutrition and Cancer*, **35**(2), 106–10.

Barber, M.D., Ross, J.A., Voss, A.C., Tisdale, M.J., and Fearon, K.C.H. (1999*b*) The effect of an oral nutritional supplement enriched with fish oil on weight-loss in patients with pancreatic cancer. *British Journal of Cancer*, **81**(1), 80–6.

Barnes, E.A. and Bruera, E. (2002) Fatigue in patients with advanced cancer: a review. *International Journal of Gynecological Cancer*, **12**, 424–8.

Beller, E., Tattersall, M., Lumley, T., Levi, J., Dalley, D., Olver, I. *et al.* (1997) Improved quality of life with megestrol acetate in patients with endocrine insensitive advanced cancer: a randomized placebo-controlled trial. *Annals of Oncology*, **8**, 277–83.

Berry, E.M. and Mechoulam, R. (2002) Tetrahydrocannabinol and endocannabinoids in feeding and appetite. *Pharmacology and Therapeutics*, **95**, 185–90.

Bing, C.H., Brown, M., King, P., Collins, P., Tisdale, M.J., and Williams, G. Increased gene expression of brown fat uncoupling protein (UCP) 1 and skeletal muscle UCP2 and UCP3 in MAC16-induced cancer cachexia. *Cancer Research*, **60**, 2405–10.

Brown, D.R., Berkowitz, D.E., and Breslow, M.J. (2001) Weight loss is not associated with hyperleptinemia in humans with pancreatic cancer. *Journal of Clinical Endocrinology and Metabolism*, **86**, 162–6.

Bruera, E. (1997) Anorexia, cachexia and nutrition. *British Medical Journal*, **315**, 1219–22.

Bruera, E., Roca, E., Cedaro, L., Carraro, S., and Chacon, R. (1985) Action of oral methylprednisolone in terminal cancer patients: a prospective randomized double-blind study. *Cancer Treatment Reports*, **69**, 751–4.

Bruera, E., Brenneis, C., Michaud, M., Jackson, F., and MacDonald, R.N. (1987*a*) Association between involuntary muscle function and asthenia, nutritional status, lean body mass, psychometric assessment and tumour mass in patients with advanced cancer. *Proceedings of the American Society for Clinical Oncology*, **6**, 261.

Bruera, E., Catz, Z., Hooper, R., Lentle, B., and MacDonald, N. (1987*b*) Chronic nausea and anorexia in advanced cancer patients: a possible role for autonomic dysfunction. *Journal of Pain and Symptom Management*, **2**, 19–21.

Bruera, E., Macmillan, K., Kuehn, N., Hanson, J., and MacDonald, N. (1990) A controlled trial of megestrol acetate on appetite, caloric intake, nutritional status, and other symptoms in patients with advanced cancer. *Cancer*, **66**, 1279–82.

Bruera, E., MacEachrn, T.J., Spachynski, K.A., LeGatt, D.F., MacDonald, R.N., Babul, N. *et al.* (1994) Comparison of the efficacy, safety, and pharmacokinetics of controlled release and immediate release methoclopramide for the management of chronic nausea in patients with advanced cancer. *Cancer*, **74**, 3204–11.

Bruera, E., Seifert, L., Watanabe, S., Babul, N., Darke, A., Harsanyi, Z. *et al.* (1996) Chronic nausea in advanced cancer patients: a retrospective assessment of a metoclopramide-based antiemetic regimen. *Journal of Pain and Symptom Management*, **11**, 147–53.

Bruera, E., Neumann, C.M., Pituskin, E., Pituskin, E., Caldler, K., Ball, G. *et al.* (1999) Thalidomide in patients with cachexia due to terminal cancer: preliminary report. *Annals of Oncology*, **10**, 857–9.

Bruera, E., Belzile, M., Neumann, C., Harsanyi, Z., Babul, N., and Darke, A. (2000) A double-blind, crossover study of controlled-release metoclopramide and placebo for the chronic nausea and dyspepsia of advanced cancer. *Journal of Pain and Symptom Management*, **19**(6), 427–35.

Burman, R. and Chamberlain, J. (1996) The assessment of the nutritional status, caloric intake, and appetite of patients with advanced cancer. In: *Cachexia-Anorexia in Cancer Patients*, (ed. E. Bruera and I. Higginson). Oxford University Press, New York, pp. 83–93.

Burns, P.C., Halabi, S., and Clamon, G.H. (1999) Phase I clinical study of fish oil fatty acid capsules for patients with cancer cachexia: Cancer and Leukemia Group B Study 9473. *Clinical Cancer Research*, **5**, 3942–7.

Cabrero, A. (2000) Down-regualtion of uncoupling protein-3 and 2 by thiazolidinediones in C2C12 myotubes. *FEBS Letters*, **484**, 37–42.

Cahlin, C., Korner, A., and Axelsson, H. (2000) Experimental cancer cachexia: the role of host-derived cytokines interleukin (IL)-6, IL-12, interferon-γ and tumour necrosis factor α evaluated in gene knockout, tumour-bearing mice on C57 background and eicosanoid-dependent cachexia. *Cancer Research*, **60**, 5488–93.

Capra, S., Ferguson, M., and Ried, K. (2001) Cancer: impact of nutrition intervention outcome-nutrition issues for patients. *Nutrition*, **17**, 769–72.

Cariuk, P., Lorite, M.J., Todorov, P.T., Field, W.N., Wigmore, S.J., and Tisdale, M.J. (1997) Induction of cachexia in mice by a product isolated from the urine of cachectic cancer patients. *British Journal of Cancer*, **76**(5), 606–13.

Cerchietti, L., Navigante, A., Peluffo, G., Diament, M.J., Stillitani, I., Klein, S. *et al.* Effects of celecoxib, medroxyprogesterone and dietary intervention on systemic syndromes in patients with advanced lung adenocarcinoma: a pilot study. *Journal of Pain and Symptom Management*, **27**, 85–95.

Coats, A.J.S. (2002) Origin of symptoms in patients with cachexia with special reference to weakness and shortness of breath. *International Journal of Cardiology*, **85**, 133–9.

Collins, P., Bing, C., McCulloch, P., and Williams, G. (2002) Muscle UCP-3 mRNA levels are elevated in weight loss associated with gastrointestinal adenocarcinoma in humans. *British Journal of Cancer*, **86**, 372–5.

Costelli, P., Garcia-Martinez, C., and Llovera, M. (1995a) Muscle protein waste in tumour-bearing rats is effectively antagonized by β-2 adrenergic agonist (clenbuterol) *Journal of Clinical Investigation*, **95**, 2367–72.

Costelli, P., Llovera, M., and García Martinez, C. (1995) Enhanced leucine oxidation in rats bearing an ascites hepatoma (Yoshida AH-130) and its reversal by clenbuterol. *Cancer Letters*, **91**, 73–8.

Crown, A.L., Cottle, K., Lightman, S.L. *et al.* (2002) What is the role of the insulin-growth factor system in the pathophysiology of cancer cachexia, and how is it regulated? *Clinical Endocrinology*, **56**, 723–33.

De Wys, W.D., Begg, D., Lavin, P.T. *et al.* (1980) Prognostic effect of weight loss prior to chemotherapy in cancer patients. *American Journal of Medicine*, **69**, 491.

Di Francia, M., Barbier, D., Mege, J.L., and Orehek, J. (1994) Tumour necrosis factor-alpha levels and weight loss in chronic obstructive pulmonary disease. *American Journal of Respiratory and Critical Care Medicine*, **150**(5, Part 1), 1453–5.

Diffee, G.M., Kalfas, K., Al-Majid, S., and McCarthy, D. (2002) Altered expression of skeletal muscle myosin isoforms in cancer cachexia. *American Journal of Physiology*, **283**, C1376–C1382.

Doehner, W. and Anker, S. (2002) Cardiac cachexia in early literature: a review of research prior to Medline. *International Journal of Cardiology*, **85**, 7–14.

Downer, S., Joel, S., Allbright, A., Plant, H., Stubbs, L., Talbot, D. *et al.* (1993) A double blind placebo controlled trial of medroxyprogesterone acetate (MPA) in cancer cachexia. *British Journal of Cancer*, **67**, 1102–5.

Dunlop, R.J. and Campbell, C.W. (2000) Cytokines and advanced cancer. *Journal of Pain and Symptom Management*, **20**, 214–32.

Engelson, E.S., Pi-Sunyer, E.F., and Kotler, D. (1999) Effects of megestrol acetate and testosterone on body composition in castrated male Sprague–Dawley rats. *Nutrition*, **15**, 465–73.

Faisinger, R. (1996) Pharmacological approach to cancer anorexia and cachexia. In: *Cachexia-Anorexia in Cancer Patients*, (ed. E. Bruera and I. Higginson). Oxford University Press, Oxford, pp. 128–40.

Falconer, S., Fearon, K.C.H., Plester, C.E., Ross, J.A., and Carter, D.C. (1994) Cytokines, the acute-phase response, and resting energy expenditure in cachectic patients with pancreatic cancer. *Annals of Surgery*, **219**, 325–31.

Fallowfield, L. (2002) Quality of life: a new perspective for cancer patients. *Nature Reviews Cancer*, **2**, 873–9.

Fearon, K.C.H. and Moses, A.G.W. (2002) Cancer cachexia. *International Journal of Cardiology*, **85**, 73–81.

Ferreira, I.M., Verreschi, I.T., Nery, L.E., Goldstein, R.S., Zamel, N., Brooks, D. *et al.* (1998) The influence of 6 months of oral anabolic steroids on body mass and respiratory muscles in undernourished COPD patients. *Chest*, **114**(1), 19–28.

Filippatos, G.S., Tsilias, K., Venetsanou, K., Karambinos, E., Manolatos, D., Kranidis, A. *et al.* Leptin serum levels in cachectic heart failure patients Relationship with tumour necrosis factor a system. *International Journal of Cardiology*, **76**, 117–22.

Finch, P.M., Roberts, L.J., Price, L., Hadlow, N.C., and Pullan, P.T. (2000) Hypogonadism in patients treated with intrathecal morphine. *Clinical Journal of Pain*, **16**, 251–4.

Ghosh, S., May, M., and Kopp, E. (1998) NF-κB and REL proteins: evolutionary conserved mediators of immune responses. *Annual Review of Immunology*, **16**, 225–60.

Goldberg, R.M., Loprinzi, C.L., Mailliard, J.A. *et al.* (1995) Pentoxifylline for treatment of cancer anorexia and cachexia? A randomized, double-blind, placebo-controlled trial. *Journal of Clinical Oncology*, **13**(11), 2856–9.

Goutopoulos, A. and Makriyannis, A. (2002) From cannabis to cannabinergics: new therapeutic opportunities. *Pharmacology and Therapeutics*, **95**, 103–17.

Greenberg, D.B., Gray, J.L., Mannix, C.M., Eisenthal, S., and Carey, M. (1993) Treatment-related fatigue and serum interleukin-1 levels in patients during external beam irradiation for prostate cancer. *Journal of Pain and Symptom Management*, **8**, 196–200.

Gregory, E.J., Cohen, S.C., Oines, D.W., and Mims, C.H. (1985) Megestrol acetate therapy for advanced breast cancer. *Journal of Clinical Oncology*, **3**, 155–60.

Gustein, H.B. (2001) The biologic basis of fatigue. *Cancer*, **92**, 1678–83.

Guttridge, D.C., Mayo, M.W., Madrid, L.V., Wang, C.-Y., and Baldwin, A.S. (2000) NF-κB-induced loss of myoD messenger RNA: possible role in muscle decay and cachexia. *Science*, **289**(5488), 2363–6.

Hardman, W. (2002) Omega-3-fatty acids to augment cancer therapy. *Journal of Nutrition*, **132**(11), 3508S–3512S.

Higginson, I. and Bruera, E. (1996) Practical concepts for clinicians. In: *Cachexia-Anorexia in Cancer Patients*, (ed. E. Bruera and I. Higginson). Oxford University Press, Oxford, pp. 184–9.

Higginson, I. and Winget, C. (1996) Psychological impact in cancer cachexia on the patient and the family. In: *Cachexia-Anorexia in Cancer Patients*, (ed. E. Bruera and I. Higginson). Oxford University Press, Oxford, pp. 172–83.

Hirai, K., Hussey, H.J., Barber, M.D., Price, S.A., and Tisdale, M.J. (1998) Biological evaluation of a lipid-mobilizing factor isolated from the urine of cancer patients. *Cancer Research*, **58**, 2359–65.

Hopwood, P., Fletcher, I., Lee, A., and Al Ghazal, S. (2001) A body image scale for the use with cancer patients. *European Journal of Cancer*, **37**(2), 189–97.

Inadera, H., Nagai, S., Dong, H.-Y., and Matsushima, K. (2002) Molecular analysis of lipid-depleting factor in a colon-26-inoculated cancer cachexia model. *International Journal of Cancer*, **101**, 37–45.

Inui, A. (1999) Cancer anorexia-cachexia syndrome: are neuropeptides the key? *Cancer Research*, **59**, 4493–501.

Jatoi, A., Kumar, S., Sloan, J.A., and Nguyen, P.L. (2000) On appetite and its loss. *Journal of Clinical Oncology*, **18**(15), 2930–2.

Jatoi, A., Yamashita, J.-I., Sloan, J., Novotny, P.J., Windschitl, H.E., and Loprinzi, C.L. (2002) Does megestrol acetate down-regulate interleukin 6 in patients with cancer associated anorexia and weight loss? A North Central Cancer Treatment Group Investigation. *Supportive Care in Cancer*, **10**, 71–5.

Kardinal, C.G., Loprinzi, C.L., Schaid, D.J., *et al.* (1990) A controlled trial of cyprohepatadine in cancer patients with anorexia and/or cachexia. *Cancer*, **65**(12), 2657–62.

Karnofsky, D.A. and Burchenal, J.H. (1949) The clinical evaluation of chemotherapeutic agents in cancer. In: *Evaluation of Chemotherapeutic Agents*, (ed. C.M. Macleod). Columbia University Press, New York, pp. 191–205.

Klausner, J.D., Makon Kaw Keyoon, S., Akarasewi, P., *et al.* (1996) The effect of thalidomide on the pathogenesis of human immunodeficiency virus type I and M. Tuberculosis infection. *Journal of Acquired Immune Deficiency Syndromes and Human Retrovirology*, 11, 247–57.

Koch, J. (1998) The role of body composition measurements in wasting syndromes. *Seminars in Oncology*, 25(Supplement 6), 12–19.

Koki, A.T. and Masferrer, J.L. (2002) Celecoxib: a specific COX-2 inhibitor with anticancer properties. *Cancer Control*, 9, 28–35.

Komurku, S., Nelson, K.A., Walsh, D., Donnelly, S.M., Homsi, J., and Abdullah, O. (2000) Common symptoms in advanced cancer. *Seminars in Oncology*, 27, 24–33.

Kotler, D.P. (2000) Cachexia. *Annals of Internal Medicine*, 133, 622–34.

Kurzok, R. (2001) The role of cytokines in cancer-related fatigue. *Cancer*, 92, 1684–8.

Lambert, C.P., Sullivan, D.H., Freeling, S.A., Lindquist, D.M., and Evans, W.J. (2002) Effects of testosterone replacement and/or resistance exercise on the composition of megestrol acetate stimulated weight gain in elderly men: a randomized controlled trial. *Journal of Clinical Endocrinology and Metabolism*, 87, 2100–6.

Langer, C.J., Hoffman, J.P., and Ottery, F.D. (2001) Clinical significance of weight loss in cancer patients: rationale for the use of anabolic agents in the treatment of cancer-related cachexia. *Nutrition*, 17, S1–S18.

Lawlor, P., Faisinger, R.L., and Bruera, E. (2000) Delirium at the end of life. Critical issues in clinical practice and research. *Journal of the American Medical Association*, 284, 2427–9.

Levine, B., Kalman, J., Mayer, L., Fillit, H.M., and Packer, M. (1990) Elevated plasma levels of tumour necrosis factor in severe chronic heart failure. *New England Journal of Medicine*, 323, 236–41.

Lindmark, L., Bennegard, K., Ekman, E.L., Schersten, T., Svaninger, G., and Lundholm, K. (1984) Resting energy expenditure in malnourished patients with and without cancer. *Gastroenterology*, 87, 402–8.

Lissoni, P., Paolorossi, F., Tancinini, G., Tancini, G., Aridzzoia, A., Barni, S. *et al.* (1996) Is there a role for melatonin in the treatment of neoplastic cachexia? *European Journal of Cancer*, 32A, 1340–3.

Loewe, R., Holnthoner, W., and Groger M. (2002) Dimethylfumarate inhibits TNF-induced nuclear entry of NF-κB/p65 in human endothelial cells. *Journal of Immunology*, 168, 4781–7.

Loo, F.D., Palmer, D.W., Soergel, K.H., Kalbfleish, J.H., and Wood, C.M. (1984) Gastric emptying in patients with diabetes mellitus. *Gastroenterology*, 86, 485–94.

Loprinzi, C.L., Michalak, J.C., Schaid, D.J., Mailliard, J.A., Athmann, L.M., Goldberg, R.M. *et al.* (1993) Phase III evaluation of four doses of megestrol acetate as therapy for patients with anorexia and/or cachexia. *Journal of Clinical Oncology*, 11, 762–7.

Loprinzi, C.L., Kuross, S.A., O'Fallon, J.R., *et al.* (1994*a*) Randomized placebo-controlled evaluation on hydrazine sulphate in patients with advanced colorectal cancer. *Journal of Clinical Oncology*, 12, 1121–5.

Loprinzi, C.L., Goldberg, R.M., Su, J.Q., *et al.* (1994*b*) Placebo-controlled trial of hydrazine sulphate in patients with newly diagnosed non-small-cell lung cancer. *Journal of Clinical Oncology*, 12, 1126–9.

Lorite, M.J., Cariuk, P., and Tisdale, M.J. (1997) Induction of muscle protein degradation by a tumour factor. *British Journal of Cancer*, 76(8), 1035–40.

Lorite, M.J., Smith, H.J., Arnold, J.A., Morris, A., Thompson, M.G., and Tisdale, M.J. (2001) Activation of ATP-ubiquitin-dependent proteolysis in skeletal muscle in vivo and murine myoblasts in vitro by a proteolysis-inducing factor (PIF) *British Journal of Cancer*, **85**, 297–302.

Lundholm, K., Gelin, J., and Hyltander, A. (1994) Anti-inflammatory treatment may prolong survival in undernourished patients with metastatic solid tumours. *Cancer Research*, **54**, 5602–6.

MacDonald, N., Alexander, H.R., and Bruera, E. (1995) Cachexia–anorexia–asthenia. *Journal of Pain and Symptom Management*, **10**, 151–5.

Magnusson, A.E., Nias, D.K.B., and White, P.D. (1996) Is perfectionism associated with fatigue? *Journal of Psychosomatic Research*, **41**, 377–83.

Majumdar, S., Lamothe, B., and Aggarwal, B.B. (2002) Thalidomide supresses NF-κB activation induced by TNF and H_2O_2, but not that activated by ceramide, lypopolysaccharides, or phorbol ester. *Journal of Immunology*, **168**, 2644–51.

Malik, U.R., Makower, D.F., and Wadler, S. (2001) Interferon-mediated fatigue. *Cancer*, **92**(6), 1664–8.

Maltoni, M., Nanni, O., Scarpi, E., Rossi, D., Serra, P., and Amadori, D. (2001) High-dose progestins for the treatment of cancer anorexia-cachexia syndrome: a systematic review of randomized clinical trials. *Annals of Oncology*, **12**, 289–300.

Mantovani G. (2002) Does megestrol acetate down-regulate interleukin-6 in patients? Supportive care in cancer **10**, 566–7.

Mantovani, G., Maccio, A., Esu, S., Lai, P., Santona, M.C., Massa, E. *et al.* (1997) Medroxyprogesterone acetate reduces the in vitro production of cytokines and serotonin involved in anorexia/cachexia and emesis by peripheral blood mononuclear cells of cancer patients. *European Journal of Cancer*, **33**, 602–7.

Mantovani, G., Maccio, A., Lai, P., Massa, E., Ghiani, M., and Santoria, M.C. (1998) Cytokine activity in cancer-related anorexia/cachexia: role of megestrol acetate and medroxyprogesterone acetate. *Seminars in Oncology*, **25**(Supplement 6), 45–52.

Mantovani, G., Maccio, A., Mura, L., Mudu, M.C., Mulas, C., Lusso, M.R. *et al.* (2000) Serum levels of leptin and proinflammatory cytokines in patients with advanced-stage cancer at different sites. *Journal of Molecular Medicine*, **78**, 554–61.

Mantovani, G., Maccio, A., Massa, E., and Madeddu C. (2001) Managing cancer-related anorexia/cachexia. *Drugs*, **61**(4), 499–514.

Masferrer, J.L., Leahy, K.M., and Koki, A.T. (2000) Antiangiogenic and antitumour activities of cyclooxigenase-2 inhibitors. *Cancer Research*, **60**, 1306–11.

May, P., Barber, A., D'Olimpio, J.T., Hourihane, A., and Abumrad, N.N. (2002) Reversal of cancer-related wasting using oral supplementation with a combination of [beta]-hydroxy-[beta]-methylbutyrate, arginine, and glutamine. *American Journal of Surgery*, **183**(4), 471–9.

McCarthy, H.D., Crowder, R.E., Dryden, S., and Williams G. (1994) Megestrol acetate stimulates food and water intake in the rat: effects on regional hypothalamic neuropeptide Y concentrations. *European Journal of Pharmacology*, **265**, 99–102.

Mendoza, T.R., Wang, X.S., Cleeland, C.S., *et al.* (1999) The rapid assessment of fatigue severity in cancer patients: use of the Brief Fatigue Inventory. *Cancer*, **85**, 1186–96.

Mitch, W.E. and Price, S.R. (2001) Transcription factors and muscle cachexia: is there a therapeutic target? [commentary]. *The Lancet*, **357**, 734–5.

Mock, V. (2001) Fatigue management. Evidence and guidelines for practice. *Cancer*, **92**, 1699–707.

Moertel, C.G., Schutt, A.J., Reitemeier, R.J., and Hahn, R.G. (1974) Corticosteroid therapy of preterminal gastrointestinal cancer. *Cancer*, **33**, 1607–9.

Morrow, G.R., Andrews, P.L.R., Hickok, J.T., Roscoe, J.A., and Matteson, S. (2002) Fatigue associated with cancer and its treatment. *Supportive Care in Cancer*, **10**, 389–98.

NCI (National Cancer Institute) (1999) Common toxicity criteria from the CTEP (Cancer Therapy Evaluation Program) http://ctep.cancer.gov/reporting/ctc.html

Needham, P.R., Daley, A.G., and Lennard, R.F. (1992) Steroids in advanced cancer: survey of current practice. *British Medical Journal*, **305**, 999–1000.

Nelson, K.A. and Walsh D. (2002) The cancer anorexia-cachexia syndrome: a survey of the prognostic inflammatory and nutritional index (PINI) in advanced disease. *Journal of Pain and Symptom Management*, **24**, 424–8.

Nelson, K.A. (2000) The cancer anorexia-cachexia syndrome. *Seminars in Oncology*, **27**, 64–8.

Newenschwander, H. and Bruera, E. (1996) Asthenia-cachexia. In: *Cachexia-Anorexia in Cancer Patients*, (ed. E. Bruera and I. Higginson). Oxford University Press, New York, pp. 57–75.

Neuenschwander, H. and Bruera, E. (1998) Pathophysiology of cancer asthenia. *Topics in Palliative Care*, **2**, 171–81.

Norcross, J.C., Guadagnoli, E., and Prochoska, J.O. (1984) Factor structure of the profile of mood states (POMS): two partial replications. *Journal of Clinical Psychology*, **40**(5), 1270–7.

Oster, M.H., Enders, S.H., Samuels, S.J., Cone, L.A., Hooston, T.M., Browder, H.P. *et al.* (1994) Megestrol acetate in patients with AIDS and cachexia. *Annals of Internal Medicine*, **121**(6), 400–8.

Peuckmann, Fisch, M., and Bruera, E. (2000) Potential novel uses of thalidomide. *Drugs*, **60**(2), 273–92.

Pinkney, J. and Williams, G. (2002) Ghrelin gets hungry [commentary]. *The Lancet*, **359**, 1360–1.

Piper, B.F., Dibble, S.L., Dodd, M.J., Weiss, M.C., Slaughter, R.E., and Paul, S.M. (1998) The revised Piper Fatigue Scale: psychometric evaluation in women with breast cancer. *Oncology Nursing Forum*, **25**, 677–84.

Quesada, J.R., Talpaz, M., Rios, A., Kurzor, C.K., and Gutterman, J.U. (1986) Clinical toxicity of interferons in cancer patients: a review. *Journal of Clinical Oncology*, **4**, 234–43.

Regelson, W., Butler, J.R., and Schulz J. (1976) Delta-9-tetrahydrocannabinol as an effective antidepressant and appetite stimulating agent in advanced cancer patients. In: *Pharmacology of Marihuana: a Monograph of the National Institute of Drug Abuse*. Raven Press, New York, pp. 763–76.

Rex, S., Kukuruzinska, M.A., and Istfan, N.W. (2002) Inhibition of DNA replication by fish oil-treated cytoplasm is counteracted by fish oil-treated nuclear extract. *American Journal of Cell Physiology*, **283**, C1365–C1375.

Richardson A. (1995) Fatigue in cancer patients: a review of the literature. *European Journal of Cancer Care*, **4**, 20–32.

Richardson, P., Hideshima, T., and Anderson K. (2002) Thalidomide: emerging role in cancer medicine. *Annual Review of Medicine*, **53**, 629–57.

Robustelli Della Cuna, G., Pellegrini, A., and Piazzi M. (1989) Effect of methylprednisolone sodium succinate on quality of life in preterminal cancer patients: a placebo-controlled, multicenter study. *European Journal of Cancer and Clinical Oncology*, **25**, 1817–21.

Roubenoff, R., Freeman, L.M., Smith, D.E., *et al.* (1997) Adjuvant arthritis as a model of inflammatory cachexia. *Arthritis and Rheumatism*, **40**, 534–9.

Rowland, K.M., Loprinzi, C.L., Shaw, E.G., Maksymiuk, A.W., Kuross, S.A., Jung, S.H. *et al.* (1996) Randomized double-blind placebo-controlled trial of cisplatin and etoposide plus megestrol acetate/placebo in extensive-stage small-cell lung cancer: a North Central Cancer Treatment Group Study. *Journal of Clinical Oncology*, **14**, 135–41.

Sauer, L.A., Dauchy, R.T., and Blask, D.E. (2000) Mechanism for the antitumour and anticachectic effects of n-3 fatty acids. *Cancer Research*, **60**, 5289–95.

Schwartz, S.A., Hernandez, A., and Evers, B.M. (1999) The role of NF-κB/IκB proteins in cancer: implications for novel treatment strategies. *Surgical Oncology*, **8**, 143–53.

Scott, H.R., McMillan, D.C., Watson, W.S., Milroy, R., and McArdle, C.S. (2001) Longitudinal study of resting energy expenditure, body cell mass and the inflammatory response in male patients with non-small cell lung cancer. *Lung Cancer*, **32**, 307–12.

Seligman, P.A., Fink, R., and Massey-Seligman, E.J. (1998) Approach to the seriously ill or terminal cancer patient who has a poor appetite. *Seminars in Oncology*, **25**(Supplement 6), 33–4.

Servaes, P., Verhagen, C.A.H.H.V.M., and Bleijenberg, G. (2002) Relations between fatigue, neuropsychological functioning, and physical activity after treatment for breast carcinoma. Daily self-report and objective behavior. *Cancer*, **95**, 2017–26.

Shureiqui, I., Chen, D., and Lee J. (2000) 15-LOX-1: a novel molecular target of nonsteroidal anti-inflammatory drug-induced apoptosis in colorectal cancer cells. *Journal of the National Cancer Institute*, **92**, 1136–42.

Simons, J.P., Aaronson, N.K., Vansteenkiste, J.F., ten Velde, G.P., Muller, M.J., Drenth, B.M. *et al.* (1996) Effects of medroxyprogesterone acetate on appetite, weight, and quality of life in advance-stage non-hormone-sensitive cancer: a placebo-controlled multicenter study. *Journal of Clinical Oncology*, **14**, 1077–84.

Sivesind, D. and Baile, W.F. (2001) The psychologic distress in patients with cancer. *Nursing Clinics of North America*, **36**, 809–25.

Smith, I.E. and de Boer, R.H. (2002) Paraneoplastic syndromes other than metabolic. In: *Oxford Textbook of Oncology*, (ed. R.L. Souhami, I. Tannock, P. Hohenberg, and J.-C. Horiot). Oxford University Press, New York, pp. 936–7.

Staal-van den Brekel, A., Dentener, M.A., Schols, A.M.W.J., Buurman, W.A., and Wouters, E.F.M. (1995) Increased resting energy expenditure and weight loss are related to a systemic inflammatory response in lung cancer patients. *Journal of Clinical Oncology*, **13**(10), 2600–5.

Stone, P., Richards, M., and Hardy J. (1998) Fatigue in patients with cancer. *European Journal of Cancer*, **34**, 1670–6.

Stone, P., Hardy, J., Huddart, R., Hern, R.A., and Richards M. (2000) Fatigue in patients with prostate cancer receiving hormone therapy. *European Journal of Cancer*, **36**, 1131–41.

Straisser, F. and Bruera, E.D. (2002) Update on anorexia and cachexia. *Hematology/Oncology Clinics of North America*, **16**(3), 579–88.

Strawford, A., Barbieri, T., Van Loan, M., Parks, E., Catlin, D., Barton, N. *et al.* (1999) Resistance exercise and supraphysiologic androgen therapy in eugonadal men with HIV-related weight loss. A randomized controlled trial. *Journal of the American Medical Association*, **281**, 1282–90.

Takabatake, N., Nakamura, H., Abe, S., Hino, T., Saito, H., Yuki, H. *et al.* (1999) Circulating leptin in patients with chronic obstructive pulmonary disease. *American Journal of Respiratory and Critical Care Medicine*, **159**, 1215–19.

Taylor, A.E., Olver, I.N., Sivanthan, T., Chi, M., and Purnell C. (1999) Observer error in grading performance status in cancer patients. *Supportive Care in Cancer*, **7**, 332–5.

Tchekmedyian, N.S., Tait, N., Moody, M., and Aisner J. (1987) High-dose megestrol acetate. *Journal of the American Medical Association*, **257**, 1195–8.

Thea, D.M., Porat, R., Nagimbi, K., *et al.* (1996) Plasma cytokines, cytokine antagonists and disease progression in African women infected with HIV-1. *Annals of Internal Medicine*, **124**, 757–62.

Tilignac, T., Temparis, S., Combaret, L.,Taillandier, D., Pouch, M.-N., Cervek, M. *et al.* (2002) Chemotherapy inhibits skeletal muscle ubiquitin-proteosome-dependent proteolysis. *Cancer Research*, **62**, 2771–7.

Tisdale, M.J. (1997) Cancer cachexia: metabolic alterations and clinical manifestations. *Nutrition*, **13**, 1–6.

Tisdale, M.J. (2000) Protein loss in cancer cachexia. *Science*, **289**, 2293–4.

Tisdale, M.J. (2002) Cachexia in cancer patients. *Nature Reviews Cancer*, **2**, 862–71.

Todorov, P.T., Field, W.N., and Tisdale, M.J. (1999) Role of a proteolysis-inducing factor (PIF) in cachexia induced by a human melanoma (G361) *British Journal of Cancer*, **80**(11), 1734–7.

Twycross, R. (1992) Corticosteroids in advanced cancer. If they are not working stop them. *British Medical Journal*, **305**(6860), 969–70.

Uefuji, K., Ichikura, T., and Mocizuki, H. (2000) Cyclooxygenase-2 expression is related to prostaglandin biosynthesis and angiogenesis in human gastric cancer. *Clinical Cancer Research*, **6**, 135–8.

Vainio, A. and Auvinen, A. (1996) Prevalence of symptoms among patients with advanced cancer: an international collaborative study. *Journal of Pain and Symptom Management*, **12**, 3–10.

Venner, P.M., Klotz, P.G., Klotz, L.H., Stewart, D.J., Davis, I.R., Orovan, W.L. *et al.* (1988) Megestrol acetate plus minidose diethylstilbestrol in the treatment of carcinoma of the prostate. *Seminars in Oncology*, **15**(2, Supplement 1), 62–7.

Verhelst, A.R., Maeyaert, J., Van Buyten, J.P., Opsomer, F., Adriaensen, H., Verlooy, J. *et al.* (2000) Endocrine consequences of long-term intrathecal administration of opioids. *Journal of Clinical Endocrinology and Metabolism*, **85**(6), 2215–22.

Vignano, A. and Bruera E. (1996) Enteral and parenteral nutrition in cancer patients. In: Cachexia-Anorexia in Cancer Patients (ed. I. Higginson and E. Bruera), Oxford University Press, Oxford, pp. 172–83.

Vigano A., Bruera, E., Jhangri, G.S., Newman, S.C., Fields, A.L., and Suarez-Almazor, M.E. (2000) Clinical survival predictors in patients with advanced cancer. *Archives of Internal Medicine*, **160**, 861–8.

Visser, M.R. and Smets, E.M. (1998) Fatigue, depression and quality of life in cancer patients: how are they related? *Supportive Care in Cancer*, **6**, 101–8.

von Haehling, S., Genth-Zotz, S., Anker, S.D., and Volk, H.D. (2002) Cachexia: a therapeutic approach beyond cytokine antagonism. *International Journal of Cardiology*, **85**, 173–83.

Walsh, D., Donnelly, S., and Ribicky L. (2000) The symptoms of advanced cancer: relationship to age, gender, and performance status in 1000 patients. *Supportive Care in Cancer*, **8**, 175–9.

Watanabe, S. and Bruera E. (1994) Corticosteroids as adjuvant analgesics. *Journal of Pain and Symptom Management*, **9**, 442–5.

Whitehouse, A.S., Smith, H.J., Drake, J.L., and Tisdale, M.J. (2001) Mechanism of attenuation of skeletal muscle protein catabolism in cancer cachexia by eicosapentaenoic acid. *Cancer Research*, **61**, 3604–9.

Wigmore, S.J., Falconer, J.S., and Plester, C.E. (1995) Ibuprofen reduces energy expenditure and acute-phase protein production compared with placebo in pancreatic cancer patients. *British Journal of Cancer*, **72**, 185–8.

Wigmore, S.J., Ross, J.A., Falconer, S.F., Plester, C.E., Tisdale, M.J., Carter, D.C. *et al.* (1996) The effect of polyunsaturated fatty acids on the progress of cachexia in patients with pancreatic cancer. *Nutrition*, **12**, S27–S30.

Witte, K.K.A. and Clark, A.L. (2002) Nutritional abnormalities contributing to cachexia in chronic illness. *International Journal of Cardiology*, **85**, 23–31.

Wray, C.J., Mammen, J.M.V, and Hasselgren, P.-O. (2002) Catabolic response to stress and potential benefits of nutrition support. *Nutrition*, **18**, 971–7.

Young, A., Topham, C., Moore, J., Turner, J., Wardle, J., Downes, M. *et al.* (1999) A patient
preference study comparing raltitraxed ('Tomudex') and bolus or infusional 5-fluorouracil
regimens in advanced colorectal cancer: influence of side-effects and administration attributes.
European Journal of Cancer Care, **8**, 154–61.

Zhang, B., Berger, J., Hu, E., Szalkowski, D., White-Carrington, S., Spiegelman, B. *et al.*
(1996) Negative regulation of peroxisome proliferated activated receptor γ gene expression
contributes to the antiaipogenic effects to tumour necrosis factor α. *Molecular
Endocrinology*, **10**, 1457–66.

Part 2

The experience of fatigue

Chapter 5

Fatigue in lay conceptualizations of health and illness

Meinir Krishnasamy and David Field

Introduction

In Chapters 1 and 2 the incidence and prevalence of fatigue as a facet of the cancer experience has been clearly stated. Its complex, multidimensional nature has been explored and challenges inherent to its management will be alluded to in Chapter 12. Nevertheless, despite an acknowledgement of its multifaceted nature and its propensity to impact on numerous domains of quality of life (see Chapters 6 and 13) little has been written of lay conceptualizations of fatigue within the context of cancer and cancer treatment. Meaning attributed to a symptom or illness has been shown to be more likely to explain perceptions of distress than disease-oriented or illness-related factors (Woodgate and McClement 1998). Therefore, if advances in healthcare provision are to be successful in minimizing the suffering and distress caused by fatigue, an understanding of how people communicate its impact to family, friends, and healthcare professionals, and what meanings they ascribe to it, appear to be centrally important (Hinds *et al.* 1992).

This chapter is structured around four key areas important to an appreciation of fatigue in lay conceptualizations of health and illness. It begins with a consideration of the potential for improvements in healthcare utilization and provision through an appreciation of lay perceptions. A brief overview of fatigue as a facet of health and well-being follows, and then factors likely to shape lay conceptualizations of the experience of cancer-related fatigue are discussed. Finally a tentative model of the complex and dynamic nature of lay constructions of this phenomenon is presented. The interactions outlined in the proposed model shed light on how such an approach may help practitioners discover the meaning a symptom may hold for an individual, and how that depth of understanding may, in turn, be translated into appropriate practice opportunities. Recommendations for future research and practice development draw the chapter to a close.

Throughout, the terms symptom and problem are used interchangeably to refer to the phenomenon of cancer-related fatigue, and are used to convey an unpleasant symptom, inaccessible to others, which leads to a departure from normal functioning

(Lobchuk 1999). Although the term 'fatigue' is acknowledged as being problematic when used with people with cancer and their family members (Krishnasamy 2000), it is employed here for the sake of brevity.

Lay perceptions and the potential for contextually relevant healthcare

An appreciation of the potential of 'lay conceptions of health and illness' to inform clinical practice is dependent on an understanding of what is meant by that term. Lay perceptions of states of ill-health are dynamic and multifaceted constructions. They are shaped and influenced by physiological, psychological, and spiritual domains, as well as by social status and societal norms relating to appropriate and legitimized health behaviour. They potentially provide a valuable source of information to inform clinical decision-making, providing clinicians with insights into the ways in which disease impact, treatment, and self-care requirements will (or will not be) be assimilated into an individual's life and that of his or her social network. An awareness of what an illness means to a person and the ways in which that individual's life will be affected by it (and subsequent treatments) may provide essential information to professionals. This involves considering what it means to be ill or well, the influence of cultural or religious beliefs, moral or ethical attributes that may shape a person's attitudes to suffering, illness and sick-role behaviour, and ultimately the legitimacy they confer on their state of ill-health or perceive others to confer on it. In short, an appreciation of lay conceptions of health and illness may make the difference between acceptance or rejection of professional recommendations for recovery or sustenance of optimal quality of life (health behaviours), by enabling the construction and provision of relevant, acceptable healthcare interventions which are received by individuals as pertinent to their values and belief systems. As such, they have the potential to directly influence health outcomes and, therefore, constitute a long underexamined and undervalued aspect of professional healthcare decision-making.

The ways in which people construct their views of and talk about their health or illness are much more than mere disclosures of physiological aberration. People are known to draw on a range of ideas and unique definitions about health to make sense of the physiological as well as the emotional impact of illness. They reflect instead peoples' beliefs about the nature of health and illness, the legitimacy of a given symptom or problem and, consequently, a person's worthiness to receive help (Radley and Billig 1996).

Given this complex dynamic, the potential for miscommunication regarding the nature, severity, and impact of an illness between professional carers and the lay public is both considerable and commonplace. Evidence indicates (Goffman 1963; Field *et al.* 1993) that such miscommunication leads to:

- ◆ poor cooperation between professionals and the public,
- ◆ apportioning of blame,

- labelling,
- stigmatization,
- lack of compliance with treatment,
- over- or underuse of services,
- failure of generally successful interventions at an individual level'
- rejection of health education and health promotion messages.

How do lay conceptions differ from professional constructions of illness? Traditionally a biomedical model of disease has been resistant to the view that illness is both personal and social, and that to be ill is not simply to be in a physically altered state, but also to be in a socially altered condition (Field *et al.* 1993). It has largely excluded people's accounts of their illness experience, and been unheeding of the potential of the complex constructions of these accounts for successful intervention and individuals' feelings of well-being (Baker *et al.* 1996). Illness or disease has predominantly been understood as a physiological or biological abnormality, complicated by inconsistencies and unpredictable responses to standardized interventions. As stated above, an appreciation of lay perspectives of health and illness has the potential to improve compliance with, and efficient uptake of, services, clinical effectiveness, and health promotion. Within the context of serious illness, such as a diagnosis of cancer, it has the fundamentally important potential to make individuals feel heard, valued, and cared for, irrespective of the stage of disease and outcome of their illness (Lupton 1996; Murphy 1990).

Fatigue, health, and well-being

> Air, rest and sleep, pleasure and food
> If taken in moderation, keep man in good health

> (Loux and Richard in Pierret 1995, p. 186)

Limited energy reserves and inability to undertake valued daily activities have been identified as key manifestations of cancer-related fatigue and ill-health (see Chapters 1 and 6). Herzlich's (1973) influential study of social representations of illness and health was one of the earliest studies to demonstrate the extent to which individuals associate the absence of fatigue as being synonymous with well-being. Energy, vitality, and strength were identified not only as central facets of well-being but were also depicted as fundamental to sustaining health. Furthermore, being in receipt of adequate energy reserves to be able to take and sustain an active role in society conferred on one not only the vestiges of a normal, healthy individual but also implied a moral attribution, where health is good and ill-health is bad. William's study of older Aberdonians (Williams 1990) also emphasized the moral dimension of lay views of health, where sustaining functional capacity and vitality were inextricably linked with preventing ill-health and sustaining independence (Blaxter 1990; Williams 1990). 'Abiding vitality' was identified as a core theme to emerge from a synthesis of 35 qualitative studies (involving 787 sick and healthy informants) examining meanings inherent in health and disease (Jensen and Allen 1993). Informants reported that feeling energized and vigorous were central to feeling healthy, but that illness brought with it feelings of being 'drained', 'run down', or no longer having energy or time to face responsibilities or relationships. This vitality, referred to by Herzlich (1973) as 'the capital asset' of the healthy, has latterly been reinforced by Blaxter (1990), who found that younger people had vitalistic and athletic views of health in which keeping fit was related to a greater sense of personal responsibility for health. Older people who took part in Blaxter's survey were found to stress the importance of functional capacity and sustaining independence as the basis of good health. Similar beliefs were reported by Pierret (1995), based on a study of over 100 people who took part in interviews and completed self-report questionnaires, aimed at discovering their behavioural patterns and beliefs regarding health and healthcare. One out of two people in the study talked of fatigue as a central construct of health where being healthy meant being able to work, while others differentiated between 'healthy fatigue', that is physical tiredness associated with manual work, and 'nervous fatigue' which was associated with office and factory work:

> for me, health is everything, if you haven't got your health, you can't work......for example, if you study, when your health is bad you don't have the energy to study. For manual work it's the same, you need energy.

> (Pierret 1995, p. 201)

Analysis of Blaxter's (1990) survey data provided by 9000 adults living in the UK between 1984 and 1985 clearly highlights people's beliefs about the importance of adequate energy levels and the ability to perform valued roles and pursuits as facets of well-being. Nine general categories of 'health' were elicited from the data (Blaxter 1990, pp. 20–30), including:

◆ Health as not ill.
◆ Health as absence of disease/health despite disease.
◆ Health as a reserve.
◆ Health as behaviour/healthy lifestyle.
◆ Health as physical fitness.
◆ Health as energy, vitality.
◆ Health as social relationships.
◆ Health as function.
◆ Health as psychosocial well-being.

In Table 5.1 examples are provided to illustrate the extent to which absence of fatigue was linked to feelings of well-being or health by the survey respondents. Alongside the survey examples, quotes are presented from cancer-specific literature to show how the

Table 5.1 Fatigue as a major quality of life issue

Blaxter (1990)	Cancer fatigue literature
Health as not ill: 'Healthy is when you don't feel tired and short of breath' (p. 21)	Health as not ill: 'Some days you wake up feeling fine, and others, just terrible.' (Krishnasamy 1997, p. 76)
Health as physical illness: 'Being healthy is when my skin is good and my hair isn't greasy and I can do all the things I want without feeling tired' (p. 25)	Health as physical illness: 'All I do is rest and sleep. That's it. That's a typical day. I just don't have any energy.' (Hilfinger Messias et al. 2000, p.46) 'At this point of treatment, quality of life to me has very little meaning. Coping with the physical effect consumes all train of thought to function and accomplish even the simplest task' (Ferrell et al. 1996, p. 1543)
Health as energy: 'Health is when I feel I can do anything.... Nothing stops you in your tracks' (p. 25)	Health as energy: 'My level of energy affects my quality of life. I'm generally energetic so anything that affects my energy levels affects my life.' (Ferrell et al. 1996, p. 1543) 'I want to take my loved one dancing and can't do it, and that bothers me. We try to plan at least one day a weekend to do something not physically straining' (Holley 2000, p. 92)
Health as psychosocial well-being: 'Energetic, outgoing. I can cope with more pressure ... whereas if I'm less healthy, tired ...' (p. 29)	Health as psychosocial well-being: 'some days I think I must be going mad ... I think I could understand someone saying they could commit suicide ... but then you have to get on with it ... find the energy to' (Krishnasamy 1997, p. 60) 'It's this anxiety, all this worry and expectation, you keep waiting for the lab test results, that makes you tired.' (Magnusson et al. 1999, p. 228) 'Feelings like uncertainty, dread, powerlessness, loss of control, possible hopelessness, disease puts you into this frame of mind and gives you those feelings. The fatigue will highlight these feelings.' (Holley 2000, p. 92)

broad concepts of health, presented by Blaxter (1990), have an affinity with the way in which people with cancer and their family members have talked about the impact of fatigue on their lives (Ferrell *et al.* 1996; Hilfinger-Messias *et al.* 1997; Glaus 1998; Jacobsen *et al.* 1999; Magnusson *et al.* 1999; Holley 2000).

These quotes begin to illustrate the extent to which people with cancer associate fatigue with deteriorating health and diminishing energy reserves, whilst also highlighting the central role of 'fatigue' as an influential component shaping an individual's conception of his or her own state of health. Nevertheless what lies behind the words as they communicate the impact of this complex problem on their lives, and on that of their family and friends, has received little empirical study. It is difficult, therefore, to appreciate how lay constructions of fatigue are shaped as a result of different contextual cues depending on diagnosis, perception of well-being, and quality of life. Further work is needed in this area if contextually relevant supportive care strategies are to be developed and evaluated.

The experience and course of an illness can be understood as a product of both the illness itself and the social responses to it (Karp 1994), and individuals are known to construct their state of health as part of their ongoing identity in relation to others (Radley and Billig 1996). An acute awareness on the part of people of the value placed on vigour, productivity, and usefulness within modern Western society (Libbus 1996; Richman *et al.* 2000) may therefore further add to the plethora of values, beliefs, and attitudes that shape an individual's conceptualization of cancer-related fatigue. As such, fatigue and its impact on ability to function and contribute to society may present profound threats to identity:

> I've only known him for about two months and already I can see a big change in him ... he's dying and they all know it, he looks exhausted all the time and moves about very little now. When I first went in he could at least still get about a bit but he's close to death now no question and they can talk about him in those terms which I think has helped them to put things in perspective.
>
> (Krishnasamy 1997, p. 7)

> I know cancer patients are chronically ill or terminally ill people but I feel useless because I can't do anything any more. I can't work properly.
>
> (Mathieson and Stam 1995, p. 294)

What is evident both from data reported by 'well' populations and individuals with cancer is that fatigue is associated with a deviation from the norm, where normality implies a state of health, and assumes moral overtones associated with wellness and goodness (Ferrell *et al* 1996; Tishelman and Sachs 1998). In talking about their fatigue, individuals are potentially making explicit claims about themselves as 'worthy' or 'fit' participants within a cultural group (Radley and Billig 1996). Acknowledging that one is restricted by a symptom shrouded by potentially negative stereotypical images (e.g. malingerer, 'yuppie flu', being of weak or insufficient stamina or character, someone who gives up or doesn't try hard enough) may be particularly difficult and painful, even within the context of a diagnosis of cancer. Little is known of these issues for individuals with serious illness, and as such they constitute an important area for future research:

> ... live till you die they say, that's what all this palliative care's about ... when they were selling this hospice to me she [the nurse] said well they can help you to keep well to do the things that you really want to ... God that would be good, instead, they can't do much and I feel more and more like everyone has to do everything for me, and that bothers me, I've never been like that, always done for myself never believed that you should let other people do things you can do yourself, plenty of that kind about, never thought I'd be one ... yes I know you're going to say it's not the same, but that's it for me, that's what it's like somedays.
>
> (Krishnasamy 1997, p. 34)

Fatigue, perhaps more so than any other cancer problem, captures the interface between body, self, and identity.

Constructing the fatigue experience

'Fatigue' is a nebulous concept. As a word, it seems to be unhelpful when used to ask people, whether well or ill, to describe it. People instead tend to complain of tiredness, lack of energy, general lethargy, weakness, depression, anxiety, exhaustion, inability to sustain exertion, impaired mobility, motivation and concentration span, sleepiness, drowsiness, heaviness, apathy, an inability to carry on, as well as many other sensations (Hilfinger Messias *et al.* 1997; Ream and Richardson 1997; Glaus 1998; van der Linden *et al.* 1999). Nevertheless the majority of empirical work undertaken in this area continues to use the term both for brevity and convenience, despite general agreement that as a term 'fatigue' is inadequate to capture the essence of the phenomenon (Lenz *et al.* 1997). For individuals with cancer it fails to capture or convey the magnitude of its impact on their lives (Krishnasamy 2000). Part of the difficulty in capturing and articulating constructs such as cancer-related fatigue lies with their resistance to being captured in words. As such they remain invisible to others, including healthcare professionals, who consequently overlook them as potential areas for research and therapy. Therefore, enabling people to articulate their views or concerns about cancer-related fatigue in a language pertinent to them is likely to be important both as a therapeutic endeavour and as a means of contributing to practice development (Giardino and Wolf 1993).

The process of shifting from an individual's language of ill-health (often internalized), where problems such as cancer-related fatigue are 'felt' rather than objectively manifested (for example vomiting), to a professional language amenable to the development and evaluation of care strategies, is a complex undertaking liable to misinterpretation and individual bias (Bailey 1999). The danger is that the process of translating internalized accounts via in-depth exploration or clinical assessment of a particular phenomenon such as cancer-related fatigue merely results in a professional terminology that matches patients' descriptions of the phenomenon (Wenger 1993). In other words the undertaking becomes little more than an exercise in exchanging one set of descriptors for another, without the corresponding and fundamental shift in research or therapeutic ethos, where a patient's construction shapes the essence of the research or therapeutic approach taken. The success of such a 'translational' endeavour (Wenger 1993) rests with an ability to listen and ask questions that facilitate in-depth description of an individual's experience in a language that is meaningful to them. However, this is not to suggest that the process of communicating beliefs about fatigue within the context of ill-health should or can occur without recourse to biomedical language. Indeed, Bury (1982) argues that medical parlance provides certainty and objectivity during period of uncertainty (Bury 1982, p. 179), and exposure to health jargon and a disease semantic through multimedia sources has meant that for many lay people 'telling it as it is', within the context of symptomatology, involves an amalgam of subjective, holistic, and biomedical concepts. The result is a portrayal of aspects of ill-health or well-being which may at the same time be complex, subtle, superficial, and sophisticated (Blaxter 1990). Evidence presented below indicates that this is certainly the case for individuals living with, and witnessing the impact of, cancer-related fatigue.

Fatigue, perhaps even more so than pain, appears to belong to a private domain (Radley and Billig 1996), in so much as those of us standing on the periphery are reliant on the individual experiencing it to convey its impact to us. Only once it has been communicated does it become a public construction (Radley and Billig 1996), a facet of ill-health potentially amenable to intervention. And yet the process of communicating its impact does not appear to be an easy undertaking. Evidence from studies undertaken with people with cancer and their lay carers indicate that constructing the experience in such a way as to make it accessible to others appears to be easier through physical or functional descriptors, for example heaviness, weakness, no energy to walk, need to sit down, and can't do the things I used to be able to (Krishnasamy 1997; Richardson and Ream 1997; Glaus 1998). Capturing and conveying the emotional or psychosocial impact appears to be more difficult:

> It's hard to tell you or tell really anyone what it's like because it's something that you feel all over, inside and outside … it's like a pulling down inside when you have to fight even to stand up. Some days it's hard to imagine I will ever be able to do anything again and I can feel myself in danger of just giving up, that's what it's like, but I don't know if that makes sense to you or anyone but me … [interviewer:] 'you talked about it being inside and out …' yes well, no I'm not sure I can but outside it's um like a feeling on your skin, like your skin is really sensitive to any touch, not all the time just when it's really bad … that probably sounds mad but on the outside it's more my body than my mind or how I feel mood wise'.

> (Krishnasamy 1997, p. 20)

Part of the reason for the difficulty in conveying the emotional aspects of the symptom may be that in attempting to do so individuals try to talk about those aspects of life which still really matter within the context of their redefined lives (Mathieson and Stam 1995). It may be that lay constructions concentrating on the physical retain a focus on the situation (I have cancer, am receiving treatment, therefore am tired), whereas conceptualizations focusing on emotional dimensions are focused on the self (Karp 1994):

> I remember going home and I just lay down in bed. I saw my baby but couldn't appreciate him. Sometimes, it was like I couldn't be around him. I couldn't be near him because he would cry. He would irritate me. All I wanted to do was sleep.
>
> (Ferrell *et al.* 1996, p. 1545)

Lay perceptions of cancer-related fatigue: an emergent model

The model outlined in Fig. 5.1 attempts to capture ways in which people assimilate cues that shape their dynamic experience of cancer-related fatigue as it changes with time and alternating cues. It endeavours to indicate how people's varied constructions in turn impact on their well-being and ability to respond to the challenge of living with cancer and its treatment. Furthermore it attempts to respond to and support Wenger's (1993) assertion that nursing's care agenda should be broader than an illness episode *per se*, taking account of an individual's day-to-day life concerns and associated cultural constructions, rather than limited to biomedically defined illness boundaries. Wenger suggests that research and practice directed at developing culturally sensitive care reflect the following guidelines (Wenger 1993, p. 27):

- That those experiencing a symptom or problem are most knowledgeable about it and are most appropriate to teach the researcher or practitioner (who takes on the role of learner) about the symptom experience.
- That words and phrases are recognized as 'culture bearers', and that it is important therefore not to assume that words contain similar meanings across cultures (e.g. professional, organizational, or people-oriented cultures).
- That no value judgements are made by a researcher or clinician during the process of listening to and learning about an individual's account of his/her symptom experience.
- That the researcher/practitioners' understanding of the symptom as experienced is fed back to the individual for confirmation or reflection.
- That an amalgam of research/clinical and lay constructions of the problem being explored are constructed and agreed amongst all involved so that culturally coherent care strategies can be developed.

As stated at the outset of the chapter, the interactions outlined in the proposed model begin to indicate how such an approach may help practitioners discover the 'real' meaning a symptom may hold for an individual. This appreciation, in turn, provides an opportunity for developments in client-centred supportive care strategies (see Box 5.1). For example, data from a case study undertaken by Krishnasamy (1997)

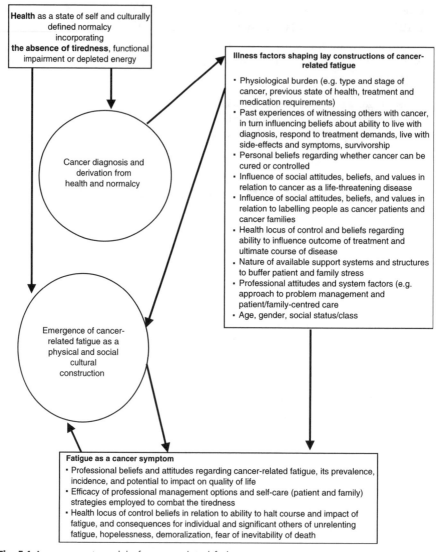

Fig. 5.1 An emergent model of cancer-related fatigue.

indicated that perceptions of severity of fatigue were not necessarily associated with perceptions of distress. That is, for some of the participants, distress associated with cancer-related fatigue may have been scored as being high but its severity was rated as low, or vice versa. Teel *et al.* (1997) argue that the naming of a symptom as severe may not be sufficient to enable the symptom experience to be comprehended, and that reports of severity or frequency should be understood merely as aspects of the experience in its totality (Rhodes and Watson 1987).

Box 5.1 Future areas for research

Recommendations for research and practice:

◆ Establishing mutual understanding between professionals, patients, and the lay public is a basic element in effective healthcare and as such should be integrated into future practice development research into cancer-related fatigue.

◆ The development of psychometrically sound clinical assessment tools and research measures can only be achieved when conceptual clarity of concepts being assessed, measured, and evaluated is established (Ream and Richardson 1996; Visser and Smets 1998; Krishnasamy 2000).

◆ The development of relevant patient and lay carer self-help information is reliant on an amalgam of patient (emic) and professional (etic) care knowledge (Wenger 1993).

◆ Given the complex nature of cancer-related fatigue, attempts at understanding its physiological and psychosocial domains via lay constructions may prove to be a fruitful way of diversifying the search for associated correlates.

◆ Shared meaning increases understanding and the potential for ethical, humanistic care and research (Hinds *et al.* 1992; Reason 1996). Cancer-related fatigue belongs to the world of those attempting to live with, and make sense of, a life-threatening illness. To restrict future practice development initiatives to predominantly professionally constructed knowledge and intuition is to exclude those with most to contribute and benefit.

What may be behind the apparent dichotomy between reports of fatigue severity and resultant distress may in part be understood in context of the information provided in Chapter 1. There, Hotopf reminds us that fatigue in the general population is more common in women than men (although this is not unequivocally supported in studies of patients reporting cancer-related fatigue), becomes increasingly prevalent in adolescence and early adulthood, and then tends to decline with advancing age. The picture in relation to age and prevalence or severity of cancer-related fatigue is not clear (see Chapter 1). Social circumstances have also been shown to play a part in an individual's construction of illness. People from lower social classes are more likely to rate their health as poor (Blaxter 1990), while an inverse relationship has been demonstrated between fatigue and social class (Meltzer *et al.* 1995). In Fig. 5.1 the impact of age, gender, and social class are included as influences that may account, in part, for the complex interactions between perception of fatigue severity and distress as described in the literature. Age, gender, or social class may bring essentially important values to bear on lay conception of fatigue, where women may report the distress associated with it more freely than men, or where people with fewer social resources may experience it more acutely than those who are financially well-supported.

References

Bailey, C. (1999) Derrida, de Man, Habermas: implications for qualitative analysis of interviews in cancer nursing research. A methodological study. Unpublished Master's Dissertation. Institute of Cancer Research, University of London.

Baker, P., Yoels, W., and Clair, J. (1996) Emotional expression during medical encounters: social disease and the medical gaze. In: *Health and the Sociology of Emotions* (ed. V. James and J. Gabe). Blackwell Publishers, Oxford, pp. 173–200.

Blaxter, M. (1990) *Health and Lifestyles*. Routledge, London.

Bury, M. (1982) Chronic illness as a biological disruption. *Sociology of Health and Illness*, 4(2), 167–82.

Ferrell, B., Grant, M., Dean, G., Funk, B., and Ly, J. (1996) 'Bone tired': the experience of fatigue and its impact on quality of life. *Oncology Nursing Forum*, 23(10), 1539–47.

Field, D., Minkler, M., Falk, R.F., and Leino, E.V. (1993).The influence of health on family contacts and family feelings in advanced old age: a longitudinal study. *Journal of Gerontology*, 48(1), 18–28.

Giardino, E. and Wolf, Z. (1993) Symptoms: evidence and experience. *Holistic Nurse Practitioner*, 7(2), 1–12.

Glaus, A. (1998) Fatigue in patients with cancer. Analysis and assessment. *Recent Results in Cancer Research*, 145, i–ix, 1–172.

Goffman, E. (1963) *Stigma. Notes on the Management of Spoiled Identity*. Simon and Schuster, New York.

Helman, C.G. (1994) *Culture, Health and Illness*, 3rd edn. Butterworth-Heinemann, Oxford, pp. 179–93.

Herzlich, C. (1973) Modern medicine and the quest for meaning. illness as a social signifier. In: *The Meaning of Illness. Anthropology, History and Sociology*, (ed. M. Auge and C. Herzlich). Harwood Academic Publishers, Luxembourg, pp. 151–73.

Hilfinger Messias, D.K., Yeager, A., Dibble, S., and Dodd, M. (1997) Patients' perspectives of fatigue while undergoing chemotherapy. *Oncology Nursing Forum*, 24(1), 43–8.

Hinds, P., Chaves, D., and Cypess, S. (1992) Context as a source of meaning and understanding. *Qualitative Health Research*, 2(1), 61–74.

Holley, S. (2000) Cancer-related fatigue. Suffering a different fatigue. *Cancer Practice*, 8(2), 87–95.

Jacobsen, P., Hann, D., Azzarello L., Horton, J., Balducci, L., and Lyman, G. (1999) Fatigue in women receiving adjuvant chemotherapy for breast cancer: characteristics, course, and correlates. *Journal of Pain and Symptom Management*, 18(4), 233–42.

Jensen, L. and Allen, M. (1993) Wellness: the dialectic of illness. *Image Journal of Nursing Scholarly Inquiry*, 25(3):220–4.

Karp, D. (1994) Living with depression: illness and identity turning points. *Qualitative Health Research*, 4(1), 6–30.

Krishnasamy, M. (1997) *An exploration of the Nature and Impact of fatigue in Patients with Advanced Cancer: a Case Study*. London: Macmillan Practice Development Unit, Centre for Cancer and Palliative Care Studies, Institute of Cancer Research.

Krishansamy, M. (2000) Fatigue in advanced cancer. Meaning before measurement? *International Journal of Nursing Studies*, 37(5), 401–14.

Lenz, E.R., Pugh, L.C., Milligan, R.A., Gift, A., and Suppe, F. (1997) The middle-range theory of unpleasant symptoms: an update. *Advances in Nursing Science*, **19**(3), 14–27.

Libbus, M. (1996) Women's beliefs regarding persistent fatigue. *Issues in Mental Health Nursing*, **17**(6), 589–600.

Lobchuk, M.M. (1999) Symptoms as meaningful 'family culture' symbols in palliative care. *Journal of Palliative Care*, **15**(4), 24–31.

Lupton, D. (1996) Your life in their hands: trust in the medical encounter. In: *Health and the Sociology of Emotions*, (ed. V. James and J. Gabe). Blackwell Publishers, Oxford, 157–72.

Magnusson, K., Moller, A., Ekman, T., and Wallgren, A. (1999), A qualitative study to explore the experience of fatigue in cancer patients. *European Journal of Cancer Care*, **8**, 224–32.

Mathieson, C. and Stam, H.J. (1995) Renegotiating identity: cancer narratives. *Sociology of Health and Illness*, **17**(3), 283–306.

Meltzer, H., Gill, B., and Petticrew, M. (1995) The prevalence of psychiatric morbidity among adults aged 16–64, living in private households, in Great Britain. *OPCS Surveys of Psychiatric Morbidity in Great Britain*, Bulletin 1. Office of National Statistics, London.

Murphy, R. (1990) *The Body Silent*. WW Norton, London.

Pierret, J. (1995) The social meanings of health: Paris, the Essonne, the Herault. In: *The Meanings of Illness. Anthropology, History and Sociology*, (ed. M. Auge and C. Herzlich). Harwood Academic Publishers, Luxembourg. pp. 175–206.

Radley, A. and Billig, M. (1996) Accounts of health and illness: dilemmas and representations. *Sociology of Health and Illness*, **18**(2), 220–40.

Reason, P. (1996) Reflections on the purposes of human inquiry. *Qualitative Inquiry*, **2**(1), 15–28.

Ream, E. and Richardson, A. (1997) Fatigue in patients with cancer and chronic obstructive airways disease: a phenomenological enquiry. *International Journal of Nursing Studies*, **34**(1), 44–53.

Rhodes, V. and Watson, P. (1987) Symptom distress: the concept past and present. *Seminars in Oncology Nursing*, **3**(4), 242–7.

Richardson, A. and Ream, E. (1997) Self-care behaviours initiated by chemotherapy patients in response to fatigue. *International Journal of Nursing Studies*, **34**, 35–43.

Richman, J., Jason, L., Taylor, R., and Jahn, S. (2000) Feminist perspectives on the social construction of chronic fatigue syndrome. *Health Care Women International*, **21**(3), 173–85.

Teel, C., Meek, P., McNamara, A., and Watson L. (1997) Perspectives unifying symptom interpretation. *Image Journal of Nursing Scholarship*, **29**(2), 175–81.

Tishelman, C. and Sachs, L. (1998) The diagnostic process and the boundaries of normality. *Qualitative Health Research*, **3**(1), 48–60.

van der Linden, G., Chalder, T., Hickie, I., Hoschera, A., Sham, P., and Wessely, S. (1999) Fatigue and psychiatric disorder: different or the same' *Psychological Medicine*, **29**(4), 863–8.

Visser, M.R.M. and Smets, E.M. (1998) Fatigue, depression and quality of life in cancer patients: how are they related? *Supportive Care in Cancer*, **6**(2), 101–8

Wenger, A.F. (1993) Cultural meaning of symptoms. *Holistic Nurse Practitioner*, **7**(2), 22–35.

Williams, R. (1990) *A Protestant Legacy: Attitudes to Death and Illness Among Older Aberdonians*. Oxford: Clarendon Press.

Woodgate, R. and McClement, S. (1998) Symptom distress in children with cancer: the need to adopt a meaning-centred approach. *Journal of Paediatric Oncology Nursing*, **15**(1), 3–12.

Chapter 6

The experience of cancer-related fatigue

Jo Armes

Introduction

Fatigue is a common complaint, experienced both in health and in illness, as indicated by Hotopf (see Chapter 1) and Krishnasamy and Field (see Chapter 5). Among cancer patients it has been identified as one of the most common symptoms experienced (Nail 2002), and over the last 15 years there has been a growing recognition of its deleterious impact on those affected. Fatigue, however, is a vague and elusive symptom that has defied precise definition and conceptualization, thus hindering the development of theoretical frameworks to guide its assessment, measurement, and management (Wu and McSweeney 2001) (see Chapter 9). This has led Lewis and Wessely (1992, p. 92) to 'repeat an earlier plea for more precise information on the phenomenology of fatigue'. That is, an appreciation of how it is experienced by individuals within the context of their day to day lives, and what the implications may be of its impact on their physical, mental, emotional, spiritual, and social selves. By asking questions such as:

(1) how is fatigue experienced and interpreted within the context of a life-threatening illness?

(2) in what way does cancer-related fatigue (CRF) contribute to the emotional distress associated with cancer and its treatment?

(3) how is the experience of CRF articulated?

the way in which cancer-related fatigue (CRF) contributes to an individual's suffering may be better understood. Consequently healthcare professionals may be able to use these insights to develop and target meaningful intervention strategies to help patients and family members take on and sustain engagement in self-care strategies that ultimately contribute to emotional well-being. This may be particularly important in the context of a cancer diagnosis that, in and of itself, has the potential to cause considerable distress and suffering.

This chapter draws on qualitative studies conducted to explore how those experiencing CRF describe it, and considers the potential of CRF to contribute to an individual's suffering. Throughout this chapter the term suffering is used to denote the experience of a whole person to a real or perceived threat, and the meaning(s) that they attribute to it (Kahn and Steeves 1986). Ten studies that met predefined inclusion criteria (namely using a qualitative methodology and whose focus was CRF) were retrieved and reviewed. In Table 6.1 the setting, aims, methods, and findings of each are presented.

A number of common themes emerged from the papers reviewed. These included:

* the nature of fatigue
* the physical effects of fatigue
* the cognitive effects of fatigue
* the social effects of fatigue
* the emotional effects of fatigue
* the effect of fatigue on 'self'
* coping with fatigue.

A review of the key themes indicated that much of the nature of the sensations experienced by people and the dimensions of their lives affected by CRF have previously been identified. However, whilst it is generally acknowledged that CRF is not seen as being a discrete entity (Armes 1995; Glaus *et al.* 1996; Krishnasamy 1996; Pearce and Richardson 1996; Messias *et al.* 1997; Ream and Richardson 1997) the domains it affects seem to have been treated as such. For example, most studies state that participants described how fatigue affected them physically, mentally, socially, and emotionally. But little attempt has been made to explore the relationships between these dimensions. Instead they tend to be presented as isolated components of individuals' experiences, rather than as dynamic parts of an interactive whole. This, in part, may be explained by a tendency of authors of these studies to simply describe peoples' experiences of CRF rather applying rigorous analytic processes of interpretation, which result in 'interpretive explanations' of how the phenomena connect and interact (Turner 1980). This may be an artefact of the difficulties of presenting qualitative studies in peer-reviewed journals, where the ability to provide enough data with which to indicate the level of interpretation is hampered by word limits. Nevertheless this presents qualitative researchers with an important challenge. If exploratory studies are to promote a greater understanding, not only of what cancer-related fatigue is and how it affects people, but also of what it means to them and why they find it so problematic, authors must find a way of presenting the necessary detail in accessible and credible ways.

This chapter attempts to evaluate the findings of the studies retrieved within a framework drawing on sociological literature around chronic illness, embodiment, and suffering. The potential of physical, mental, and social effects of fatigue to create feelings of loss of self and to cause suffering will be discussed. The centrality of these two meta-themes in shaping and being shaped by an individual's experience of CRF will be considered. Fatigue, however, is not the only factor that can cause a sense of loss

Table 6.1 Overview of the reviewed studies

Study and setting	Sample, age, gender, and diagnosis	Aim	Methodology	Findings	Comments
Armes (1995): UK hospice day unit.	Purposive sample of 10 patients Mean age = 58.4. Male = 2, female = 8. Diagnoses, mixed: breast = 4, colorectal = 2, other = 4	To describe the lived experience and meaning of fatigue for those suffering from cancer	Three focus groups—open ended questions. Analysis: interpretative phenomenology	Nature of fatigue: difficult to describe, unpleasant, abnormal, overwhelming, unpredictable, uncontrollable. Physical effect. Cognitive effect. Emotional effect. Social effect. Effect on self. Meaning of CRF: disease progression and death	Small sample with small numbers in some of the focus groups. Mainly female sample
Ferrell et al. (1996). US national medical centre	Convenience sample of 910 cancer survivors. Approximate mean age = 48. Male not given, female not given. Diagnoses, mixed: breast = 332, ovary = 152, thyroid = 34, other = 392	To present fatigue data compiled from several studies focusing on QOL of cancer survivors	Secondary analysis of data from four QOL studies. Data collected by a mixture of interviews, focus groups and mailed surveys. Analysis: content analysis guided by the use of a QOL model	Nature of fatigue: overwhelming Physical effect. Emotional effect. Social effect. Meaning of CRF: sign of cancer or recurrence	Secondary analysis of data collected for another reason, therefore fatigue not specifically asked about. Mainly female sample. It is not clear how many of the total sample of 910 discussed fatigue
Glaus et al. (1996).	Purposive sample of 20 cancer patients and 20 people	To explore the concept of fatigue	Individual unstructured interviews. Analysis:	Nature of fatigue: difficulty finding	Relationships between the

Table 6.1 (continued) Overview of the reviewed studies

Study and setting	Sample, age, gender, and diagnosis	Aim	Methodology	Findings	Comments
Swiss teaching hospital– oncology unit	without cancer within a sampling frame of age and gender. Mean age = 66. Male = 45%, female = 55%. Diagnoses: mixed	from the native's perspective and to generate theoretical knowledge	grounded theory—constant comparative method. Thematic and pattern analysis. Descriptive statistics for each theme	words, unpleasant, overwhelming, abnormal and chronic. Physical effect. Cognitive effect. Motivational effect. Emotional effect	themes not discussed
Krishnasamy (1996). UK specialist oncology teaching hospital—palliative care unit	Purposive sample of 15 palliative care patients. Mean age = 63.5. Male = 7, female = 8. Diagnoses: breast = 5, prostate = 4, lung = 5, ovary = 1	To explore the nature and impact of fatigue in patients with advanced cancer	Multiple case study of patient, main carer, and a health professional. Semistructured individual interviews. Analysis: grounded theory approach—generation of categories	Nature of fatigue: difficult to describe, intangible, oppressive, overwhelming, abnormal, unpredictable, persistent. Physical effect. Emotional effect. Social effect. Effect on self. Meaning of fatigue: progression towards death	Limited by one-off interactions with participants. Patients had advanced cancer and disentangling the experience of fatigue from the distress of imminent death was problematic
Pearce and Richardson (1996). UK teaching hospital—oncology unit	Purposive sample of 6 cancer patients. Mean age not given. Gender not given. Diagnoses not given	To understand and describe the meaning of fatigue	Open-ended individual interviews. Analysis: phenomenological analysis following the steps described by Giorgi. Thematic analysis. Data collection and analysis were simultaneous	Nature of fatigue: unable to describe and explain fatigue, unpredictable, and chronic. Physical effect. Emotional effect. Social effect. Effect on self.	Small sample size

				Meaning of fatigue: deterioration	
Messias et al. (1997). USA, 18 hospital sites—outpatient units	127 cancer patients receiving chemotherapy. Mean age = 52. Male = 31%, female = 69%. Diagnoses: breast = 43%, lung = 15%, ovary = 9%, bladder = 7%, other = 27%	To explore the descriptions of fatigue as experienced by a group of cancer patients undergoing chemotherapy	Secondary analysis of data collected to test the impact of a nursing intervention on the practice of self-care behaviours and morbidity of patients receiving chemotherapy. Completed a battery of questionnaires and a semistructured interview. However, the interview did not specifically ask about fatigue. Analysis: grounded theory approach—thematic analysis and analytic expansion	Nature of fatigue: overwhelming, differed from normal tiredness, variation, and duration. Physical effect. Emotional effect. Social effect. Effect on self	Mainly female sample. Predominant diagnosis was breast cancer. Secondary analysis of data collected for another reason
Ream and Richardson (1997). UK teaching hospital—outpatient unit	9 cancer patients and 6 patients with chronic obstructive airways disease. Mean age = 50. Male = 1, female = 8. Diagnoses: breast = 5, colorectal = 2, NHL = 2	To elicit, record, and describe patients' experiences of fatigue in cancer and chronic obstructive airways disease	Semistructured individual interviews. Analysis: phenomenological following the steps described by Moustakas. Only textual description provided	Nature of fatigue: very difficult to describe, nebulous, ubiquitous, unpleasant, overpowering, unpredictable, and difficult to control. Physical effect. Cognitive effect. Emotional effect. Effect on self	Small mainly female sample. Predominant diagnosis was breast cancer
Magnusson et al. (1999).	Theoretical sample of 15 cancer patients receiving chemotherapy as an outpatient.	To explore the experience of fatigue and to describe the	Unstructured individual interviews. Analysis: grounded theory—constant	Nature of fatigue: abnormal and hard to verbalize. Physical effects.	

Table 6.1 (continued) Overview of the reviewed studies

Study and setting	Sample, age, gender, and diagnosis	Aim	Methodology	Findings	Comments
Swedish university hospital—oncology unit	Mean age = 49.6. Male = 7, female = 8. Diagnoses, mixed: lymphoma = 5, breast = 3, gastrointestinal = 2, ovarian = 2, other = 3	categories and dimensions of the symptom	comparative method	Cognitive effects. Emotional effects. Social effects. Effect on self	
Holley (2000). US hospital—cancer centre	Purposive sample of 17 cancer patients receiving cytotoxic treatment. Mean age = 58.9. Male = 12, female = 5. Diagnoses, mixed: breast = 4, melanoma = 2, lung cancer = 2, colon = 2, other = 7	To describe, from the patients' perspectives, the experience of CRF, and the impact of CRF on patients' lives	Theoretical framework: symbolic interactionism. Interviews—probably individual. Five patients were interviewed twice. Analysis: content analysis	Nature of fatigue: different from normal, persistent, unexpected. Physical effect. Cognitive effect. Emotional effect. Social effect. Meaning of CRF: decline in health	It is not clear why some people were interviewed twice and what influence this had on the findings presented
Barsevick et al. (2001) USA	Convenience sample of 8 patients with cancer. Gender: majority were female. Age range = 33–70. Diagnoses: ovary = 2, other = 6	To describe CRF from the perspective of individuals experiencing it and examine the fit of their descriptions with the Common Sense Model	Secondary analysis of data from two focus groups on supportive interventions for CRF. Three patients attended both focus groups. Analysis: content analysis using the Common Sense Model as an analysis guide. Descriptive statistics for each theme	Nature of fatigue: different between people, cumulative, chronic, and unpredictable. Physical effect. Cognitive effect. Emotional effect. Meaning of fatigue: symptom of cancer	Secondary analysis of data collected for another reason Small sample size. It's not clear why some people only took part in one focus group and what effect that this had on the group discussions and the findings presented

Abbreviations: CRF, cancer-related fatigue; QOL, quality of life; NHL, non-Hodgkin lymphoma.

of self and suffering and so the relationship between them is circular rather than simply that of cause and effect; loss of self and suffering can also induce fatigue.

The nature of fatigue

It is generally agreed that fatigue is difficult to describe and participants in these studies were no exception to the rule (Armes 1995; Glaus *et al.* 1996; Krishnasamy 1996; Pearce and Richardson 1996; Ream and Richardson 1997; Magnusson *et al.* 1999). Ream and Richardson (1997) suggest that CRF has a 'nebulous' quality', whilst Krishnasamy (1996) interprets it as being 'intangible'. As a consequence many authors highlighted the varied colloquial descriptive expressions used to describe it (Armes 1995; Ferrell *et al.* 1996; Glaus *et al.* 1996; Pearce and Richardson 1996; Messias *et al.* 1997). Some authors reported that participants in their studies used metaphorical descriptions (Armes 1995; Ferrell *et al.* 1996; Krishnasamy 1996; Ream and Richardson 1997; Magnusson *et al.* 1999) and Table 6.2 provides examples of these. Brown (1977) suggests that metaphors are used because a phenomenon cannot be conveyed directly; however, through the medium of language, a new experience is transformed into something we have experienced and understand (Martin 1975). Radley (1993) concurs with this, suggesting that metaphors consist of subtle descriptions that help to illuminate, assess, and, at times, make sense of experience. Thus, Armes (1995) interprets the metaphorical descriptions in her study (see Table 6.2) as indicating that participants felt that their once-contained bodies were now out of control. However, in general, little attempt has been made in published accounts of these studies to interpret the usage and meaning of these metaphorical descriptions and assess whether they might represent the severity and differing dimensions of CRF.

Table 6.2 Metaphorical descriptions of cancer-related fatigue

Study	Metaphorical descriptions
Armes (1995)	'like water pouring out of a bottle', 'I just feel as though I want to melt', 'a bit like being drunk'
Ferrell *et al.* (1996)	'bone tired', 'wet cement'
Krishnasamy (1996)	'It's so heavy, like a weight coming down on you', 'It feels as though my back isn't supporting me'
Messias *et al.* (1997)	'I feel like someone let the plug out', 'I feel like someone beat me up', 'I felt deathly hung over'
Ream and Richardson (1997)	'as if the stuffing had been taken out of them', 'a clockwork toy whose spring has been wound down', 'a jointed doll whose elastic has slackened'
Magnusson *et al.* (1999)	'my feet feel like lead', 'I couldn't run, my legs felt like spaghetti'

In most of the studies, CRF was reported by participants as being of a longer duration than previously experienced 'normal' fatigue. This has been interpreted as implying that CRF is 'chronic' in nature (Armes 1995; Glaus *et al.* 1996; Krishnasamy 1996; Messias *et al.* 1997; Holley 2000; Barsevick *et al.* 2001), and as being 'abnormal' (Armes 1995; Glaus *et al.* 1996; Krishnasamy 1996; Messias *et al.* 1997; Magnusson *et al.* 1999; Holley 2000). Three studies (Ferrell *et al.* 1996; Glaus *et al.* 1996; Holley 2000) proposed the reason for this is its intensity which is reported as being 'one that consumed their whole bodies' (Ferrell *et al.* 1996). It is this notion of all-consuming intensity that seems to be embodied in the interpretation of fatigue as 'overwhelming' or 'overpowering' (Armes *et al.* 1995; Ferrell *et al.* 1996; Glaus *et al.* 1996; Krishnasamy 1996; Messias *et al.* 1997; Ream and Richardson 1997). Moreover Holley (2000) and Armes (1995) both note that participants in their studies stated that the intensity of CRF was not related to the amount or type of activity performed and was unrelieved by rest.

Some authors have suggested that fatigue can be perceived as being 'unpredictable' or 'unexpected' (Armes 1995; Krishnasamy 1996; Pearce and Richardson 1996; Ream and Richardson 1997; Holley 2000; Barsevick *et al.* 2001), and this has been allied to the notion of CRF being 'uncontrollable' (Armes 1995; Ream and Richardson 1997). All or some of these properties led many of the researchers to deduce that CRF was experienced as being unpleasant (Armes 1995; Glaus *et al.* 1996; Ream and Richardson 1997).

The unpleasant, abnormal, chronic, overwhelming, and all-encompassing nature of fatigue has previously been identified in some definitions, as has the idea that CRF is unrelated to activity and rest (Potempa 1986; Piper *et al.* 1987; Carpenito 1995; NANDA 1993; Ream and Richardson 1997; Atkinson *et al.* 2000). However, there are two indicators of CRF that are not included in the definitions: its unpredictable and uncontrollable nature. These perhaps are the most salient properties when it comes to explaining the effects of, and distress caused by, CRF.

Cancer-related fatigue and alterations in bodily awareness

Freund and McGuire (1995) suggest that illnesses—and by association symptoms—that are perceived as being overwhelming, unpredictable, and uncontrollable are especially damaging as they impede a person's ability to manage life, to plan, and to act. As the body is seen as a medium for action (Corbin and Strauss 1987; van Manen 1998), a loss of bodily integrity, as in the case of an unpredictable or uncontrollable symptom, leaves people no longer feeling able to perform their usual activities (Conrad 1987). As such, they may feel that mind and body are no longer working in harmony. The taken-for-granted relationship that a person has with their body, which results in an almost unconscious relationship between person as self and person as embodied self, has been disrupted (Bury 1982) by the impact of a symptom that forces acknowledgement of physical incapacity. The body becomes less biddable and so the person becomes more aware of it in their encounters with what used to be their easily negotiated world.

This is the state of 'disembodiment', as one participant notes in the study by Ferrell *et al.* (1996, p. 1543): '...coping with the physical effect consumes all train of thought to function and accomplish even the simplest task'. An important element in the taken-for-granted relationship between a person and their body is the ability to control the body in order to fulfil the tasks that the person requires of it (Corbin and Strauss 1987). With illness, the body becomes 'an 'other'—at best an unpredictable ally' (Freund and McGuire 1995, p. 145). One of the respondents in Ferrell *et al.*'s (1996) study remarks on this 'I used to rule my body, now my body rules me. It tells me when to lie down and relax and there's no more pushing my body' (p. 1544) and from Armes' (1995) study: 'It's not nice something else being in control of my body' (p. 62). This would seem to confirm that the bodily limitations imposed by the body as a result of CRF fractures the synergistic relationship between person and body and, as will be shown below, hinders the ability to carry out everyday tasks.

Physical and cognitive effects of cancer-related fatigue

Most of the studies mentioned the cognitive and motivational effects of CRF in some form or another. The most commonly identified aspects being loss of concentration (Glaus *et al.* 1996; Ream and Richardson 1997; Magnusson *et al.* 1999; Barsevick *et al.* 2001) and a loss of motivation (Armes 1995; Glaus *et al.* 1996; Messias *et al.* 1997; Ream and Richardson 1997; Magnusson *et al.* 1999; Holley 2000). However, in the latter case this was variously described as 'loss of initiative' (Magnusson *et al.* 1999), 'lacking get up and go' (Ream and Richardson 1997), and 'can't be bothered' (Armes 1995). This was viewed as being 'frightening' (Holley 2000; see also Chapter 11, this volume).

Two authors comment on how frequently participants discussed CRF in relation to loss of physical functioning (Armes 1995; Barsevick *et al.* 2001). Typically it was reported that respondents' level of physical functioning had diminished and that this interfered with many aspects of everyday life: self-care, housework, work, and strenuous physical activity (Armes 1995; Ferrell *et al.* 1996; Glaus *et al.* 1996; Krishnasamy 1996; Pearce and Richardson 1996; Messias *et al.* 1997; Ream and Richardson 1997; Barsevick *et al.* 2001). This was frequently seen as upsetting 'I'd get very annoyed because I couldn't do the things I was used to doing' (Ferrell *et al.* 1996, p. 1544). It is for this reason that Charmaz (2000, p. 282) says that: 'People learn what illness is through their experience of it. Lessons in chronicity come in small everyday experiences such as opening a can, bending over to pick up a newspaper, folding bedsheets, and weeding the garden. Comparisons with past effortless performance can be shocking' (see Chapter 13, this volume).

Within the sociological literature there is a recognition of the central role of experience and control of the body and mind, working harmoniously, in the creation of social identity and self-conception (Corbin and Strauss 1987; Freund and McGuire 1995; Kelly and Field 1996; Charmaz 2000). That is, we are what we do and we use our body to express the person we are through the performance of a range of tasks. Whilst these can be viewed simply as physical activities, they coalesce to represent enactments of chosen social roles (Corbin and Strauss 1987). If we are physically unable to perform these roles our social relationships and place in society may alter, which is when illness can be at its most threatening (Freund and McGuire 1995).

Social effects of fatigue

Many of the researchers highlighted how participants' social lives had been affected by CRF (Armes 1995; Ferrell *et al.* 1996; Krishnasamy 1996; Pearce and Richardson 1996; Magnusson *et al.* 1999; Holley 2000). This included limited social activities and contacts (Armes 1995; Ferrell *et al.* 1996; Krishnasamy 1996; Ream and Richardson 1997; Magnusson *et al.* 1999; Holley 2000), and loss of valued activities (Armes 1995; Krishnasamy 1996; Ream and Richardson 1997; Magnusson *et al.* 1999). In addition, the invidious impact fatigue made on family life and relationships was described (Armes 1995; Ferrell *et al.* 1996; Krishnasamy 1996; Pearce and Richardson 1996; Holley 2000). This was interpreted by some authors as inducing feelings of 'isolation' (Armes 1995; Ferrell *et al.* 1996; Krishnasamy 1996; Pearce and Richardson 1996), feeling 'excluded' or like an 'outsider' (Magnusson *et al.* 1999), or that the person had become 'socially disengaged' (Holley 2000). This occurs because, when physical incapacity results in failure to carry out tasks required of selected social roles, it is likely that this will have a negative effect on people's view of themselves, as is evidenced by the following quotations:

> I was the kind of person that never missed a day of work. I never stayed at home, never got the 'flu. I had the ordinary things. It was my selling point. I never missed work. And now, two and a half years later I became a liability and not an asset. I feel that way anyhow. You find that you are sick all the time. It just wears you out. The idea that your body has failed you.
>
> (Barsevick *et al.* 2001, p. 1367)

> I have the desire to contribute. The hardest thing is for me to find ways I can participate in the lives of my husband and children in a more passive way.... They do not need me to be with them at functions and so someone else can drive them, so I am less and less part of their lives. At work I now do lots at the computer so I feel good about my ability to contribute. At home, the job is physical so I feel less adequate.
>
> (Ferrell *et al.* 1996, p. 1545)

When we are healthy much of our social interaction is based on the notion of reciprocity, whereby all give and receive, and no one person is completely dependent on others (Freund and McGuire 1995). In the case of illness, loss of independence as a result of bodily limitations can create the possibility of others seeing us in a differing light, calling into question our personal competence and integrity (Conrad 1987) (see Chapter 5). Not being seen as a whole person makes people vulnerable to discrimination by others as they assign them new identities based on their physical capabilities. Charmaz (1983) suggests that this occurs because the greater the loss of control and extent of the embarrassment from an unpredictable illness, the more their self-concept suffers and so the more likely the person is to voluntarily restrict their life, as one woman describes below:

> Purely and simply because I couldn't plan anything 'cos I know that I would fall asleep half way through whatever I'd gone to, which then of course would make me feel embarrassed, and I mean you don't know what other people would think of you.

(Armes 1995, p. 67)

There are times, however, when people do not feel physically capable of coping with social interaction. This is echoed in the following quotation:

> I was forced to focus mainly on my own needs and just getting through each day.... I did not have the physical or emotional energy to give to anyone else. It was a very humbling and isolating experience.

(Ferrell *et al.* 1996, p. 1543)

Kelly and Field (1996) make the point that, in order to cope with illness, coping with the physical body has to precede coping with relationships. Thus it possible to see that CRF may hinder people as social beings at a number of levels. It is important, therefore, to acknowledge the primacy that valued roles and pursuits play in preserving a coherent sense of self (Charmaz 2000).

Effect of cancer-related fatigue on perceptions of self

An important effect of CRF detected in half of the qualitative studies was that participants reported it changed their view of themselves (Armes 1995; Krishnasamy 1996; Pearce and Richardson 1996; Messias *et al.* 1997; Ream and Richardson 1997; Magnusson *et al.* 1999). Feelings of a loss of control (Armes 1995; Krishnasamy 1996; Ream and Richardson 1997; Holley 2000), disempowerment (Krishnasamy 1996), and reduced self-confidence (Ream and Richardson 1997) seemed to induce lowered self-efficacy (Armes 1995) and self-esteem (Armes 1995; Krishnasamy 1996; Magnusson *et al.* 1999). As a consequence of this, participants developed an altered perception of themselves (Armes 1995; Messias *et al.* 1997) and grieved for their old self and previous life (Krishnasamy 1996; Ream and Richardson 1997):

> I am just not myself.

(Messias *et al.* 1997, p. 45)

> Why can't I be me again? That's all I want to be me again.

(Ream and Richardson 1997, p. 49)

Corbin and Strauss (1987) have identified that when people are unable to carry out activities they associate with different aspects of self then these are, 'metaphorically, "lost". Since the integration of these various aspects of self forms the more inclusive self, with that loss comes an accompanying sense of a loss of wholeness' (Corbin and

Strauss 1987, p. 264). The extent of this will depend on what the loss means to the person, whether it is permanent, and their ability to adapt and create new identities (Corbin and Strauss 1987). This encapsulates the notion that the person is in a state of flux or change; fluctuations in conceptions of self are seen as the link between the biological and social effects of illness (Kelly and Field 1996):

> I don't think you're ever ready to let go ... when you have to sit about all day you think well, what's the point .... I think sometimes, how long can this go on?

> (Krishnasamy 1996, p. 19)

In the studies in Table 6.1 participants frequently identified that they saw themselves as dependent (Armes 1995; Krishnasamy 1996; Ream and Richardson 1997) and so it is not surprising that, as a result, they reported that they felt 'childlike', 'old before their time' or like an 'invalid' (Armes 1995):

> It's like these girls here making me cups of tea, I mean, as I walk in ... and that's when you know that your are an invalid sort of thing.

> (Armes 1995, p. 80)

These constitute new self-concepts and they are all synonymous with the more helpless and marginalized members of society. They have not been generated purely as a result of the fissure between body and self; identities reflected back to them from their social relationships and interactions have also been influential. Thus the questions 'What can I do?' and 'How do others see me?' are mediated by 'Who am I?' (Robinson 1988). This is echoed in the following quotation:

> it must be difficult for them because they know me as a sparky character full of fun and now I'm this rather quiet, slow character.

> (Krishnasamy 1996, p. 19)

This consequence is possibly the most damaging aspect of CRF for individuals and it is likely to be one of two meta-effects of fatigue. All the other effects of fatigue combine to force the person to take stock of their capabilities, see what they are no longer able to do, and re-evaluate not only their view of themselves as agents in their life and world, but also how those around them perceive them. Freund and McGuire (1995) suggest that an empowered self experiences both a sense of wholeness and health, whilst a dispirited self lacks a sense of control, feels overwhelmed, and experiences anxiety and depression. This emotional impact of fatigue will now be considered.

The emotional experience of cancer-related fatigue: suffering

Most studies identified the emotional impact that CRF made on the participants. A wide range of adjectives for differing emotions were extracted from eight of the studies in Table 6.1 (Armes 1995; Ferrell *et al.* 1996; Glaus *et al.* 1996; Krishnasamy 1996; Pearce and Richardson 1996; Messias *et al.* 1997; Ream and Richardson 1997;

Magnusson *et al.* 1999). Those most frequently cited were 'frustration' (Armes 1995; Krishnasamy 1996; Messias *et al.* 1997; Ream and Richardson 1997; Magnusson *et al.* 1999), anxiety (Armes 1995; Ferrell *et al.* 1996; Magnusson *et al.* 1999), and depression (Armes 1995; Ferrell *et al.* 1996; Ream and Richardson 1997). Also present were feelings of anger and resentment, irritability, displeasure, disappointment, guilt, confusion and bewilderment, loss and emptiness, uncertainty and insecurity, and finally boredom.

> With the feeling tired you feel kind of depressed … . I feel down all the time to a certain degree … . You know sometimes you think 'What's the point' … 'What's the point in life?
>
> (Ream and Richardson 1997, p. 49)

Mathieson and Stam (1995) have suggested that whilst classifications of psychosocial difficulties have been developed, this has not been translated into an exploration of what this means to cancer patients. Certainly, little attempt has been made in the studies reviewed, and the CRF literature in general, to try and account for these feelings and explain why they occur, except to try and establish whether anxiety and depression cause fatigue.

Within the clinical setting the feelings outlined above are described either as distress or signs of psychopathology; however, there may be considerable merit in considering them as expressions of suffering. Cassell (1992) has defined suffering as 'the state of distress induced by the threat of the loss of intactness or the disintegration of a person from whatever cause. Suffering is a consequence of personhood—bodies do not suffer, persons do' (Cassell 1992, p. 3). The extent of the suffering depends on the meaning of the loss (Kahn and Steeves 1995). In the quotations below there is a real sense of anguish when participants discuss how their life has changed as a result of CRF and what this means to them:

> It's a horrible feeling you don't belong anymore … life goes on without me.
>
> (Pearce and Richardson 1996, p. 113)

> I feel worthless, so much has been taken away from me.
>
> (Magnusson *et al.* 1999, p. 228)

> You see this is what hurts you. You think 'Oh God! Life's passing by' … . You see all these real old ladies trotting along to the bus, and sometime I could and cry when I see them … . I should be doing that, going and standing in the bus stop as I've done in the past but I cannot do that now.
>
> (Armes 1995, p. 82).

Kahn and Steeves (1995) have identified that suffering, although unique to each person, has a common basic structure. It:

- alters experiences of embodiment
- constricts social world and lived space
- changes the relationship with time.

Cassell (1992) has stated that for suffering to occur there must be a concept of the future. 'The future onto which suffering is projected must contain an idea of the person's identity and that must have arisen in the past and be cohesive from the past through the present and into the future' (Cassell 1992, p. 4). Conrad (1987) has identified cancer as a 'mortal' illness, that is one that threatens to rob people of their future by taking their life away. In the studies reviewed it was reported that participants interpreted their fatigue as a sign of cancer, a deterioration in their health, of disease progression, or that they were dying (Armes 1995; Ferrell *et al.* 1996; Krishnasamy 1996; Pearce and Richardson 1996). Ellis-Hill and Horn (2000) suggest that when individuals cannot create a clear sense of a future self they experience anxiety and are unsure how to act.

Coping with cancer-related fatigue

In many of the studies participants described how they tried to deal with the CRF. These strategies are outlined in Table 6.3. Whilst the most popular strategies employed were resting/sleeping and conserving energy, people experimented with a wide range of strategies, such as acceptance, distraction, exercise, and thinking differently. What is not clear is how effective they find them, although evidence (Richardson and Ream 1997) indicates that they provide little relief (see Chapter 12). Many of these strategies

Table 6.3 Coping strategies used to combat cancer-related fatigue

Coping strategy	Authors
Rest/sleep	Barsevick *et al.* (2001), Magnusson *et al.* (1999), Messias *et al.* (1997), Pearce and Richardson (1996), Armes (1995)
Conserve energy	Holley (2000), Messias *et al.* (1997), Pearce and Richardson (1996), Ferrell *et al.* (1996), Armes (1995)
Planning/pacing	Magnusson *et al.* (1999), Messias *et al.* (1997), Ream and Richardson (1997)
Acceptance	Magnusson *et al.* (1999), Pearce and Richardson (1996), Ferrell *et al.* (1996)
Think differently	Holley (2000), Magnusson *et al.* (1999), Armes (1995)
Distraction	Barsevick *et al.* (2001), Magnusson *et al.* (1999), Armes (1995)
Withdraw/disengage	Holley (2000), Ferrell *et al.* (1996), Armes (1995)
Adapt	Magnusson *et al.* (1999), Armes (1995)
Medication	Barsevick *et al.* (2001), Holley (2000)
Fight it	Messias *et al.* (1997), Armes (1995)
Exercise	Magnusson *et al.* (1999), Messias *et al.* (1997)
Alter priorities	Magnusson *et al.* (1999)
Nutrition	Holley (2000)
Denial	Pearce and Richardson (1996)
Social support	Pearce and Richardson (1996)

(offered within the context of promoting self-care through information) are advocated by health professionals as potentially effective management techniques and are becoming the focus of increasing numbers of experimental intervention studies.

The importance of tailoring self-care strategies to the needs of individual patients within their unique social context is described by Robinson (1988), who suggests that the crucial factor in the promotion of self-efficacy is the re-creation of a sense of personal and social order. This is achieved by developing a detailed plan for each day of what activities will be performed and when, ideally spreading them out through the day, and reorganizing the environment within which one enacts social roles. He says that this 'involves making harsh decisions about what is achievable in the light of competing objectives. These decisions may involve making complex calculations, for example about the use of a limited supply of energy before fatigue sets in' (Robinson 1988, p. 116). Kelly and Field (1996) concur with this, saying 'coping with chronic illness involves coping with bodies' (Kelly and Field 1996, p. 247), but this is particularly difficult work and may be emotionally draining as an individual struggles to accept that life will never be the same again, and that previously held life-long values about their ability to participate in social roles have to be renegotiated on a continuous basis. Corbin and Strauss (1987) have defined this as 'biographical work', where the emphasis is placed on coming to terms with illness and integrating it into a reconstituted self.

Kahn and Steeves (1995) have pointed out that the expression of suffering is more accessible than the experience. They suggest that clinicians listen very carefully to the language used by patients to talk about their circumstances and recommend that they resist the temptation to translate it into professional terminology. Being able to speak about the fatigue experience can assist people in making sense of what has happened to them, how that fits into their life and view of themselves, and provides a chance to explore what it means for them in the future. This, Mathieson and Stam (1995) state, 'is crucial to a life that is circumscribed by social and bodily limitations' (Mathieson and Stam 1995, p. 302) and so they have called for the psychosocial framework of cancer care to focus more on patients' continual readjustment of self and identity in the face of chronic illness and its symptoms, such as fatigue.

Implications for practice and research

There has been a growing recognition among health professionals of the deleterious impact that CRF makes on those affected by it (Stone *et al.* 2002). Much of the nature of CRF has been described and included in definitions and CRF measures; however, this review of the qualitative studies exploring CRF indicates that it is also perceived as being unpredictable and uncontrollable. These properties should now be included in fatigue measures and clinical assessments as they may be important indicators of severity and predictors of the impact that it makes on people.

The effect CRF has on people's view of themselves has received little in attention in research studies conducted to date. This may prove to be a fruitful line of enquiry when attempting to explain the relationship between severity and distress and the level of functional and social restrictions experienced. In addition, it may well be a useful outcome measure in future studies. Interventions should be developed that not only aim to provide advice and information on cancer-related fatigue and the best ways of managing it, but that try to maintain and restore people's sense of self and personal identity.

Within clinical practice it may be helpful to listen as closely as possible to what patients say about their CRF and the language they use to describe it and the impact it makes on them. Moreover, it may be illuminating to ask them to describe how they see themselves at the moment and what they were like prior to their cancer diagnosis, as this can give some indication of the extent of disruption caused by the fatigue as well as an opportunity to explore this further (see Box 6.1).

Conclusion

It is clear from the qualitative studies reviewed in this chapter that fatigue is perceived by those who experience it to be a vague and elusive symptom, as is evidenced both by their comments that it is difficult to describe, and their attempts to shed more light on it using metaphorical descriptions. Nevertheless, despite the differing samples studied and methodologies used, most of the studies consistently identified a number of properties that seemed to differentiate cancer-related fatigue from normal fatigue. These are

Box 6.1 Implications for research and practice

◆ The unpredictable and uncontrollable properties of cancer-related fatigue should be included into assessments and measures designed to assess it, as, along with its overwhelming characteristics, these may be better indicators of its severity and predictors of the impact it makes on people.

◆ Measures of self-conception and suffering should be included in future studies and relationships between these and the functional and social restriction should be explored.

◆ Interventions aimed at maintaining and restoring people's sense of self and identity should be carried out.

◆ Clinicians should enable people to talk about cancer-related fatigue and listen carefully to the language used when they explain how it has affected them in order to assist them to make sense of the experience and assimilate it into their life story and sense of self.

Box 6.2 Summary points

- The nature of cancer-related fatigue has been identified as being unpleasant, chronic, abnormal, overwhelming, unpredictable, and uncontrollable.
- Cancer-related fatigue fractures the harmonious, taken-for-granted relationship between a person and their body, creating an awareness of bodily limitations.
- Functional and social restrictions, as a result of cancer-related fatigue, combine to induce a loss of self as a whole person and altered self-conceptions.
- The potential threat cancer-related fatigue poses to a person's sense of 'wholeness' is distressing and can cause suffering.
- People experiencing cancer-related fatigue experiment with a variety of strategies for managing it; many of these are aimed at maintaining a sense of personal and social order.

that it is seen as: unpleasant, abnormal, chronic, overwhelming, unrelated to rest and activity, unpredictable, and uncontrollable. And, as such, it fractures the harmonious taken-for-granted relationship between a person and their body, creating an awareness of bodily limitations. Resulting functional and social restrictions combine to induce a loss of self as a whole person and altered self-conceptions, which can be distressing and cause suffering. Patients describe a number of strategies for trying to manage their fatigue, many of which are now being advocated as potentially effective management techniques for CRF. Evidence presented in this chapter suggests that interventions may be helpful if they are aimed at helping those affected maintain a sense of personal and social order as well as enabling them to make sense of fatigue, as a symptom of cancer and its treatments, and the disruption that they are facing to their lives as a result of it (see Box 6.2).

References

Armes, P.J. (1995) Cancer patients experiences of fatigue. Unpublished BSc Thesis, University of Hull.

Atkinson, A., Barsevick, A., Cella, D., Cimprich, B., Cleeland, C., Donnelly, J., *et al.* (2000) National Comprehensive Cancer Network. NCCN practice guidelines for cancer-related fatigue. *Oncology,* **14**(11A, Supplement 10), 151–61.

Barsevick, A., Whitmer, K., and Walker, L. (2001) In their own words: using the common-sense model to analyze patient descriptions of cancer-related fatigue. *Oncology Nursing Forum,* **28**(9), 1368–9.

Brown, R. (1977) *A Poetic for Sociology,* Cambridge University Press, New York.

Bury, M. (1982) Chronic illness as biographical disruption. *Sociology of Health and Illness,* **4**, 167–82.

Carpenito, L. (1999) Fatigue. In: *Handbook of Nursing Diagnosis.* Lippincott, Philadelphia, pp. 135–9.

Cassell, E. (1992) The nature of suffering: physical, psychological, social and spiritual aspects. In: *The Hidden Dimension of Illness: Human Suffering* (ed. P. Starck and J. McGovern), National League for Nursing Press, New York, pp. 1–10.

Charmaz, K. (1983) Loss of self: a fundamental form of suffering in the chronically ill. *Sociology of Health and Illness*, **5**, 168–95.

Charmaz, K. (2000) Experiencing chronic illness. In: *Handbook of Social Studies in Health and Medicine* (ed. G. Albrecht, R. Fitzpatrick, and S. Scrimshaw), Sage Publications, London, pp. 230–42.

Conrad, P. (1987) The experience of illness: recent and new directions. *Research in the Sociology of Health Care*, **6**, 1–31.

Corbin, J. and Strauss, A. (1987) Accompaniments of chronic illness: changes in body, self, biography and biographical time. *Research in the Sociology of Health Care*, **6**, 249–81.

Ellis-Hill, C. and Horn, S. (2000) Change in identity and self-concept: a new theoretical approach to recovery following a stroke. *Clinical Rehabilitation*, **14**, 279–87.

Ferrell, B., Grant, M., Dean, G., Funk, B., and Ly, J. (1996) 'Bone tired': the experience of fatigue and its impact on quality of life. *Oncology Nursing Forum*, **23**(10), 1539–47.

Freund, P. and McGuire, M. (1995) *Health, Illness and the Social Body*. Prentice Hall, Englewood Cliffs, NJ.

Glaus, A., Crow, R., and Hammond, S. (1996) A qualitative study to explore the concept of fatigue/tiredness in cancer patients and in healthy individuals. *European Journal of Cancer Care*, **5**(2, Supplement), 8–23.

Holley, S.K. (2000) Evaluating patient distress from cancer-related fatigue: an instrument development study. *Oncology Nursing Forum*, **27**(9), 1425–31.

Kahn, D. and Steeves, R. (1986) The experience of suffering: conceptual clarification and theoretical definition. *Journal of Advanced Nursing*, **11**, 623–31.

Kahn, D. and Steeves, R. (1995) The significance of suffering in cancer care. *Seminars in Oncology Nursing*, **11**(1), 9–16.

Kelly, M. and Field, D. (1996) Medical sociology, chronic illness and the body. *Sociology of Health and Illness*, **18**(2), 241–57.

Krishnasamy, M. (1996) *An Exploration of The Nature and Impact of Fatigue in Patients With Advanced Cancer*. The Institute of Cancer Research, London.

Lewis, G. and Wessely, S. (1992) The epidemiology of fatigue: more questions than answers. *Journal of Epidemiology and Community Health*, **46**, 92–7.

Magnusson, K., Moller, A., Ekman, T., and Wallgren, A. (1999) A qualitative study to explore the experience of fatigue in cancer patients. *European Journal of Cancer Care*, **8**(4), 224–32.

Martin, G. (1975) *Language, Truth and Poetry*. Edinburgh University Press, Edinburgh.

Mathieson, C. and Stam, J. (1995) Renegotiating identities: cancer narratives. *Sociology of Health and Illness*, **17**(3), 283–306.

Messias, D., Yeager, K., Dibble, S., and Dodd, M.J. (1997) Patients' perspectives of fatigue while undergoing chemotherapy. *Oncology Nursing Forum*, **24**(1), 43–8.

Nail, L.M. (2002) Fatigue in patients with cancer. *Oncology Nursing Forum*, **29**, 537–44.

NANDA (North American Nursing Diagnosis Association) (1993) Fatigue. In: *Nursing Diagnosis and Intervention* (ed. G. McFarland and E. McFarland), Mosby, St Louis, MO, pp. 288–93.

Pearce, S. and Richardson, A. (1996) Fatigue in cancer: a phenomenological perspective. *European Journal of Cancer Care*, **5**(2), 111–15.

Piper, B.F., Lindsey, A.M., and Dodd, M.J. (1987) Fatigue mechanisms in cancer patients: developing nursing theory. *Oncology Nursing Forum*, **14**(6), 17–23.

Potempa, K. (1986) Chronic fatigue. *Image: Journal of Nursing Scholarship,* **18**(4), 165–9.

Radley, A. (1993) The role of metaphor in adjustment to chronic illness. In: *Worlds of Illness* (ed. A. Radley). Routledge, New York, pp. 109–23.

Ream, E. and Richardson, A. (1997) Fatigue in patients with cancer and chronic obstructive airways disease: a phenomenological enquiry. *International Journal of Nursing Studies,* **34**(1), 44–53.

Richardson, A. and Ream, E. (1997) Self-care behaviours initiated by chemotherapy patients in response to fatigue. *International Journal of Nursing Studies,* **34**(1), 35–43.

Robinson, I. (1988) Managing symptoms in chronic disease: some dimensions of patients' experiences. *International Disability Studies,* **10**(3), 112–18.

Stone, P., Ream, E., Richardson, A., Thomas, H., Andrews, P., Campbell, P. *et al.* (2002) Cancer-related fatigue—a difference of opinion? Results of a multicentre survey of healthcare professionals, patients and caregivers. *European Journal of Cancer Care,* **12**, 20–7.

Turner, S. (1980) *Sociological Explanation as Interpretation.* Cambridge University Press, New York.

van Manen, M. (1998) Modalities of body experience in health and illness. *Qualitative Health Research,* **8**(1), 7–24.

Wu, H.-S. and McSweeney, M. (2001) Measurement of fatigue in people with cancer. *Oncology Nursing Forum,* **28**(9), 1371–84.

Chapter 7

Carers, caring, and cancer-related fatigue

Meinir Krishnasamy and Hilary Plant

Introduction

Despite an acknowledgement of the prevalence of fatigue as a facet of the lives of individuals living with and caring for people with cancer (Zarit 1994; James 1998), little is known of the ways in which carers experience or articulate the physical and emotional dimensions of fatigue associated with their caring role. In addition, ways in which family members perceive and interpret fatigue as a manifestation of cancer, and its treatment, have largely been overlooked. Overwhelming tiredness or loss of energy have been described by patients with cancer as forcing them to withdraw from family, work, social, and recreational activities (Ferrell *et al.*1996; Glaus *et al.* 1996; Ream and Richardson 1997; Berger 1998); activities identified as being important aspects of constructions of self-worth and self-esteem (Radley and Billig 1996; van Manen 1998). Relinquishing social and occupational roles may lead patients to experience intense feelings of isolation, a lack of motivation to continue to try to undertake daily activities (Greene *et al.* 1994; Ferrell *et al.* 1996; Smets *et al.* 1998), and feelings of 'spoiled identity' (Goffman 1963) or loss of self (Mathieson and Stam 1995). Supporting those who experience these profound feelings as a result of the diagnosis of a life-threatening illness demands enormous reserves of physical and emotional energy (Biegel *et al.* 1991; Holicky 1996). Furthermore, observing the slow deterioration of a partner has been described as the most difficult aspect of caregiving (Stetz and Hanson 1992), while caring for an individual with high functional impairment (as is often the case with people with advanced cancers) has been shown to be positively correlated with depression and fatigue in the caregiver (Clarke 2002). Nevertheless, there has been an assumption that carers can and will be able to sustain this demanding work largely unaided (Northouse 1984; Corbin and Strauss 1988; Kuyper and Wester 1998; Northouse *et al.* 2002). Evidence presented below suggests that caring for people incapacitated by cancer-related fatigue may lead to strong feelings of isolation, a forced relinquishing of valued roles, and a renegotiation of identity on the part of carers. Coupled with demanding physical care responsibilities, this may contribute to the development and experience of fatigue amongst carers (Teel and Press 1999).

This chapter draws on empirical data from qualitative studies focusing on the experiences of carers of people with cancer. It begins with a consideration of lay caring and then moves on to explore the impact of a cancer diagnosis on carers. The impact of cancer-related fatigue on patients and the subsequent consequences of this for carers are then discussed. Key factors shaping carers' experiences of their own fatigue, and their perceptions of cancer-related fatigue as it affects patients, are presented. In conclusion, recommendations for practice development are highlighted.

Caring and carers

Caring is a complex and much defined concept (Pasacreta and McCorkle 2000; Thomas *et al.* 2002). Within the context of social support networks, it has been defined as being concerned with helping, supporting, protecting, and practical tending, as well as attending to social and familial responsibilities (Twigg and Atkin 1994). Key components of informal or lay caring have been summarized as helping another, usually a family member living with the carer, perform tasks not normally shared between adults, such as washing, dressing, or toileting. These acts of caring have largely and, sometimes erroneously, been associated with a readiness, ability, and moral imperative to care, based on assumptions of love or affection (James 1998). However defined, these acts, provided away from professional healthcare settings, have traditionally been hidden, undervalued, and overlooked (James 1998).

The task of defining 'carers' is acknowledged as being problematic. A number of government policy documents published in the UK (DOH 1995, 1999, 2000) have used the term 'informal carers' to convey unwaged caring, provided out of love by family, friends, or neighbours and largely in the patient or dependant's own home. These definitions, however, are largely devoid of any indication of the considerable psychosocial costs or physical burden of caring. Clear distinctions are drawn between formal and informal caring, with the latter depicted as the mainstay of community care, backed up, during times of crisis or when carers are in need of respite, by formal care networks (Twigg and Atkin 1994). However, the term 'informal carer' is problematic. James (1998) describes it as 'whimsical' (p. 216) and misleading, implying that carers have some form of choice as to whether they wish to undertake or sustain a caring role. Others view the term more favourably (Thomas *et al.* 2002), believing it to be a way of distinguishing between individuals providing care within and away from the professional, voluntary, or charitable sectors. The term 'caregivers' offers no overt distinction between professional carers or family members providing care, and again suggests little in terms of carer choice. It does, however, suggest an active caregiving role and conveys the physically supportive ethos of caring for a family member or friend. Although widely used, the term 'lay carers' has also been criticized on the grounds that it has the potential to devalue skilled caring activities often developed over prolonged periods of time (James 1998). This downgrading of the skills inherent to 'care by the community' may denigrate the contribution of carers, adding further to their isolation and altered self-concept (Holicky 1996).

James (1998) advocates the use of the term 'unwaged carer', as it serves to remind us of the many possible costs to non-professional providers of care. Nevertheless, she acknowledges that this term also has its limitations, as it may imply that cost of care, rather than its value, should be the prime focus for those involved and affected. Arksey *et al.* (1998), in a study of the needs of young adults with complex disabilities, found that carers did not identify with the label 'carer', preferring instead to describe themselves in relation to their relationship to the young adult. That is, as mother, father, brother, or friend. This raises important questions about the future utility of the term 'carer' within the context of family-oriented care.

The term 'involved other' is sometimes used to describe lay, informal, or unwaged carers. It is helpful in that it allows for the inclusion of any member of one's social support network as a carer. The word 'involvement' also conveys a sense of the commitment required to provide the physical (care for) and emotional (care about) work necessary to support patients with cancer (Thomas *et al.* 2002). Being involved, willingly or otherwise, highlights how a permanent aspect of 'others' lives are affected by a cancer diagnosis (Grbich *et al.* 2001; Thomas *et al.* 2002), mirroring language used by carers in qualitative studies undertaken to explore their needs (Wilson 1991; Ferrell *et al.* 2002; Thomas *et al.* 2002): 'This is not just her disease, it is mine too' (husband in Wilson 1991, p. 248). Each of the terms considered has its strengths and limitations. However, for the sake of brevity and convenience, the term 'carer' is used throughout the remainder of this chapter.

Cancer and caring

Greater numbers of patients with cancer are living longer with treatments often provided during short hospital admissions or on an outpatient basis. Consequently, the need for carers to look after dependent or very sick individuals, who require physical and emotional care for extended periods of time, is increasing. Carers are known to take on practical and emotional care work, often at considerable personal, physical, and emotional health costs to themselves (Teel and Press 1999; Plant 2000; Harden *et al.* 2002). They report experiencing one or more of the following (Wilson 1991; Holicky 1996; Krishnasamy 1997*a*; Kuyper and Wester 1998; Enyert and Burman 1999; Plant 2000; Grbich *et al.* 2001; Thomas *et al.* 2002):

- greater vulnerability to physical illness
- insomnia
- exhaustion
- anxiety
- depression
- frustration
- resentment
- fear

- social isolation
- role conflict
- financial hardship.

However, these findings do not imply that the experience of caregiving is universally negative. Nijboer *et al.* (2000) and Koop and Strang (2003) found that, as consequences of taking on a caring role, family members of people with cancer reported a sense of accomplishment, improved family relationships, comfort, and fulfilment.

Factors affecting carers' perceptions of fatigue

The relief of debilitating and distressing symptoms is described as an essential feature of quality cancer and palliative care, and has been shown to be crucial to an individual's ability to cope with the challenges of a caregiving role (Stetz and Hanson 1992). Unrelieved symptoms are not only known to induce patient reports of reduced quality of life, but are also increasingly recognized as having profound effects on the psychological well-being of carers (Payne *et al.* 1999). When symptoms are regarded as being poorly defined and understood, as is the case with cancer-related fatigue (see Chapter 4), attempts at minimizing the functional and emotional impact is further complicated. The repercussions for those observing the effects of unresolved symptoms on the lives of patients may be especially stressful, particularly if they are also attempting to take on the tasks and roles that their relative is no longer able to undertake. The extent to which the resultant distress may affect carers' well-being, contributing to feelings of tiredness or exhaustion, are considered below.

Carers of patients experiencing cancer-related fatigue have been found to report lower levels of functioning and well-being than the patients themselves (Sneeuw *et al.* 1997; Vogelzang *et al.* 1997). Sneeuw *et al.* (1997) concluded that these findings might be due, in part, to carers' proximity to patients, making them acutely aware of the magnitude of the effect of fatigue on patients' lives and the subsequent impact on their own. Findings from studies by Addington-Hall *et al.* (1991); Krishnasamy (1997a, 2000); Payne *et al.* (1999), and Plant (2000), appear to confirm Sneeuw *et al.*'s (1977) findings, where the burden of care shouldered by carers as a result of patients' increasing dependency was repeatedly shown to be a major source of physical and emotional stress. For carers, having to absorb tasks previously undertaken by the patient at a time when their own energy reserves and coping strategies may be stretched to the limit, has been show to lead to intense feelings of frustration and even anger at the person with cancer (Kuyper and Wester 1998; Krishnasamy 2000; Plant 2000): 'When he is in pain, it just irritates me. Well damn, I walk around healthy and he's always in pain; that really is hard to bear, you know' (wife in Kuyper and Wester 1998, p. 247).

Table 7.1 provides a summary of factors likely to contribute to carers' own tiredness and its likely consequences. Following this, insights from empirical studies undertaken

Table 7.1 Factors contributing to fatigue

Factors contributing to fatigue	Potential consequences
Fatigue is often viewed as a symptom of, or antecedent to, anxiety and depression (see Chapters 1 and 4). Feelings of anxiety, sadness, anticipation of loss, or fear of loss have repeatedly been identified as sources of stress and unmet need amongst carers of people with cancer (Plant 2000)	Loss of social roles caused by increased caregiver responsibilities may lead to intense feelings of isolation on the part of the carer. When this affects employment there may also be considerable negative financial repercussions, which contribute to feelings of anxiety and fatigue
Certain variables influence an individual's resistance and response to stress. They include, the source of the stress (physiological, psychological, or situational), the impact of the stress, stress resistance, available coping mechanisms, and duration of the stress response (Aistars 1987; Weiner and Dodd 1993). The hypothesis that prolonged stress causes fatigue can readily be applied to people with cancer and their carers, who often experience extreme stress that continues for prolonged periods of time. For some carers cancer may initially have been perceived as a disease of short duration, necessitating an intense but time-limited care burden. The reality for many, however, is that the role of primary caregiver may last several months or years, considerably outstripping their physical and emotional energy reserves (Payne et al. 1999).	Overexertion has been identified as a cause of fatigue, specifically with younger patients with cancer who try to maintain busy, active lives, during chemotherapy and radiotherapy (Irvine et al.1994). For carers trying to balance family responsibilities, work commitments, financial stability, and physical care tasks the potential for exhaustion is apparent
Problems with relationships, loss of partners, or social roles all impact negatively on self-esteem and feelings of well-being (Mathieson and Stam 1995). Negative perceptions of self-worth have been linked to feelings of fatigue, depression, and anxiety. Often undisclosed feelings such as resentment or anger towards the patient as a result of the severe limitations imposed on the carer's life may further contribute to their sense of low self-worth and subsequently contribute to feelings of fatigue (Holicky 1996; Kuyper and Wester 1998)	The period around waiting for diagnostic tests and results, suspicion and confirmation of recurrence of disease, or commencement of new treatments, can be highly anxiety-provoking for patients and carers. Fatigue may be exacerbated at these crisis points when carers have described themselves as being ill-informed, excluded, or overlooked by healthcare professionals (Holicky 1996; Plant 2000)

(continued)

Table 7.1 (continued) Factors contributing to fatigue

Factors contributing to fatigue	Potential consequences
Observing the effects of poorly controlled symptoms have been identified by carers as sources of considerable distress (Addington-Hall et al. 1991; Wilson 1991; Payne et al. 1999; Krishnasamy et al. 2000). Given the lack of proven interventions for managing the fatigue and its related distress, watching its impact on sick individuals (Krishnasamy 1997a) may exacerbate feelings of fatigue and distress amongst carers.	A reluctance, or inability, to turn to others, whether family, friends, or neighbours, for practical or emotional support has been identified as a feature of carers' coping strategies (Payne et al. 1999; Krishnasamy et al 2001). This may contribute further to feelings of isolation and fatigue
Grief, anticipation of loss, and bereavement impact significantly upon emotional, physiological, cognitive, and behavioural dimensions of an individuals' life and are known to be associated with increased feelings of fatigue. (Jensen and Given 1993) (see Chapter 10)	Low self worth resulting from feelings of powerlessness and lack of recognition by others have been identified as major sources of stress for carers. Reports on the lack of awareness of carers' needs by patients, coupled with feelings of being overlooked by healthcare professionals, have been identified as being distressing to carers, and thus potentially contribute to feelings of fatigue (Holicky 1996; Kuyper and Wester 1998; Plant 2000)
Complaints of nausea, loss of appetite, weight loss, tightness in chest, broken sleep, and insomnia are all common reactions to emotional distress amongst carers of patients with cancer (Plant 2000; Grbich et al. 2001; Thomas et al. 2002). Each in its own way is known to contribute feelings of tiredness. In addition, many carers will themselves to be living with ongoing or long-standing illnesses, many of which will be associated with fatigue, for example cardiac or renal diseases	

with carers of people with cancer are presented to elaborate on ideas presented in Table 7.1.

Emotions: sustaining caring and emotion work

During interviews undertaken by Plant (2000), in a study of carers of people with a common cancer, many relatives cried and gave voice to feelings previously undisclosed. However, there was a strong sense that the majority felt that they must keep some control over their emotions—at least for most of the time. One participant, who described herself as being 'tough' in order to get her husband through his lung cancer treatment, found an outlet when she was on her own:

> ... when I was on my own, took the dogs for a walk, which I do every morning. I'm out in a field, and it's all quiet and you think ... it was just terrible .... I used to have awful sort of sessions ... tears running down my face ... and quickly used to wipe them before Arthur could see me ... because you've got to put on this very brave front the whole time.

> (wife in Plant 2000, p. 5)

Similar coping strategies were described by participants in studies by Wilson (1991), and Thomas *et al.* (2002):

> Somebody said it must be hard for you, I said no it's not hard for me, it's J, J's got the problem not me .... Well I just sort of feel in a way I had to look as though I wasn't being reached, for the sake of the kids as well. You know, I don't mind admitting in the meantime, in the farm buildings, I cried my eyes out.

> (husband in Thomas *et al.* 2002, p. 540)

> When things bothered me, I suffered in silence. I accepted it, and I dealt with it alone.

> (husband in Wilson 1991, p. 265)

Throughout most of the studies reviewed, diagnosis was the time of greatest emotional impact for carers, characterized by initial feelings of being physically shocked, although for many, this resolved with time: 'I couldn't get warm for weeks. I was cold, you know ... really a shock' (Grbich *et al.* 2001, p. 33). However, for some there were longer-term chronic health problems, particularly associated with sleeping or eating. Following the first interview, over half of the relatives in Plant's (2000) study indicated, in the post interview questionnaire, that their sleep was disrupted, and exactly one-half still had sleep disturbance at the third interview (see Chapter 4). In addition, during the initial interview, relatives reported that their eating had been affected by the illness—many of them lost substantial amounts of weight. Jade, the wife of one patient explained:

> But I suppose really your health does deteriorate, you feel tired, you feel irritable, in my case you lose weight, you find it hard to put it back on, you're tired, but you can't sleep, and it does catch up with you in the end.

> (Plant 2000, p. 28)

The daughter of one patient in Grbich *et al.*'s study of 12 bereaved carers explained:

> I think it is very stressful on people who care for people .... I went to the doctor a few weeks ago. I had this tightness in my stomach area and they said it's probably an ulcer, or a lot of stomach acid build up.

> (Grbich *et al.* 2001, p. 33)

Sabo *et al.* (1986) found that the husbands of women with breast cancer reported increased moodiness, loss of energy, and growing fears about their own health and death. They attribute this to the men denying their own feelings and placing those of their wives in the foreground of their thoughts, thus intensifying their deeper anxieties. The wife of a patient who took part in Krishnasamy's (1997*a*) case study explained the intense and complex feelings that this could engender:

> Diane [district nurse] said to me do you feel cross at him because he just can't do anything and sleeps and I just cried it was such a relief ... but I know now that it's OK and we talked a lot about why I feel cross about David getting ill and then being so tired not doing anything and dying.

> (Krishnasamy 1997*a*, p. 3)

Increasing physical dependence leading to a reliance on carers for often very basic daily activities has been identified as a major source of stress for carers (Hull 1990; Holicky 1996; Kuyper and Wester 1998; Enyert and Burman 1999):

> Some days you just want to forget about it all and just be able to do things like you used to without having to think will she be ok if I go out for an hour or so.

> (husband in Krishnasamy 1997*a*, p. 8)

> I've got the feeling that you are a kind of prisoner. I don't know exactly how to say this .... If you want to go somewhere, it is: just let me know ... but before you just did it. Now you've got to ... well, you don't have to, but you want as much as possible to take each other into account, and that, I sometimes find that rather difficult.

> (wife in Kuyper and Wester 1998, p. 242)

With the change in a patient's physical and emotional well-being, normal relationships, roles, and patterns of interaction can all be disrupted, further reinforcing the impact of a cancer diagnosis, and its side-effects, on the whole family (Hull 1990; Given *et al.* 1993; Beach 1995). These disruptions were evident in the lives of carers as a consequence of fatigue on the patients:

> Well it's just a nightmare I know everyone says that but you feel like it's all just fallen apart all around you and just when you are um falling away, in a big hole and trying not to show ... he's got no energy to do anything so you have to find some extra strength to pick up all the things he'd normally do and then lots of other things get left and I suppose it doesn't matter but it's all upside down you know ... it feels not all the time but it feels like there's nothing right anywhere.

> (wife in Krishnasamy 1997*a*, p. 7)

> I was already exhausted, physically and emotionally. It was not easy to switch gears and summon whatever reserves still existed inside of me, but I knew it was absolutely necessary to do so.

> (family carer in Brown and Stetz 1999, p. 195)

Taking on additional responsibilities, which alter a person's long-established daily routines, has been reported to result in feelings of resentment or frustration directed at the ill person (Stetz and Hanson 1992). Subsequent feelings of guilt were commonly reported (Hull 1990; Kristjanson and Ashcroft 1994; Krishnasamy 1997*b*; Thomas *et al.* 2002):

> I counted up one day—because she lies on here and I sit over there—and within 10 minutes I was up 15 times. Just put me pillow right, just pick me up, just put me down, you know, frustration really.

> (Thomas *et al.* 2002, p. 536)

> God you think how much longer can I keep doing everything and then I feel terrible like I'm only worried about me, but some days … I could scream at him and say for God sake make an effort … then I feel absolutely washed out because I'm tired from the effort of it and then getting myself into such a state.

> (wife in Krishnasamy 1997*a*, p. 9)

> It troubled me a great deal, the anger, resentment. It's a very mixed-up time, you don't know what your emotions are.

> (husband in Wilson 1991, p. 249)

A consideration of the experiences presented above suggests that the physical and psychological manifestations described as accompanying a diagnosis of cancer set in motion a process that impacts on carers' emotional and physical reserves of energy. As the disease progresses the increasing demands on the carers' energy reserves affect their ability (but often not their willingness or desire) to care, sometimes leading to feelings of being overwhelmed by the caring role, whilst at other times giving rise to feelings of fulfilment and satisfaction as described below.

Caring in isolation

Work by Wellard (1998) and Mishel (1988) has identified uncertainty as a facet of chronic illness, noting that unpredictability, in relation to the impact illness and its treatments make on patients' lives, may be particularly difficult to cope with. However, unpredictability allows room for hope and scope for ongoing reconstruction of one's situation, and this may be particularly beneficial during the early stages of a serious illness. For the friends and relatives of patients with advancing disease this may be more difficult to accept, as lack of clarification of the contextual significance of problems witnessed may only add further to the pressures of caring or lead to feelings of ambivalence towards professional carers:

> It really seems to me he [the doctor] meant: stay out of this will you? You're not the patient, are you? .... Finally you think I'll keep my mouth shut.

> (partner in Kuyper and Wester 1998, p. 246)

A lack of information from professionals as to the nature and course of illness, or ways of minimizing illness-related problems, has been described as a key source of distress to carers (Krishnasamy 1997*b*; Kuyper and Wester 1998; Rogers *et al.* 2000; Plant 2000; Grbich *et al.* 2001): 'It's the not knowing, the not knowing was the most stressful' (Wilson 1991, p. 244). And:

> ... we were never invited to discuss his condition .... I felt that we were gathering information from several people, squirreling it out of them.

> (Rogers *et al.* 2000, p. 770)

In Krishnasamy's study (1997*a*) each of the carers interviewed volunteered explanations of how they had 'worked out' for themselves the effect of fatigue on the patient, and what its presence and unrelenting nature came to convey about the patient's prognosis:

> I suppose when you see someone having to just sleep more and more you can't keep pretending, well not pretending perhaps you just stop hoping for because it's just not like there's any way back now well that's what I think about it, it's like the last thing just taking over ... in a way it's like you know what to expect.

> (wife in Krishnasamy 1997*a*, p. 12)

The process of having to work out for oneself what the tiredness or exhaustion meant, whilst struggling with feelings an inability to protect the patient from the impact of functional limitations, and the emotional distress associated with it, were described as an unnecessary additional source of stress. As a result, carers reported that their own energy levels were diminished and their ability to sustain the caring role jeopardized. Providing practical support for patients was particularly difficult when there were other demands on the carer's time:

> ... people say well you've only got to get a prescription ... but you go back 'cos in between you've got to empty a commode, you've got to pick your children up from school, you've got to get your house work done ... so you can't hang around waiting for a prescription, you're backwards and forwards.

> (daughter in Plant 2000, p. 16)

In studies undertaken by Oberst *et al.* (1989), Carey *et al.* (1991), McCorkle *et al.* (1993), Holicky (1996), and Thomas *et al.* (2002) emotional support was described as requiring the most effort for carers. Only 7% of the bereaved families surveyed in Addington-Hall *et al.*'s (1995) study found caring for their dying relative burdensome, whilst 53% found it rewarding. Such was the case for carers in Plant (2000) and Grbich *et al.*'s (2001) studies:

> I think I get ... not pleasure, you can't say that ... I feel I'm doing something if I'm doing it for him ... you know I can do it ... so I'd rather not have people do it for him, because I can do it.

(wife in Plant 2000, p. 12)

> It felt good I was able to manage, and I was happy that I managed and I enjoyed managing. I mean I did get ... it gave me a good feeling inside and she appreciated it.

(Grbich *et al.* 2001, p. 33)

This could nevertheless prove exhausting and the wife in Plant's (2000) study (cited above) fractured both her wrists during the study period (about 13 months), however she consistently refused any outside help from friends, family members, or professionals. This was a recurrent theme throughout many of the papers reviewed:

> ... you don't like to ask other people to help they've got their own families ... so you carry on

(wife in Krishnasamy 1997*a*, p. 3)

The interviews in Plant's (2000) study illustrated high levels of tension in the carers' situation. The need to 'do' something to combat the more existential concerns was further illustrated by the frantic cleaning undertaken by some to get through a difficult time. This could be seen as a way of creating some order in the external, if not the internal, world. Certainly the carers in the early stages of the illness expressed little ability to relax or to be able to think about doing anything for themselves:

> Stephen was gonna be operated on the Friday morning ... so I pulled my house apart Friday morning, I cleaned every nook and cranny possible.

(wife in Plant 2000, p. 4)

Most of these relatives, despite operating within reasonably cohesive family structures, appeared to be isolated and had little support, understanding, or advice from the health professionals concerned. They were invariably emotionally and physically exhausted, with few means of resting, relaxing, reflecting, or sharing the tensions. Evidence suggests that the needs of lay carers are hidden, both from professional carers and indeed patients themselves, with as few as 29% (61) of patients identifying that the lay carers also had needs (Kuyper and Wester 1998: Krishnasamy *et al.* 2001). In a qualitative study of family caregivers of women diagnosed with ovarian cancer carers expressed little concern for their own physical well-being, despite reporting limited support, feelings of isolation, and considerable anxiety in relation to the nature of the disease (Ferrell *et al.* 2002). In the absence of any professional, cohesive, supportive care strategy directed specifically at their needs, their ability to sustain the caring role appeared to rely, almost exclusively, on personal strength and a commitment to the sick relative:

> I was desperate a couple of times for someone to talk to ... you'd like to have been able to talk to somebody or just you know, just to be reassured.

(Grbich *et al.* 2001, p. 34)

The exhaustion of uncertainty

A diagnosis of cancer has been described as creating a world of experiences (Feigenberg 1995), one in which all of those affected by it are bombarded with fluctuating emotions, reactions, and realities. The majority of participants in Plant's (2000) study found it difficult to think carefully about what the diagnosis of cancer in someone close meant to them personally. Although in the past participants may have thought about death in the abstract, they were now faced with a real threat to someone they cared about. Despite some improvements in treatment and survival rates, cancer appears to have a unique ability to inspire fear and dread—and the participants in each of the studies were no exception to this. For example in Plant's (2000) study, despite being assured that her husband's testicular cancer was curable, Debra was deeply distressed and unable to tell her husband, with whom she usually shared her worries, of her great fear that he might die. With her parents telling her that she must 'be braver', Debra felt very isolated by the experience. She described how she saw things:

> You've got this black tunnel and that's all you can see is that black tunnel, nothing else.

> (Debra in Plant 2000, p. 7)

Similarly the wife of a patient with colorectal cancer in Thomas *et al*.'s (2002) study stated:

> And he [the personnel officer] said ... well you've got to be strong ... and I thought afterwards ... well why have I got to be strong, because I'm as vulnerable as anyone else? And I feel like I'm taking it all on my shoulders.

> (Thomas *et al.* 2002, p. 540)

Carers often described not knowing where they could take their own distress, talking about it was difficult and invariably suppressed by their need to protect the patient's well-being. They did not feel supported by any of their own current support systems particularly as, for many, the person with cancer had been the central to these:

> I was not able to tell him about my work anymore, I couldn't speak to him anymore because he was exhausted; that just wasn't possible anymore. He could not be open for that anymore and I found that difficult. If you can't talk about things like that, what is left?

> (Kuyper and Wester 1998, p. 244)

For many, their world was turned upside down but they felt that their role in this was to keep everything going as 'normally' as possible, without revealing too much of their own inner turmoil. Hence they experienced feelings of loneliness, lack of control, and fear. Rosenblatt (1988) uses symbolic interaction theory to try to understand the effect of grief (actual or threatened) on individuals, and states:

> ... part of the social context for understanding, organising, validating, and defining feeling, action, values, and priorities is removed .... Thus grief can be seen as arising not only because of a loss of a person but also because of losing part of the foundation for dealing with loss and with all of experience.

> (Rosenblatt 1988, p. 68)

From the studies reviewed it was evident that, for many carers, there is a deep 'existential' element to this experience which may be difficult to identify or talk about. In essence it is a sense of unreality and fundamental loss of bearings created by the threat to the life of a loved one:

> When you first get to know … gosh, you feel as though you're the only one, you know. Shock at finding she had it [cancer], because the first diagnosis was anaemia, and immediate shock after that and then rather dull [when it became clear the tumour was inoperable and death inevitable]
>
> (Grbich *et al.* 2001, p. 32)

For many the opportunity to relax and enjoy things was, at least, temporarily banished. If the patient's condition deteriorated this was exacerbated. A sense of not being able to *do* anything to change what was happening was one of the most difficult experiences for many of the relatives, as the following quotation illustrates:

> … it's a waiting game, and in the meantime Jonathan is deteriorating. And that's the hardest thing to do, is to sit and wait, and to watch, it's a watching game. And when you see someone you love deteriorating … well it's heart wrenching, see.
>
> (wife in Plant 2000, p. 5).

In Krishnasamy's (1997*a*) study, with the increasing realization that the fatigue was becoming ever more pervasive carers began to piece together the reality of the patient's situation as the inevitability of death was conveyed through the physical demise and emotional withdrawal of the individual before them:

> … you know there's no cure right from the start … I was looking for things to change for David to become weaker and so when he started to have less energy and lose weight I thought well here we go, you know, it's all part of it … for David it says I'm dying.
>
> (wife in Krishnasamy 1997*a*, p. 2)

For some, this was a 'boundary' time, living with an increasing recognition of the imminence of death:

> it's like being at a boundary between wanting him to pick up but not wanting him to keep going like this, like I said, this isn't Tom
>
> (wife in Krishnasamy 1997*a*, p. 12).

The fatigue observed by carers in Krishnasamy's (1997*a*) study was not described as a discrete symptom, with contained boundaries and distinct properties. Instead they talked of a problem that affected all aspects of the patient and family's life, forcing changes in perceptions of self as husband, wife, mother, or father, to cancer patient, cancer relative, friend, and carer, and ultimately to terminally ill patient or bereaved lay carer. Similarly painful redefinitions have been described elsewhere:

> At one time I was lifting, doing all the shopping, doing all the bags, I found I was having to do everything. Whereas I used to rely on [him] for doing things … . But I suppose our life has changed [in] a matter of three months, it's just totally changed.
>
> (wife in Thomas *et al.* 2002, p. 536)

Recommendations for research and practice

The following recommendations are adapted from Plant (2001, p. 96) (see also Box 7.1):

- There is an urgent requirement to develop and evaluate supportive care strategies targeted at meeting the explicit needs of carers of patients with cancer. This can be achieved by listening to and acknowledging what is important for relatives as they try to care for people affected by cancer-related fatigue.

- Those involved in practice and research initiatives should not assume that they know who constitutes the 'family'.

- There is a need to provide a supportive environment where relatives can recount their own experiences of living with, and witnessing, cancer-related fatigue, and where they can express distress.

- Cancer-related fatigue is a complex and unpredictable symptom that may give rise to feelings of frustration and resentment. Professionals need to be aware of the possible need to facilitate family communication around this challenging problem.

- Cancer-related fatigue affects people differently. The importance of attending key consultations with the family, and an awareness of the need to tailor information to each family's needs, is vital to promote self-efficacy in the management and prevention of fatigue for patients and carers.

- Cancer-related fatigue requires multi-professional input if it is to be effectively managed. Ensuring that family members know how to contact key professionals, when they are available, and making referrals to other relevant professionals is essential where necessary.

Box 7.1 Future areas for research

- Identifying and evaluating strategies to support carers of patients with cancer present important areas of research hitherto overlooked.

- Designing collaborative, exploratory studies to elicit behaviours and services perceived to be helpful should be undertaken in the first instance.

- Studies to elicit the constraints that exist on carers to support patients to the best of their (desired) capacity are urgently needed.

- Intervention studies, designed in response to data elicited from exploratory needs assessment projects, focusing on identifying pragmatic ways of introducing, resourcing, and sustaining lay carer-oriented initiatives in primary and acute care settings should be undertaken.

Conclusion

A large body of research now exists to indicate that lay carers are dramatically affected by a diagnosis of cancer and the subsequent caring roles associated with it (see Box 7.2). However, this reality seems to be slow to be translated into healthcare practice, with the majority of services continuing to be almost unilaterally directed at patients, with little or no evidence of attempts at reconfiguration of services to meet, or empirical studies to address, the needs of this large and important body of people (Yates 1999; Krishnasamy *et al.* 2001; Thomas *et al.* 2002).

In order to provide support for those close to someone with cancer there are many practical concerns that need to be addressed, both for professionals and for carers. Regardless of the individual's social circumstances, there are certain barriers (often psychological) to providing help and information for them. Healthcare is largely reactive, so where a problem is not immediately apparent it is less likely to be addressed. In a climate of stretched resources, the focus of professional care has to be with the person who is sick. Indeed this is what carers themselves would want. Some are able to make their needs known to professional carers but, as has been illustrated here, many may not.

The carers' ways of managing the situation, emotionally and practically, need to be worked *with*. Effective support requires careful listening and sensitive negotiation. However, as Cribb (2001) acknowledges, the immeasurable issues of caring, which are often 'informal and invisible' even when undertaken by health professionals, are often neglected by influential policy makers, or even in the day-to-day running of a ward.

Box 7.2 Summary points

- Lay carers are an integral part of a cancer patient's care from diagnosis through to the conclusion of treatment or death.

- Carers bring with them their own values, beliefs, attitudes, and emotions, all of which may affect their ability or desire to care for the individual with cancer as well as impact on the patient's own psychosocial outcomes.

- The needs of carers continue to be an overlooked and neglected aspect of professional healthcare provision—often at considerable emotional and physical cost to the caregivers.

- Lay carers have considerable emotional and practical support needs.

- Carers often have an immense knowledge of the needs and preferences of the patients, information crucial to the delivery of meaningful, expert healthcare.

References

Addington-Hall, J., MacDonald, L., Anderson, H., and Freeling, P. (1991) Dying from cancer: the views of bereaved family and friends about the experiences of terminally ill patients. *Palliative Medicine*, **5**, 207–14.

Aistars, J. (1987) Fatigue in the cancer patient: a conceptual approach to a clinical problem. *Oncology Nursing Forum*, **14**(6), 25–30.

Arksey, H., Heaton, J., and Sloper, P. (1998) Carers tell it like it is. *Health Services Journal*, **108**(5588), 32–3.

Beach, D.L. (1995) Caregiver discourse: perceptions of illness-related dialogue. *The Hospice Journal*, **10**(3), 13–25.

Berger, A. (1998) Patterns of fatigue and activity and rest during adjuvant breast cancer chemotherapy. *Oncology Nursing Forum*, **25**(1), 51–62.

Biegel, D.E., Sales, E., and Schultz, R. (1991) *Family Care Giving in Chronic Illness: Alzheimer's Disease, Cancer, Heart Disease, Mental Illness, and Stroke.* Sage, Newbury Park, CA.

Brown, M.A. and Stetz, K. (1999) The labor of caregiving: a theoretical model of caregiving during potentially fatal illness. *Qualitative Health Research*, **9**(2), 182–97.

Carey P., Oberst M., McCubbin M., and Hughs S. (1991) Appraisal and caregiving burden in family members caring for patients receiving chemotherapy. *Oncology Nursing Forum*, **18**, 1341–8.

Clarke, P.C. (2002) Effects of individual and family hardiness on caregiver depression and fatigue. *Research in Nursing and Health*, **25**(1), 37–48.

Corbin, J.M. and Strauss, A. (1988) *Unending Work and Care: Managing Chronic Illness at Home.* Jossey-Bass, San Francisco.

Cribb, A. (2001) Knowledge and caring: a philosophical and personal perspective. In: *Cancer Nursing: Care in Context* (ed. J. Corner and C. Bailey), pp. 12–25. Blackwell Science, Oxford.

Department of Health. (1995) Carers (recognition and services) Act. HMSO, London.

Department of Health. (1999) Caring about carers. A national strategy for carers. http://www.doh.gov.uk/carers.htm

Department of Health. (2002) Carers and disabled children's act. The Stationery Office, London.

Enyert, G. and Burman, M.E. (1999) A qualitative study of self-transcendence in caregivers of terminally ill patients. *American Journal of Hospice and Palliative Care*, **16**(2), 455–62.

Feigenberg, L. (1985) *Psychosocial Aspects of Cancer and Cancer Care.* Stockholm: The Swedish Cancer Society.

Ferrell, B., Ervin, K., Smith, S., Marek, T., and Melancon, C. (2002) Family perspectives of ovarian cancer. *Cancer Practice*, **19**(6), 269–76.

Ferrell, B., Grant, M., Dean, G., Funk, B., and Ly, J. (1996) 'Bone tired': the experience of fatigue and its impact on quality of life. *Oncology Nursing Forum*, **23**(10), 1539–47.

Given, C.W., Stommel, M., Given, B., Osuch, J., Kurtz, M.E., and Kurtz, J.C. (1993) The influence of cancer patients' symptoms and functional states on patients' depression and family caregivers' reaction and depression. *Health Psychology*, **12**(4), 277–85.

Glaus, A., Crow, R., and Hammond, S. (1996) A qualitative study to explore the concept of fatigue/tiredness in cancer patients and in healthy individuals. *European Journal of Cancer Care*, **5**(Supplement 2), 8–23.

Goffman, E. (1963) *Stigma. Notes on the Management of Spoiled Identity.* Simon and Schuster, New York.

Greene, D., Nail, L., Fieler, V., Dudgeon D., and Jones, L. (1994) A comparison of patient-reported side effects among three chemotherapy regimes for breast cancer. *Cancer Practice*, **2**(1), 57–62.

Grbich, C., Parker, D., and Maddocks, I. (2001) The emotions and coping strategies of caregivers of family members with a terminal cancer. *Journal of Palliative Care*, **17**(1), 30–6.

Harden, J., Schafenacker, A., Northouse, L., Mood, D., Smith, D., Pienta, K. *et al.* (2002) Couples' experiences with prostate cancer: focus group research. *Oncology Nursing Forum*, **29**(4), 701–9.

Holicky, R. (1996) Caring for the caregivers: the hidden victims of illness and disability. *Rehabilitation Nursing*, **21**(5), 247–52.

Hull, M.M. (1990) Sources of stress for hospice caregiving families. *Hospice Journal*, **6**(2), 29–54.

Irvine, D., Vincent, L., Graydon, J., Bubela, N., and Thompson, L. (1994) The prevalence and correlates of fatigue in patients receiving treatment with chemotherapy and radiotherapy. A comparison with the fatigue experienced by healthy individuals. *Cancer Nursing*, **17**(5), 367–78.

James, V. (1998) Unwaged carers and the provision of health care. In: *Sociological Perspectives on Health, Illness and Health Care* (ed. D. Field and S. Taylor), pp. 211–29. Blackwell Science, Oxford.

Jensen, S. and Given B. (1993) Fatigue affecting family caregivers of cancer patients. *Supportive Care in Cancer*, **1**(6), 321–5.

Koop, P.M. and Strang, V.R. (2003) The bereavement experience following home-based family caregiving for persons with advanced cancer, *Clinical Nursing Research*, **12**(2), 127–44.

Krishnasamy, M. (1997a) *An Exploration of the Nature and Impact of Fatigue in Advanced Cancer. A Case Study*. Macmillan Practice Development Unit, Centre for Cancer and Palliative Care Studies, Institute of Cancer Research, London.

Krishnasamy, M. (1997b) An exploration of the nature and impact of fatigue in advanced cancer. *International Journal of Palliative Nursing*, **3**(3), 126–31.

Krishnasamy, M. (2000) Fatigue in advanced cancer-meaning before measurement? *International Journal of Nursing Studies*, **37**, 401–14.

Krishnasamy M., Wilkie E., and Haviland J. (2001) Lung cancer health care needs assessment: Patients' and informal carers' responses to a national mail questionnaire survey. *Palliative Medicine*, **15**(3), 213–27.

Kristjanson, L.J. and Ashcroft, T. (1994) The family's cancer journey: a literature review. *Cancer Nursing*, **17**(1), 1–17.

Kuyper, M.B. and Wester, F. (1998) In the shadow: the impact of chronic illness on the patient's partner. *Qualitative Health Research*, **8**(2), 237–53.

Mathieson, C.M. and Stam, H.J. (1995) Renegotiating identity: cancer narratives. *Sociology of Health and Illness*, **17**(3), 283–306.

McCorkle, R., Shegda Yost, L., Jepson, C., Malone, D., Baird, S., and Lusk, E. (1993) A cancer experience: relationship of patient psychosocial responses to care-giver burden over time. *Psycho-Oncology*, **2**, 21–32.

Mishel, M.H. (1988) Uncertainty in illness. *Image: Journal of Nursing Scholarship*, **20**(4), 225–32.

Nijboer, C., Triemstra, M., Tempelaar, R., Mulder M., Sanderman R., and van den Bos, G.A. (2000) Patterns of caregiver experiences among partners of cancer patients. *Gerontologist*, **40**(6), 738–46.

Northouse, L. (1984) The impact of cancer on the family: an overview. *International Journal of Psychiatry in Medicine*, **14**, 215–42.

Northouse, L., Mood, D., Kershaw, T., Scafenacker, A., Mellon, S., Wall, J. *et al.* (2002) Quality of life of women with recurrent breast cancer and their family members. *Journal of Clinical Oncology*, **20**(19), 4050–64.

Oberst, M., Thomas, S., Gass, K., and Ward, S. (1989) Caregiving demands and appraisal of stress amongst family caregiverss. *Cancer Nursing*, **12**, 209–15.

Pasacreta, J.V. and McCorkle, R. (2000) Cancer care: impact of interventions on caregiver outcomes. *Annual Review of Nursing Research*, **18**, 127–48.

Payne, S., Smith, P., and Dean, S. (1999) Identifying the concerns of informal carers in palliative care. *Palliative Medicine*, **13**(1), 37–44.

Plant, H. (2000) Living with cancer. Understanding the experiences of close relatives of people with cancer. Unpublished Ph.D. thesis, University of London.

Plant, H. (2001) The impact of cancer on the family. In: *Cancer Nursing: Care in Context* (ed. J. Cornerand C. Bailey), pp. 86–99. Blackwell Science, Oxford.

Radley, A. and Billig, M. (1996) Accounts of health and illness: dilemmas and representations. *Sociology of Health and Illness*, **18**(2), 220–40.

Ream, E. and Richardson, A. (1997) Fatigue in patients with cancer and chronic obstructive airways disease: a phenomenological enquiry. *International Journal of Nursing Studies*, **34**(1), 44–53.

Rogers, A., Karlsen, S., and Addington-Hall, J. (2000) Dying for care: the experiences of terminally ill cancer patients in hospital in an inner city health district. *Palliative Medicine*, **14**(1), 53–4.

Rosenblatt, P. (1988) Grief: the social context of private feelings. *Journal of Social Issues*, **44**, 67–78.

Sabo, B., Brown, J., and Smith, C. (1986) The male role and mastectomy: support group sand men's adjustment. *Journal of Psychosocial Oncology*, **4**, 19–31.

Sandelowski, M. (1986) The problem of rigor in qualitative research. *Advances in Nursing Science*, **8**(3), 27–37.

Smets, E., Visser M., Garssen, B., Frijda B., Oosterveld, P., and deHaes, J. (1998) Understanding the level of fatigue in cancer patients undergoing radiotherapy. *Journal of Psychosomatic Research*, **45**(3), 277–93.

Sneeuw, K.C.A., Aaronson, K.N., and Sprangers, M.A.G. (1997) Value of caregiver ratings in evaluating the quality of life of patients with cancer. *Journal of Clinical Oncology*, **15**, 1206–17.

Stetz, K.M. and Hanson, W.K. (1992) Alterations in perceptions of caregiving demands in advanced cancer during and after the experience. *Hospice Journal*, **8**(3), 21–34.

Teel, C.S. and Press, A.N. (1999) Fatigue amongst elders in caregiving and non-caregiving roles. *Western Journal of Nursing Research*, **21**(4), 498–514.

Thomas, C., Morris, S.M., and Harman, C. (2002) Companions through cancer: the care given by informal carers in cancer contexts. *Social Science and Medicine*, **54**(4), 529–44.

Twigg, J. and Atkin, K. (1994) *Carers Perceived: Policy and Practice in Informal Care*. Open University Press, Buckingham.

van Manen, M. (1998) Modalities of body experience in illness and health. *Qualitative Health Research*, **3**(1), 7–24.

Vogelzang, N.J., Breitbart, W., Cella, D., Curt, G.A., Groopman, J.E., Horning, S.J. *et al.* (1997). Patient, caregiver, and oncologists perceptions of cancer-related fatigue: results of a tripart assessment survey. *Seminars in Hematology*, **34**(3, Supplement 2), 4–12.

Weiner, C.L. and Dodd, M.J. (1993) Coping amid uncertainty: an illness trajectory perspective. *Scholarly Inquiry for Nursing Practice: an International Journal*, **7**(1), 17–31.

Wellard, S. (1998) Constructions of chronic illness. *International Journal of Nursing Studies*, **35**, 49–55.

Wilson, S. (1991) The unrelenting nightmare: husbands experiences during their wives chemotherapy. In: *The Illness Experience, Dimension of Suffering* (ed. J. Morse). Sage, London, pp. 237–314.

Yates, P. (1999) Family coping: issues and challenges for cancer nursing. *Cancer Nursing*, **22**(1), 63–71.

Zarit, S. (1994) Research perspectives on family caregiving. In: *Family Caregiving: Agenda for the Future* (ed. M.H. Cantor), pp. 35–9. American Society on Aging, San Francisco.

Chapter 8

The experience of cancer-related fatigue in children, adolescents, and their families

Marilyn Hockenberry, Pamela Hinds,
Patrick Barrera, Cindy Burleson, Jami Gattuso,
Nancy Kline, Sarah Bottomley, Patricia Alcoser,
and Jill Brace O'Neill

Introduction

Living with cancer may affect every aspect of a child's or adolescent's life, disrupting relationships with family members and friends and having a negative impact on a young person's future development of important social skills (Green 1998; Weinblatt 1998). However, it is precisely these two types of relationship that are critical to the ultimate wellness of a child or adolescent who has been treated for cancer, with adjustment to the disease and to life as a survivor significantly and positively influenced by family functioning and social support (Kellerman *et al.* 1980; Teta *et al.* 1986; Rudin *et al.* 1988; Hockenberry-Eaton and Minick 1994; Hockenberry-Eaton *et al.* 1995).

The 5-year survival rates for childhood cancer approach 75%, with the 3-year survival over 80% (Pizzo and Poplack 2002). Nevertheless, the success of treatment is often attributed to aggressive chemotherapy regimens that may have numerous side-effects, which can be emotional, mental, and physical. These may result in alterations in family and social dynamics, often creating permanent changes within the family, and disrupting the social environment (Spinetta and Deasy-Spinetta 1981; Green 1998; Weinblatt 1998). Frequent absences from school and the inability to participate in physical and leisure activities (Chekryn *et al.* 1986; Bossert and Martinson 1990) have been shown to have a negative impact on a young person's psychosocial well-being. Children and adolescents with cancer experience multiple problems associated with cancer treatment, such as nausea and vomiting that may cause weight loss, nutritional deficits, electrolyte imbalances, weakness, and lethargy (Hockenberry-Eaton and Benner 1990). Infection and fever also occur commonly during treatment (Kline 2002). Although these side-effects are discussed extensively in the literature, there is only limited discussion of fatigue as a symptom experienced by children and adolescents with cancer, and only recently has fatigue been considered a side-effect and a recognized symptom experienced by them.

Prior to the research conducted by the Clinical Research Scholars in Pediatric Oncology (1996 to the present), (Hockenberry-Eaton *et al.* 1998) there was limited information available on the occurrence of fatigue in children and adolescents with cancer. [†]Consequently material presented in this chapter focuses on insights gained from this evidence base.

The research

Work undertaken by the group has contributed to a contextual understanding of fatigue through discussions with children, adolescents, parents, and staff members (Hinds and Kelly 1998; Hinds *et al.* 1999; Hockenberry-Eaton *et al.* 1998). The research was carried out in two phases with the first goal being to define the symptom of fatigue and the second being to develop valid assessment tools of fatigue. In the first phase of the fatigue research, patients and their parents were interviewed and tape-recorded in small focus groups and asked a series of questions which helped to define the symptom of fatigue. A group of expert paediatric oncology nurses then reviewed the transcribed interviews and by consensus developed a definition for fatigue and its associated physical symptoms. In the next phase, clinical assessment tools were developed from the information gathered in the focus group interviews and tested for validation in 150 children with cancer. Valid tools were developed to assess fatigue from the perspective of children, parents, and nursing staff (Hockenberry-Eaton *et al.* 1998; Hockenberry *et al.* 2003; Hockenberry-Eaton and Hinds 2000; Hinds *et al.* 1999; Hinds and Hockenberry-Eaton 2001).

Fatigue in children and adolescents with cancer: definitions, causes, and coping

Definitions and descriptions

The work undertaken by Hockenberry and colleagues has led to an appreciation of fatigue as a debilitating, functionally limiting problem for children and adolescents with cancer, which has a negative impact on the ability to participate in normal daily activities. Descriptions and reports of fatigue found in this group were similar to those identified by children with chronic fatigue syndrome (CFS) (Walford *et al.* 1993; Carter *et al.* 1995, 1996, 1999), as well as by adults with cancer (Knoff 1986; Aistars 1987; Pickard-Holley 1991; Cimprich 1992; Winningham *et al.* 1994; Irvine *et al.* 1994). Like children with CFS and adults with cancer, the children and adolescents described limitations in daily activities, lack of energy, and feelings of extreme tiredness.

[†] In 1996, a grant was obtained from the Oncology Nursing Foundation/Ortho Biotech Foundation to examine fatigue in children and adolescents with cancer.

However, the children with cancer were better able to identify specific causes of fatigue in comparison to children with CFS. In contrast, children with CFS are known to identify fatigue in relation to somatic symptoms such as abdominal pain, headaches, and myalgias, rather than the more generalized non-specific feelings of fatigue described by the children and adolescents with cancer.

Findings from the focus groups undertaken as part of our programme of research reveal that definitions of fatigue vary depending upon the child or adolescent's level of development. For example, adolescents use a comprehensive vocabulary to describe fatigue, and to discuss the differences between mental and physical symptoms. Adolescents also provide much more detailed descriptions of the causes of fatigue than those given by children (Table 8.1).

In the focus group discussions with children and adolescents with cancer, fatigue is described as having both physical and mental (psychological) characteristics (Hockenberry-Eaton *et al.* 1998). All participants discussed changes in their ability to normally perform activities they undertook prior to being diagnosed and treated for cancer. One child stated, 'because I am tired I don't have any energy, I can't run fast or anything'. Limitations in physical abilities were reported to occur and were characterized by being unable to play sports or participate in activities with friends. Some children felt they needed more quiet activities such as watching TV or reading books. Another child stated, 'When I am tired I can watch a movie, I can't read too well anymore because I can't keep my eyes open'. Children were able to identify when fatigue occurred and reported that it occurred most often in the mornings, on school days, and during the week following treatment. Adolescents within the focus groups described physical fatigue as 'you don't feel like your normal self' and mental fatigue as 'tired of everything that has happened'. Not being able to participate and function normally because of feeling tired and the lack of energy were common complaints

Table 8.1 Children's and adolescents' descriptions for fatigue

	Describing fatigue
Child	Hard to move or run Weak/tired When fatigue occurs: physical signs, not able to think, feel like lying around, makes you sad/mad, not able to play, fall asleep easily
Adolescent	Wearing away of your body All in your mind Mental and physical Physical weakness, not normal self Makes you mad Not be bothered Feeling sorry When fatigue occurs: physical symptoms, sleepy, mentally tired, feel like lying around

from adolescents. One young person stated, 'I used to play sports and play with my friends all the time, and now I am on crutches ...'. Another reported, 'you can't hang out with your friends and go to the skating rink'. Mental fatigue was described in terms of feeling sorry for yourself, being mad at the world, or just not wanting to be bothered. Adolescents were also able to describe the compounded influence mental and physical fatigue had upon them:

> you think about it, dwell on it, [and] it makes it worse. So, part of it's mental, part of it's physical.

Some adolescents expressed being mad or upset during treatment:

> ... you're in there getting chemo ... and you feel really bad ... it makes you so mad

Others were able to identify specific times when fatigue occurred stating that it usually followed chemotherapy and when their blood counts were decreased:

> I just felt tired the days I get chemo ...

> When your counts are down, it's really bad ...

Factors contributing to the experience of fatigue

Contributing and alleviating factors of fatigue (Tables 8.2 and 8.3) identified by the children, adolescents, and parents who took part in focus groups as part of Hockenberry-Eaton *et al.*'s. (1998) research fell into the following categories:

♦ environmental

Table 8.2 Causes of fatigue in children and adolescents

	Causes of fatigue	**What helps**
Child	Treatment Pain Low counts Being active Sleep changes Hospital environment	Naps/sleep Fun/activities Visitors
Adolescent	Chemotherapy Hospital environment Sleep position changes Sleep pattern changes Young children making noise Going for treatment Doing too many things Nurses making noise Being bored Treatment side-effects Fear Worry	Going outside Protected rest time Need for medication Physical therapy Having fun Rest/naps Keep busy Blood transfusion

Table 8. 3 Example of a parental diary format used to detect patterns in the ill child's fatigue

	Course 1	Course 2	Course 3
Day 1 (Date):	(Wake/sleep activities)	(Wake/sleep activities)	(Wake/sleep activities)
7–11 a.m.			
11–3 p.m.			
3–7 p.m.			
7–11 p.m.			
11–7 a.m.			
Day 2 (date) etc.			
Day 3 (date) etc.			

- ◆ treatment-related indicators
- ◆ family
- ◆ personal/behavioural.

The environment

Any intervention developed for managing fatigue will therefore need to be inclusive of the needs and perspectives of patients, parents, and healthcare professionals, and be cognisant of the need to target specific aspects of an intervention at the diverse elements of fatigue, that is, the physical, mental, emotional, and spiritual domains. The hospital environment was identified as a frequent cause of fatigue because of the constant interruptions and noises that led to lack of sleep. For example, noises from the nurses' station, younger patients, intravenous infusion pumps, telephones, shutting of doors, and frequent interruptions. Children commented that the hospital environment caused fatigue because of frequent disruptions in sleep:

> When I am in the hospital, I am just so drained when I get home.

Frequent disruptions in sleep whilst in the hospital led to alterations in sleep patterns for some young people, for example, going to sleep late or being woken in the middle of the night. One adolescent described being in the hospital as, 'it's like jet lag'. Another discussed not wanting to sleep while in the emergency room for fear of what might happen while she was asleep.

Worrying about the future and forced lifestyle changes was also found to have an impact upon the adolescents' normal sleep patterns. Young people who were on home-bound education programmes discussed staying up late at night and sleeping late into the morning. This made getting up early in the morning a problem and caused them to be fatigued. When at home, parents described attempts to modify noise levels and other behaviours to decrease the disruptive stimuli around the ill child, chastising family members to control their voice volume in conversations, and limiting the number of friends allowed inside the home at any one time.

Treatment-related indicators

Treatment and the associated side-effects were frequently described as causes of fatigue:

> that's the worst, knowing what's going to happen ... knowing that you have to go do it [chemotherapy], that it's going to wear you out

Treatment-related fatigue was described as altering family plans, as was exposure to typical family activities that could place the ill child at risk for injury or infection, due to abnormal chemistry or haematology values associated with cancer-related treatment and fatigue. The resultant danger appeared to be that the ill child might be excluded from certain scheduled activities or events because of treatment-related fatigue, and families report carefully monitoring the ill child's clinical laboratory reports before determining whether it was safe and prudent to schedule a family outing.

Impact of the child's fatigue on the family

To date, the research and clinical assessments of fatigue in children and adolescents with cancer have focused on the impact of the fatigue on parents and family schedules, but have not directly included the impact on siblings. Therefore, the content in this section is primarily derived from the perspectives of parents regarding their child's fatigue, and its repercussions for the family. The parental perspectives have been derived from data with parents who participated in focus groups, individual interviews, and questionnaires on their child's fatigue (Hockenberry-Eaton *et al.* 1998; Hinds *et al.* 1999).

The perspective of parents

Parents offered their impressions of the causes of their child's fatigue and tended to specify from three to seven causes, suggesting that they recognize the confusing nature of this symptom (Hinds *et al.* 1999). Examples of their perceived causes include environmental characteristics such as noise, altered sleep patterns, treatment effects such as lowered haematocrit, and inadequate nutrition. Furthermore, the parental context of observing and prioritizing fatigue in a sick child has been defined as including multiple layers of demands that compete for parents' attention, and at times decision-making and action (Fig. 8.1), which include:

- the ill child's chances of cure and survival
- the ill child's suffering
- knowledge about the cancer and its treatment
- the drive to be a 'good parent'
- nuclear family and marital demands
- extended family, friends, and other social demands

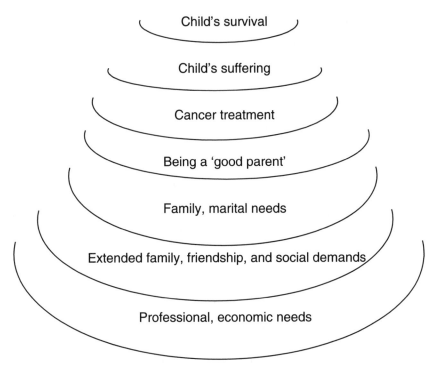

Child's survival

Child's suffering

Cancer treatment

Being a 'good parent'

Family, marital needs

Extended family, friendship, and social demands

Professional, economic needs

Fig. 8.1 Context within which parents perceive fatigue in their ill child.

- ◆ professional and economic demands
- ◆ the parents' experience with their own fatigue.

All of the layers within which the parental experience of fatigue is contextualized potentially exert great influence over parents and at least indirectly over the family. However, the first four layers are especially consuming of parents' attention and energy during the diagnosis and early treatment of their child's disease, and during subsequent intense treatment periods. As a result, without interventions initiated by healthcare professionals regarding the significance of fatigue in the child or adolescent with cancer, parental attention to their child's fatigue will vary based on competing contextual demands and fluctuating concerns. For example, parents of children who have relapsed report a predominant focus on their child's chances of surviving the disease and a lesser concern with symptoms that are secondary to the disease or its treatment (Hinds *et al.* 1996). The risk is that parents will consider fatigue to be a natural part of the cancer experience, and as result, do not spontaneously report their child's fatigue to healthcare providers. They may therefore unwittingly contribute to an underreporting of fatigue and a decreased likelihood of fatigue being treated.

Further confounding this issue is parents' experience of their own fatigue, as the mother of a 15-year-old male youth diagnosed with osteosarcoma described during one focus group meeting:

> It is not easy to keep a smile on your face and let's face it, at the same time, you are battling the fatigue yourself because you are tired, also. It puts a real strain on the entire family at points and times and a lot of it is directly attributed to not so much the medical end of it but the emotional and psychological end to it. That's where the real problem lies. I think it is the mental attitude that makes you physically tired, physically worn out.

These sentiments were emphatically corroborated by another parent in the same focus group:

> …I timed it and I got exactly eight and a half minutes of sleep in seven days, and my daughter got even less than that. So if I was that tired, I could imagine what she felt like. How long does it take your body to recover from something like that? How many months literally, because you put your body into that kind of restraint; it's going to take months for you to recover. Not just days, like I said, when you add on to it the mental stress with what they're going through, what they're facing, the mental stress of what they're doing to their families, their normal lives, their friends. All of these contribute to the fatigue, every bit of it.

(mother of a 10-year-old girl diagnosed with acute lymphoblastic leukaemia)

At the same time as attempting to deal with complexities that are new to them within the context of a serious, threatening situation, parents are in the midst of ongoing family demands, such as those related to the needs of other children, extended family members, friendships, and social and professional commitments. It is hypothesized that the parental contextual layers outlined in Fig. 8.1 are linked and sensitive to each other, such that a change in one may prompt change in one or more other layers (Hinds *et al.* 1996). This suggests that when healthcare providers give information to parents about the significance of fatigue as a facet of their child's cancer experience and about its management, other layers in the parental context are likely to be altered—examples include the following.

The contextual layer of 'being a good parent' reflects the parental sense of role responsibility to:

- promote their child's chances of survival
- protect their child from suffering
- facilitate their child's development in the midst of the cancer experience.

This represents parents' intense commitment to doing all that they possibly can to position their child for the best treatment outcomes (Hinds *et al.* 1996). When combined with the layers about child survival and suffering, it serves as a powerful motivator for parents to be mindful of their child's cancer-related symptoms by carefully observing changes in their child.

Ironically, however, the combination of these layers appears to contribute to a clouding of parents' abilities to detect and identify the type of fatigue that their child is experiencing, and to determine a reasonable method for managing the fatigue. When specifically invited to respond to the question 'Does your child experience different types of fatigue?' 22 parents (100%) in focus groups responded affirmatively. The types of fatigue identified by participating parents included mental, emotional, and treatment-related fatigue and parents appeared to apply differing strategies to managing the different types (Table 8.4). As a result, the child's fatigue seemed to have a different level of impact on the family. For example, parents reported that with mental fatigue they needed to exert additional firmness with their child to force the child into action. One parent described the efforts of another parent to intervene with her son's mental fatigue:

> the mother enters her ill child's hospital room, greets her son and warns him that within a few moments she will be opening his blinds. After a few minutes, the mother proceeds to open his blinds, turn on room lights, and tells him, 'up and out' of the bed.

This incident indicates the added parental effort involved in caring for a very fatigued child. Behaving in this way appeared to be difficult for some families as it typically included the parent getting insistent with the ill child—an approach seen as unkind by some family members and not likely to be supported by them. Additionally, some parents held themselves responsible for either not giving enough encouragement to their child to 'try', or for wrongfully forcing the child to do more than he or she could safely do.

The perspective of healthcare professionals

Staff discussed various descriptions of fatigue in children receiving treatment for cancer. These descriptions focused upon changes in the child's usual energy level, activity type, or desire to participate (Hinds *et al.* 1999). One nurse stated, 'parents say they can't even get their kids to do their mouth care … they would rather sleep than eat'. Noticeable changes in the willingness of a child to participate in activities related to patient care were discussed in all staff focus groups (Table 8.1). Staff members identified

Table 8.4 Types of fatigue identified by parents and the corresponding general management approach used by the parents

Type of fatigue experienced by ill child	General parental management approach
1. Mental fatigue: child is weary, unable to concentrate	Time-limited protection from interruptions then force participation in an activity that is easy and gives pleasure
2. Emotional fatigue: child is discouraged, sad, without energy	On-going protection from demands and stimuli, comfort-giving strategies including gentle touch and quiet talk
3. Treatment-related fatigue: child is physically unable to safely complete activities of daily living	Allowing symptoms (i.e. low haemoglobin, low platelet counts) to correct prior to encouraging the ill child to put more effort into interactions or activities

an unwillingness to communicate and participate socially as a behaviour associated with fatigue in children and adolescents. One staff nurse described this as, 'you see this dramatic change from this perky little kid … to sitting underneath the covers'. Another focus group participant stated, 'I've heard a child say that they sleep all the time and they are still tired'.

Staff described patient care activities and hospital/clinic waiting times to be a significant cause of fatigue. Many staff members found that children would become uncooperative during patient care activities when they were experiencing fatigue, and children were described as being less cooperative during times of reported fatigue. Some children were unwilling or unable to participate in patient care activities because they were too tired:

> There are only so many pills you can take and so many times you can have your temperature taken before you say 'enough'. They get the hospital doldrums.

Lack of a daily routine created more fatigue for patients who were hospitalized. The hospital environment also contributed to fatigue, with staff describing the child as being surrounded by noise, and numerous healthcare providers. Numerous interruptions occurred throughout the day and night-time hours, disrupted the child's usual sleep and eating patterns, and contributed to mental fatigue. One nurse stated:

> They get out of their normal sleep habits. They may be up half the night. We may keep them sedated in the daytime … they are just getting sporadic sleep.

Coping strategies

Children identified fewer interventions that helped decrease fatigue than adolescents. One child's description of how rest helps was, 'I usually take two naps every day and that makes me feel better'. A good night's sleep was described as something that helped the children when they were tired as indicated by one child who discussed not being tired at the time of the focus group, 'I slept good last night'. Children discussed quiet activities such as reading a book or listening to music as helpful when they experienced fatigue. 'Having someone come visit you', was one example of a child's description of how visitors can help distract them when in the hospital.

Having protected rest time in the hospital and naps when at home were identified as helpful interventions by most adolescents. One adolescent discussed how his mother provided a rest period when in the hospital:

> My mom normally will tell them not to come in and put a sign on the door … because I'm just so tired that I really can't talk to them.

Participating in activities that kept the adolescent busy and which helped take their mind off feeling tired were discussed as helpful in decreasing fatigue:

> I don't know what it does for me but I've heard people say, that if you're sick, laughter helps you … watching movies kind of relaxes you, and if it is funny and makes you laugh, then you feel better because you forget about being tired, hurting, and all that.

Going outside the hospital for a change of environment, receiving blood transfusions, and taking sleeping pills to combat the fatigue caused by lack of sleep were all cited as ways of coping with the tiredness. Several had participated in physical therapy while hospitalized and found that this decreased their fatigue.

Although parents appeared able to identify the type of fatigue their child experienced and described themselves as being willing to implement intervention strategies, two concerns were raised regarding parental perceptions of causative factors of a child's fatigue, and subsequent attempts at managing it. Firstly, given the multiple, and at times competing, explanations for the cause of a child's fatigue, parents are at risk of implementing a strategy to manage the fatigue that does not match the type of fatigue their child is experiencing. Secondly, although parents are able to identify multiple causes of fatigue (including treatment-related such as chemotherapy, radiotherapy, or surgery), they primarily hold themselves responsible for making their child's fatigue less intense. For example, parents have reported that they could improve their child's fatigue if they prevented others from waking the sleeping child, by preparing favourite foods, or by providing distraction and entertainment (Hinds *et al.* 1999). Parents also reported that attempting these strategies places strain on the family—in part because more than a single type of strategy is implemented, requiring extra energy from the family members, with little guarantee of improvement in the fatigue.

Important interventions identified by healthcare providers to alleviate fatigue included protected rest periods for children and adolescents. Nurses felt that children benefited from uninterrupted naps and sleep time and from having a plan of scheduled activities. One nurse indicated, 'not having to wake up with somebody coming into your room to get your vital sign', as being helpful.

The importance of providing emotional support and empathy was discussed in each staff focus group. One staff nurse said:

> … baby them a little more. I try to go in and talk with them to see if we could do something to help.

Providing encouragement, a positive attitude, and allowing time for the child or adolescent to awaken slowly were presented as effective interventions to explore. Staff felt that being firm while allowing for choices when possible was an important care issue:

> It helps if we make more of an attempt to normalize their lives … not letting them lie in dark rooms all day but getting up and getting dressed.

Implications for practice development

Fatigue in children and adolescents with cancer is a debilitating symptom that is often overlooked by healthcare providers as a side-effect of treatment. Children as young as seven were able to describe physical and emotional indicators of fatigue, highlighting the importance of detailed assessment based on descriptors of fatigue used by children and adolescents. Changes in participation in normal daily activities as well as in sports and games were found to be common in children and adolescents experiencing fatigue, and mental descriptions such as feeling sad or mad were identified as potential indicators of fatigue.

Several causes of fatigue described by the children and adolescents in this study are also described in the adult literature and include chemotherapy, radiation therapy, and surgery. Side-effects of treatment, such as low blood counts and fever, were also associated with fatigue. These contributing factors, while obvious causes of fatigue, were often not considered when providing education to the patients and their families regarding what to expect following treatment. It is important, therefore, that healthcare professionals discuss fatigue as a symptom likely to occur following treatment and develop awareness of interventions that will decrease fatigue while in the hospital and at home. In addition, accurate assessment of other contributing factors that are also associated with fatigue will identify areas of education needed by the patient and family regarding other lifestyle changes, for example sleep disturbances brought on by altered schedules, staying up late at night, or not sleeping in his/her own bed.

Realization that the hospital environment was a major contributor to the occurrence of fatigue in children and adolescents was an important finding. Knowledge of the impact that a noisy hospital unit has upon the sleep patterns of patients provides insight into changes that may need to occur in hospital settings. Awareness that fatigue during hospitalization occurs because of disruptions in sleep due to noises, frequent interruptions, and even the location of the patient's room should stimulate thoughts and ideas on how to make the hospital setting more conducive to rest and sleep. Grouping necessary nursing activities together in order to decrease the number of interruptions a child or adolescent may experience may be one way in which care could be reconfigured to minimize disruption to the child or adolescent. Providing protected rest periods during the day and at night was identified as helpful in decreasing fatigue by the participants interviewed in this study. Increased awareness that the nurses' station should have quiet hours at night may also impact positively on patients' ability to sleep at night.

Boredom brought on by having nothing to do was identified as another potential cause of fatigue. Children and adolescents reported that participating in fun activities helped minimize fatigue. As such, organizing activities identified by the children and young people as stimulating and worthwhile may form part of a package of fatigue interventions worthy of evaluation in future. Adolescents discussed their feelings that worry and or fear sometimes caused fatigue, providing insight into the importance of spending time with these patients, encouraging and helping them to voice their concerns.

By providing parents with information about the causes, impact, and strategies available to manage fatigue, healthcare professionals may be able to strengthen parents' contextual layer of knowledge. In turn, developments in the contextual layer of understanding may have the potential to assist parents in developing tailored interventions for their child's fatigue, while maintaining a realistic view of their responsibility for its management, potentially diminishing family strain related to the fatigue. Parents value information and particularly benefit from written teaching tools as they can be shared with extended family members, friends, teachers, or others who are aware of and/or affected by a ill child's fatigue.

Fatigue may be most noticeable on certain days of each treatment course, or during certain hours of most days. Once a pattern is recognized, family members may be better able to plan family outings or other activities around the pattern. This may allow families to maintain a more typical routine and indirectly contribute to reduced family tension. The sleep diary may be an accurate tool in detecting fatigue patterns if 4-h time blocks are used during awake periods, that is, noting the ill child's activities between 7 o'clock and 11 in the morning, and the level of fatigue experienced. The observations noted by parents (and the ill child where possible) may be shared with healthcare professionals at different times during the course of treatment, in an effort to identify a child's fatigue pattern.

Future directions for practice and research

Conceptualizing fatigue as a physical, mental, emotional, and spiritual experience in children and adolescents allows us to develop new approaches to identifying and reducing fatigue. It is important to remember that fatigue is perceived differently by children, their parents, and healthcare professionals. Fatigue has been found to be one of the most distressing symptoms experienced during childhood cancer treatment. The prevalence of this symptom confirms the need to explore the interrelationships between fatigue and other symptoms commonly experienced by children with cancer. Developments in appreciation of age-appropriate distraction activities indicate an essential challenge within this aspect of fatigue research. Finally, as discussed in detail in Chapter 9, ongoing development and evaluation of valid and reliable clinical assessment tools for fatigue constitute a priority for future research in this important area.

References

Aistars, J. (1987) Fatigue in the cancer patient: a conceptual approach to a clinical problem. *Oncology Nursing Forum*, **14**(6), 25–30.

Bossert, E. and Martinson, I.M. (1990) Kinetic family drawings–revised: a method of determining the impact of cancer on the family as perceived by the child with cancer. *Journal of Pediatric Nursing*, **5**(3), 204–13.

Carter, B.D., Edwards, J.F., Kronenberger, W.G., Michalczyk, L., and Marshall, G.S. (1995) Case control study of chronic fatigue in pediatric patients. *Pediatrics*, **95**(2), 179–86.

Carter, B.D., Kronenberger, W.G., Edwards, J.F., Michalczyk, L., and Marshall, G.S. (1996) Differential diagnosis of chronic fatigue in children: behavioral and emotional dimensions. *Journal of Development and Behaviour in Pediatrics*, **17**(1), 16–21.

Carter, B.D., Kronenberger, W.G., Edwards, J.F., Marshall, G.S., Schikler, K.N., and Causey, D.L. (1999) Psychological symptoms in chronic fatigue and juvenile rheumatoid arthritis. *Pediatrics*, **103**(5, Part 1), 975–9.

Chekryn, J., Deegan, M., and Reid, J. (1986) Normalizing the return to school of the child with cancer. *Journal of the Association of Pediatric Oncology Nurses*, **3**(2), 20–4, 34.

Cimprich, B. (1992) Attentional fatigue following breast cancer surgery. *Research in Nursing and Health*, **15**(3), 199–207.

Green, M. (1998) *Pediatric Diagnosis: Interpretation of Symptoms and Signs in Children and Adolescents*, 6th edn. WB Saunders, Philadelphia.

Hinds, P.S. and Hockenberry-Eaton, M. (2001) Developing a research program on fatigue in children and adolescents diagnosed with cancer. *Journal of Pediatric Oncology Nursing*, **18**(2), 3–12.

Hinds, P.S. and Kelly, K. P. (1998) Studying clinical decision making by patients, parents, and health care providers in pediatric oncology. *Journal of Pediatric Oncology Nursing*, **15**(3, Supplement 1), 1–2.

Hinds, P.S., Birenbaum, L.K., Clarke-Steffen, L., Quargnenti, A., Kreissman, S., Kazak, A. *et al.* (1996) Coming to terms: parents' response to a first cancer recurrence in their child. *Nursing Research*, **45**(3), 148–53.

Hinds, P.S., Hockenberry-Eaton, M., Gilger, E., Kline, N., Burleson, C., Bottomley, S. *et al.* (1999) Comparing patient, parent, and staff descriptions of fatigue in pediatric oncology patients. *Cancer Nursing*, **22**(4), 277–88.

Hockenberry, M., Hinds, P., Barrera, P., Bryant, R., Adams-McNeill, J., Hooke, C. *et al.* (2003) Three instruments to assess fatigue in children with cancer: the child, parent and staff perspectives. *Journal of Pain and Symptom Management*, **25**(4), 319–28.

Hockenberry-Eaton, M. and Benner, P. (1990) Patterns of nausea and vomiting in children: nursing assessment and intervention. *Oncology Nursing Forum*, **17**(4), 575–84.

Hockenberry-Eaton, M. and Hinds, P.S. (2000) Fatigue in children and adolescents with cancer: evolution of a program of study. *Seminars in Oncology Nursing*, **16**(4), 261–72.

Hockenberry-Eaton, M. and Minick, P. (1994) Living with cancer: children with extraordinary courage. *Oncology Nursing Forum*, **21**(6), 1025–31.

Hockenberry-Eaton, M., Dilorio, C., and Kemp, V. (1995) The relationship of illness longevity and relapse with self-perception, cancer stressors, anxiety, and coping strategies in children with cancer. *Journal of Pediatric Oncology Nursing*, **12**(2), 71–9.

Hockenberry-Eaton, M., Hinds, P.S., Alcoser, P., O'Neill, J.B., Euell, K., Howard, V. *et al.* (1998). Fatigue in children and adolescents with cancer. *Journal of Pediatric Oncology Nursing*, **15**(3), 172–82.

Irvine, D., Vincent, L., Graydon, J.E., Bubela, N., and Thompson, L. (1994) The prevalence and correlates of fatigue in patients receiving treatment with chemotherapy and radiotherapy. A comparison with the fatigue experienced by healthy individuals. *Cancer Nursing*, **17**(5), 367–78.

Kellerman, J., Zelter, L., Ellenberg, L., Dash, J., and Rigler, D. (1980) Psychological effects of illness in adolescence. I. Anxiety, self-esteem, and perception of control. *Journal of Pediatrics*, **97**(1), 126–31.

Kline, N.E. (2002) Prevention and treatment of infections. In: *Nursing Care of Children and Adolescents with Cancer*, 3rd edn (ed. C.R. Baggott, K.P. Kelly, D. Fochtman, and G.V. Foley). WB Saunders, Philadelphia, pp. 266–78.

Knoff, H.M. (1986) Gifted children and Visual Aural Digit Span test performance. *Perceptual Motor Skills*, **62**(2), 391–6.

Pickard-Holley, S. (1991) Fatigue in cancer patients. A descriptive study. *Cancer Nursing*, **14**(1), 13–19.

Pizzo, P.A., and Poplack, D.G. (2002) *Principles and Practice of Pediatric Oncology*, 4th edn. Lippincott, Philadelphia.

Rudin, M.M., Martinson, I.M., and Gillis, C.L. (1988) Measurement of psychosocial concerns of adolescents with cancer. *Cancer Nursing*, 11(3), 144–9.

Spinetta, J.J. and Deasy-Spinetta, P. (1981) *Living with Childhood Cancer*. St Louis, MO: Mosby.

Teta, M.J., Del Po, M.C., Kasl, S.V., Meigs, J.W., Myers, M.H., and Mulvihill, J.J. (1986) Psychosocial consequences of childhood and adolescent cancer survival. *Journal of Chronic Diseases*, 39(9), 751–9.

Walford, G.A., Nelson, W.M., and McCluskey, D.R. (1993) Fatigue, depression, and social adjustment in chronic fatigue syndrome. *Archives of Diseases of Childhood*, 68(3), 384–8.

Weinblatt, M.E. (1998) Leukemia. In: *Comprehensive Adolescent Health Care*, 2nd edn (ed. S. Friedman, M. Fisher, S. Schonberg, and E. Alderman) Mosby, St Louis, MO, pp. 214–24.

Winningham, M.L., Nail, L.M., Burke, M.B., Brophy, L., Cimprich, B., Jones, L.S. *et al.* (1994) Fatigue and the cancer experience: the state of the knowledge. *Oncology Nursing Forum*, 21(1), 23–36.

Part 3

The assessment and management of fatigue

Chapter 9

The assessment and measurement of fatigue in people with cancer

Horng-Shiuann Wu and Maryellen McSweeney

Introduction

Cancer-related fatigue (CRF) is a pervasive subjective experience that can affect all aspects of a person's life. Assessment of CRF is the key to recognizing and managing this distressing symptom (Bender *et al.* 2002; Patrick *et al.* 2002; Ressel 2003). Research on the assessment and measurement of CRF has many encouraging aspects. These include the initial formulation and preliminary testing of a diagnosis of CRF within the framework of ICD-10 diagnoses and the development of Cancer-Related Fatigue Guidelines (Mock *et al.* 2003) that incorporate evidence-based fatigue assessment and evaluation. The expanded development of multidimensional measures of CRF as well as simple, single-item screening measures and the more thorough psychometric study and revision of existing and new instruments to measure CRF are promising as well. In addition, there is greater receptivity of health professionals to assessing CRF (Portenoy and Itri 1999; Patrick *et al.* 2002; Mock *et al.* 2003; Daly 2003) and increased recognition of the importance of incorporating the patients' perspective in the assessment of CRF.

Despite this substantial progress, there are still problems in conceptualizing and describing fatigue and distinguishing it from its correlates and its outcomes. The studies of CRF, whether their focus is on prevalence, assessment, or treatment, are exceedingly variable in cancer aetiology, stage, or the treatment regimen considered and in instruments used to measure CRF. Only recently have there been comprehensive, published efforts to compare various measures of CRF (Meek *et al.* 2000; Wu and McSweeney 2001; Schwartz 2002; Schwartz *et al.* 2002; Stone 2002). These issues have an impact on the selection of psychometrically sound instruments and limit the meaningful interpretation of measurements of fatigue in both clinical practice and research.

This chapter discusses the clinical assessment of fatigue and weakness, with particular reference to measurement issues in practice and research settings; critiques the methods of fatigue research, with emphasis on measurement issues; and concludes with implications for practice and research.

Clinical assessment of fatigue and weakness

CRF assessment algorithm

The National Comprehensive Cancer Network (NCCN) defines CRF as 'a common, persistent, subjective sense of tiredness related to cancer or cancer treatment that interferes with usual functioning' (Mock *et al.* 2003). CRF is a multidimensional, subjective experience that is characterized by a cluster of diverse physical, psychological, and cognitive symptoms. Assessment of CRF involves evaluating these various symptoms systematically (Naughton and Homsi 2002; Mock *et al.* 2003).

In clinical practice, it is important to assess for CRF systematically rather than waiting until patients spontaneously complain of the symptoms. Patients may be afraid to distract the physician's attention from treating the cancer by complaining about symptoms (Cleeland *et al.* 2000; Wang 2002) or they may assume that the symptoms of CRF are a normal part of the disease process or treatment side-effects to be endured without professional help or discussion. Relying on the patient's spontaneous complaint may seriously underestimate the prevalence of CRF.

The NCCN Guidelines CRF Assessment Algorithm (Mock *et al.* 2003) screens for fatigue on the basis of patient self-report to a single item. It recommends a focused history and physical examination, concentrating on disease status and treatment, and an in-depth assessment of fatigue and its temporal nature in the case of fatigue rated by the patient as 'moderate' or 'severe'. Major correlates of fatigue—pain, emotional distress, sleep disturbance, anaemia, and hypothyroidism—are also assessed. (Mock 2001; Naughton and Homsi 2002; Mock *et al.* 2003; Berger *et al.* 2003). If absent, a comprehensive assessment of systems and medications, co-morbidities, nutritional/metabolic status, and activity is recommended (Mock *et al.* 2003). The assessed information should be available to the patient's healthcare providers as quickly as possible (Cleeland *et al.* 2000), to improve the communication between patients and providers and facilitate the exploration of possible interventions.

Fatigue terminology

Using the single word 'fatigue' can limit appreciation of the phenomenon and its consequences (Winningham 2001) because various other terms have been used by cancer patients to describe their CRF experience. Persons with cancer tend to describe the experience using negative expressions reflecting noticeable loss of energy (Camarillo 1992), exhaustion, increased discomfort, and inability to perform some tasks routinely done before their cancer experience (Holley 2000*a*; Winningham 2001; Curt and Johnston 2003). CRF differs from normal fatigue in its intensity, severity, duration, and inability to be relieved by adequate rest. Unlike normal fatigue, CRF is an unpleasant sensation often accompanied by frustration and cognitive and emotional distress (Pearce and Richardson 1996; Cleeland *et al.* 2000; Curt 2000; Furst and Ahsberg 2001; Sadler *et al.* 2002).

In persons with cancer, fatigue involves four prominent physical changes: decreased physical performance, unusual and extreme tiredness, feeling of weakness, and unusual need for rest (Glaus *et al.* 1996). Nail and Winningham (1995) differentiated the concepts of fatigue and weakness. Weakness is generally perceived in relation to neurological disorders and immobility and is a condition of decreased muscle strength or endurance from baseline level, while fatigue is a subjective sensation with multiple dimensions. When weakness causes increased energy expenditure and demands, fatigue may result. But isolated muscle weakness, as in an injured extremity after immobilization, can occur without fatigue. Muscle strength and size, generalized weakness, and limb heaviness are related to but can be differentiated from CRF (Kasper and Sarna 2000; Sadler *et al.* 2002). As highlighted by Ream and Richardson (1997), fatigue and weakness have discrete properties and should not be used interchangeably or assessed as the same phenomenon. The wording used to assess CRF should be viewed cautiously.

Purposes of the assessment

The choice of assessment instrument for measuring fatigue in persons with cancer should be based on the purpose of measurement and the characteristics of the particular tool. The potential reasons for using a CRF instrument in clinical practice or research are to:

1. Identify cases with CRF using diagnostic tools. This results in diagnosis in the individual case and prevalence estimates in the population.

2. Describe symptom status. This enables clinicians to monitor their patients' symptomatology and researchers to differentiate between CRF and its correlates as well as to study the impact of interventions on symptom management.

3. Identify the consequences of CRF, such as the distress caused by fatigue and interference with individuals' functional status and quality of life. This information can improve the communication between clinicians and patients, be incorporated into treatment decisions, and help manage CRF. It can aid researchers in modelling CRF and its consequences.

CRF diagnosis

CRF diagnostic criteria appear in the International Classification of Diseases, 10th revision (ICD-10) (Portenoy and Itri 1999; Cella *et al.* 2001; Sadler *et al.* 2002). The criteria for the diagnosis of CRF include:

1. Six or more out of 11 possible fatigue symptoms, with one being 'significant fatigue', have been present every day or nearly every day during the same 2-week period in the past month.

2. The symptoms cause clinically significant distress or impairment in important aspects of functioning.

3. The symptoms result from cancer or cancer treatment.

4. The symptoms are not primarily a consequence of co-morbid psychiatric disorders.

Preliminary evaluations have shown considerable promise in using these criteria for assessing CRF (Cella *et al.* 2001; Sadler *et al.* 2002). The diagnostic criteria can improve early detection of, and appropriate response to, patients' concerns and difficulties and may prevent escalation of the problem. Widespread use of the CRF diagnostic criteria will better define the clinical syndrome of CRF, facilitate clinical understanding of its severity and persistence, and support clinical management of CRF. The NCCN algorithm provides one approach to determining whether a specific individual meets the CRF diagnostic criteria. Use of uniform criteria for determining CRF will contribute to greater consistency in condition- and treatment-specific CRF prevalence estimates.

CRF symptom assessment

Many CRF instruments have been developed to quantify symptom status and provide a way to describe an individual's level of fatigue. Presence, intensity, severity, frequency, and duration of the symptoms are most frequently queried. As many of the CRF instruments used to evaluate fatigue confound its characteristics with its consequences (Winningham *et al.* 1994), potential users must be selective in choosing instruments that focus on symptomatology when the aim is to describe symptom status.

Consequences of CRF

In addition to assessing the presence and severity of CRF and its symptomatology, it is important to recognize the degree to which CRF compromises functioning and daily activity and distresses persons with cancer. NCCN CRF practice guidelines (Mock *et al.* 2003) recommend that providers evaluate the impact of fatigue on functioning, daily activity, and quality of life.

Several currently available instruments can serve this purpose. The Functional Assessment of Cancer Therapy (FACT) (Yellen *et al.* 1997) and the European Organization for Research and Treatment of Cancer–Quality of Life Questionnaire (EORTC QLQ-C30) (Aaronson *et al.* 1993; see also www.eortc.be/home/qol) have both been frequently used in assessing functioning and quality of life in cancer populations. The Cancer-Related Fatigue Distress Scale (CRFDS) (Holley 2000*b*) is an appropriate selection to assess people's distress caused by CRF.

Issues of measurement

Instrument availability and use

Clinicians may not be aware of the availability of instruments to measure CRF or that the instruments may not be clinically feasible. Findings from a survey evaluating how nurses assess CRF (Knowles *et al.* 2000) showed that 64% of the respondents reported that a standardized patient assessment tool would be useful in assessing fatigue in patients with cancer, but only 20% reported using a structured tool to assess fatigue in their cancer patients. Although more CRF instruments are available, oncologists still recognize failure to assess CRF as a major barrier to good symptom management (Cleeland *et al.* 2000; Naughton and Homsi 2002). Attention must be paid to this discordance between instrument availability and use.

Issues of questionnaires and rating scales

Chart review, elicitation by a standardized survey questionnaire or interview, and patients' spontaneous reports are three methods to recognize symptoms in clinical practice or research (Kroenke 2001). Each method can provide a different perspective of CRF. Reliance only on chart review may underestimate the burden of CRF. Fatigue is a subjective sensation best measured by self-report. Self-report questionnaires or structured interviews can capture the unrecognized problems, but may prompt over-endorsement bias from the tendency of patients to generously claim the symptoms on a symptom checklist (Kroenke 2001). Patients' complaints are directly relevant to clinical practice but their presence and level of detail may reflect factors unrelated to fatigue (for example opportunity, assertiveness, verbal fluency) as well as CRF symptoms and consequences.

Measurement scales or rating systems are the core of adequate CRF assessment (Cleeland *et al.* 2000). Numerical scaling systems produce an unweighted value reflecting the degree or extent of the person's CRF. The seven-point rating scale traditionally recommended by psychologists (Miller 1956; Lissitz and Green 1975), may be too demanding for fatigued cancer patients. Finer categories of rating may add little to the usefulness of the rating but burden patients and decrease their capacity for judgment (Sadler *et al.* 2002). Attention needs to be given to respondent burden and limitations in processing information in selecting a rating scale.

The numerical score on a self-report questionnaire is often difficult for cancer patients to supply and clinicians to employ in meaningful ways (Cella *et al.* 2002). Although categorical measures typically provide less detailed information, use of the categorical responses of 'mild', 'moderate', or 'severe' as either initial judgments or categorization of numerical judgments (that is, 1–3 = mild, 4–6 = moderate, 7–10 = severe) is common in clinical assessment of CRF (Mock *et al.* 2003).

In clinical practice, efficiency of the measure in obtaining fatigue information and detecting change is paramount. Researchers may focus on clearly differentiating fatigue from the response to fatigue, obtaining results from various instruments, and comparing different approaches to measure fatigue (Winningham *et al.* 1994; Meek *et al.* 2000). For both clinical and research uses, the CRF measure needs to be brief and simple enough not to burden patients, sensitive enough to detect change over time, and stable enough to use repeatedly.

Symptom diaries

Symptom diaries are an efficient way to recognize the severity, pattern, and impact of CRF experienced and reported by individuals. There are potential therapeutic benefits for the patients, who can describe their symptoms in more detail and express their feelings regarding their illness and its impact. Magnusson *et al.* (1997) showed that using a patient diary was helpful in managing patients' CRF. The information may be used by clinicians to assess progress and recognize changes in physical ability, mood, and actions (Krzys 1995).

Special populations

Certain populations, such as children, the elderly, and terminally ill patients, are at especially high risk for inadequate CRF assessment. The phenomenon of CRF in children is discussed in Chapter 8 of this volume. This chapter looks briefly at special assessment issues.

Hockenberry-Eaton and Hinds (2000) found that fatigue was a significant symptom in children with cancer. Like adults, children experienced physical, emotional, and mental fatigue but with different clinical indicators. For example, the research found that mental fatigue in children should be determined by the frequency of mood changes and decreased communication with others (Hockenberry-Eaton and Hinds 2000 (see Chapter 8)). Because children are not as vocal at expressing their sensations and concerns as adults are and because CRF symptom manifestation differs, structured, adult-focused self-reports and volunteered reports are less likely to be useful in assessing children. Observational records and proxy reports by parents and other family members are likely substitutes. Hockenberry-Eaton and colleagues (Hockenberry-Eaton and Hinds 2000; Hockenberry-Eaton *et al.* 2003) have developed a useful instrument specifically for evaluating CRF in children.

Symptom assessment in elderly patients is also a significant challenge. Elderly patients may be reluctant to report CRF symptoms because of a belief that some of the symptoms are an inevitable part of aging. The presence of other illnesses and/or cognitive or sensory impairments may make fatigue assessment difficult in this population. Special attention is needed when using instruments that have not been designed for or validated on older adults.

Measurement of fatigue in advanced cancer patients receiving palliative care poses conceptual and logistical challenges. The high unpredictability of their functioning at any given time as well as the enveloping progression of their fatigue are not well captured by existing tools designed to focus on fatigue associated with treatment trajectories. As Krishnasamy (2000) notes, meaning derived from open-ended interviews may need to precede or replace measurement of fatigue on standard scales. Scales that focus on symptoms and their consequences 'right now' (POMS) or 'now' (BFI) may be preferable to those asking for a long span of judgment such as 'during the past week'. Other logistical challenges pertain to respondent burden resulting from lengthy, demanding, and complex scales and to possible communication and cognitive impairments of the palliative care patients (Naughton and Homsi 2002). Proxy data provided by family caregivers and clinicians may be helpful in cases where direct self-report of the patients is impractical; however, underestimation of the pervasiveness of patients' fatigue is likely.

Temporal issues

Fatigue was found to be the longest lasting and most impairing cancer-related symptom (Curt 2000) as well as one characterized by significant temporal variability. Three temporal issues of symptom assessment—recency, episodicity, and duration—were identified as relevant by Kroenke (2001). Episodicity of CRF reflects the fact that fatigue is not present continually but rather comes and goes, somewhat in 'roller coaster' fashion, in discrete blocks of time with symptom-free periods between episodes. Duration of CRF can be for minutes, hours, or days, and CRF may persist after treatment (Berger *et al.* 2003; Cella *et al.* 2001; Flechtner and Bottomley 2003). The ICD-10 diagnostic criteria for CRF incorporate recency ('in the past month'), episodicity ('every day or nearly every day'), and duration ('persisting at least two weeks'). However, the exploration of episodicity in these criteria focuses on the day as the reporting unit and does not explore the presence of symptom-free periods during the day. Self-report measures typically specify a discrete time frame for response. Issues of episodicity and duration, if addressed, are considered in the context of longitudinal designs rather than as a part of the self-report task. The quantification of recency, episodicity, and duration can help evaluate the severity of fatigue and monitor treatment response. These three temporal factors should be considered when assessing CRF.

The validity and reliability of fatigue questionnaires

Nineteen self-report instruments available in English were identified in the CRF literature from 1980 to present. Table 9.1 summarizes their properties. They are grouped into multiple categories in the table, depending on whether they consist of a single fatigue item or multiple items, are incorporated in another instrument or are free-standing, and are uni- or multidimensional measures of fatigue. The four single-item measures of fatigue are the Rhoten Fatigue Scale (RFS) (Rhoten 1982), Visual Analog Fatigue Scale (VAFS) (Glaus 1993), the single fatigue item of the M.D. Anderson Symptom Inventory (MDASI) (Cleeland *et al.* 2000), and the single 'get tired for no reason' item of the Zung Self-Rating Depression Scale (ZSDS) (Kirsh *et al.* 2001). Multi-item measures of fatigue are incorporated in the widely used Profile of Mood States (POMS) (vigour–activity and fatigue–inertia subscales) (McNair *et al.* 1992), the EORTC QLQ-C30 Quality of Life Questionnaire (Aaronson *et al.* 1993 (see www.eortc.be/home/qol)), the MOS 36-item Short Form Survey (SF-36) (Ware and Sherbourne 1992; Ware *et al.* 1993), and the Functional Assessment of Cancer Therapy-Fatigue (FACT-F) and Fatigue Subscale (Yellen *et al.* 1997). There are two free-standing, unidimensional fatigue measures: the Brief Fatigue Inventory (BFI) (Mendoza *et al.* 1999; Radbruch *et al.* 2003; Okuyama *et al.* 2003) and the Cancer-Related Fatigue Distress Scale (CRFDS) (Holley 2000*b*). The remaining scales are all free-standing and

Table 9.1 Measurement of cancer-related fatigue by self-report instruments

Type of measure	Study	Instrument	Characteristics of measure	Reference period
Single-item measures of fatigue: free-standing and incorporated in other instruments	Rhoten (1982)	Rhoten Fatigue Scale (RFS): one-item 0–10 graphic rating scale	Fatigue severity	Present
	Glaus (1993)	Visual Analog Fatigue Scale (VAFS): 10 cm line with 2 endpoints 'I do not feel tired at all' and 'I feel totally exhausted'	Fatigue severity	Present
	Cleeland et al. (2000)	M.D. Anderson Symptom Inventory (MDASI): 19-item (13-item part I + 6-item part II); 0–10 numeric rating scale; single fatigue item (part I, item 2)	Fatigue severity	'In the last 24 hours'
	Kirsh et al. (2001)	Zung Self-Rating Depression Scale (ZSDS) item 10 'I get tired for no reason': one item 4-point Likert scale	Fatigue frequency ('none or little of the time' to 'most or all of the time')	During the preceding week
Multi-item measures of fatigue incorporated in other instruments, typically measuring functional ability or quality of life	McNair et al. (1992)	Profile of Mood States (POMS) vigour–activity and fatigue–inertia subscales (POMS-V, POMS-F): 8- and 7-item 0–4 intensity scales	Intensity/presence of trait	'During the past week including today'; 'right now'
	Aaronson et al. (1993)	EORTC Quality of Life Questionnaire (EORTC QLQ-C30) fatigue scale (items 10, 12,18): in 30-item QLQ with 5 functioning and 9 symptom subscales	Fatigue intensity (4 response levels from 'not at all' to 'very much')	'During the past week'

Reliability and validity	Population	Comment
Validity: patients' ratings on the RFS were correlated with investigators' ratings based on observations and interviews	5 adult patients admitted for abdominal surgery within 48 hours prior to interview	Strength: simple, easy to use; minimal burden to patients. Limitation: cannot be evaluated for many forms of statistical reliability; not developed to measure CRF
Validity: comparison of fatigue scores and daily profiles showed that repeated VAFS measure reflected daily fluctuations of fatigue in 3 subsamples	3 subsamples in a teaching hospital in Switzerland: 20 inpatients in cancer treatment; 12 chronic GI disease inpatients; 30 healthy adults	Strength: simple, easy to use; minimal burden to patients; can be used in non-cancer patients and healthy individuals. Limitation: cannot be evaluated for many forms of statistical reliability; unable to identify specific symptoms of CRF
Reliability: reasonable internal consistency in validation and cross-validation samples for general symptom severity, $\alpha = 0.85–0.87$ and interference scales $\alpha = 0.91–0.94$. Construct validity: factor analysis yielded 2-factor model for 13 core items; sustained in cross-validation	Adult outpatients with various cancers: 527 for scale development; 113 for cross-validation	Strength: flexible assessment system measuring CRF and other cancer-related symptoms at once with core and added items; uses interactive voice response system in assessment. Limitation: single fatigue item; can only assess severity and impact of CRF; 6-item interference subscale was not validated
Construct validity: highly correlated with ZSDS, $r = 0.63$; FACT-An, $r = -0.70$; and individual FSI items, $r = 0.41$ to 0.71	52 patients under treatment for various cancers for instrument validation	Strength: simple, easy for fatigue screening; minimal burden to patients. Limitation: cannot be evaluated for many forms of statistical reliability; not developed to measure CRF
POMS has well-established internal consistency, test–retest reliability, concurrent validity in several studies. Psychometric properties of POMS-V and POMS-F untested	Many psychiatric outpatients and normal college students	Strength: POMS-V and POMS-F are short and easy to use. Limitation: developed to measure change in mood states in psychiatric outpatients, not CRF; measures only one aspect of fatigue; inconsistent findings between fatigue and vigour and other subscales
Reliability: subscale internal consistency α ranged 0.54 to 0.86 and 0.53 to 0.89 before and during treatment; fatigue subscale $\alpha = 0.80$ and 0.85 before and after treatment. Construct validity: known-group comparisons showed differences in functioning and symptom measures (including fatigue) between patients differing in clinical status	305 patients with non-resectable lung cancer received radiotherapy or chemotherapy in 13 countries	Strength: translated into and validated in 42 languages; scale characteristics were stable across cultural and language groups; appropriate for measuring quality of life of cancer patients in multicultural clinical research settings; normative data available for interpretation. Limitation: developed to measure quality of life in cancer, not CRF

Table 9.1 (continued) Measurement of cancer-related fatigue by self-report instruments

Type of measure	Study	Instrument	Characteristics of measure	Reference period
	Ware et al. (1993)	The MOS 36-item Short-Form Survey (SF-36). Vitality Scale (items 9a, 9e, 9g, 9i): in 36-item SF-36 with 8 health concepts	Fatigue frequency (6 response levels: from 'all the time' to 'none of the time')	'During the past 4 weeks'
	Yellen et al. (1997)	Functional Assessment of Cancer Therapy-Fatigue (FACT-F): 41-item 0–4 5-point rating scale (consisting of 28-item FACT General and 13-item Fatigue subscale)	Fatigue subscale measures fatigue presence/intensity affective aspects, and interference with functioning	'During the past 7 days'
Free-standing unidimensional fatigue measures	Mendoza et al. (1999)	Brief Fatigue Inventory (BFI): 9-item 0–10 numeric rating scale	Severity and impact of fatigue	'Now' and 'during the past 24 hours'
	Holley (2000b)	Cancer-Related Fatigue Distress Scale (CRFDS): 20-item 0–10 numeric rating scale	CRF distress with 5 categories: physical, social, psychological, cognitive, and spiritual distress	'During the past 7 days'

Reliability and validity	Population	Comment
SF-36 has well established internal consistency reliability, content validity, construct validity, and criterion-related validity in many studies	Tested in various medical, surgical, psychiatric populations as well as general US population, and different age, gender, and ethnic groups	Strength: can be used for measuring general health status. Limitation: not specifically developed to measure CRF; long reference period hard to reflect CRF fluctuations; not well-tested in cancer populations
Reliability: FACT-F showed good internal consistency ($\alpha = 0.95$), good stability (test–retest $r = 0.87$ over 3–7 days). Fatigue subscale showed good internal consistency ($\alpha = 0.93$–0.95) and test–retest reliability ($r = 0.90$). Convergent–divergent validity: both FACT-F and Fatigue subscale showed negative r with POMS Fatigue and PFS, positive r with POMS Vigor; non-significant r with Marlowe–Crowne Social Desirability. Discriminant validity: both FACT-F and Fatigue subscale significantly correlated with haemoglobin	14 anaemic oncology patients and 5 medical experts for item generation; 49 oncology patients under treatment for instrument testing	Strength: to assess fatigue alone, use the fatigue subscale (brief, simple, easy to use); to assess both fatigue and its consequences, use FACT-F; sensitive to change over time; items were generated from patients' perspective. Limitation: length of FACT-F could add burden to patients; items were generated for anaemia-related symptoms
Reliability: internal consistency $\alpha = 0.96$. Construct validity: factor loadings show single factor. Concurrent validity: BFI correlated with both FACT ($r = -0.88$) and POMS ($r = 0.84$) fatigue subscales. Discriminant validity: BFI significantly different across ECOG performance status ratings	305 adult cancer inpatients and outpatients and 290 community-dwelling adults	Strength: short and easy to use; simple to translate into other languages; useful in clinical practice with a filter question to screen for the presence of CRF. Limitation: single-dimensional measure of fatigue; identifies cut points to discriminate different levels of fatigue severity, but the cut points between mild and moderate severity are unclear
Reliability: good internal consistency: $\alpha = 0.98$ for 23-item scale and $\alpha = 0.98$ for 20-item scale. Content validity: 23-item CVIs ranged from 0.60–1.00 with a mean CVI of 0.91. Construct validity: factor analysis confirmed all items loaded on only 1 factor; 20 of the 23 items had factor loading > 0.70	Item development: 23 in-depth interviews with 17 adults having CRF; item/scale testing: 5 cancer survivors assessed content validity; 221 diverse cancer patients completed 23-item CRFDS	Strength: items generated based on patient interview content and content validated by cancer survivors; good instrument to assess the impact of CRF. Limitation: measures only one aspect of CRF experience—distress

Table 9.1 (continued) Measurement of cancer-related fatigue by self-report instruments

Type of measure	Study	Instrument	Characteristics of measure	Reference period
Free-standing multidimensional fatigue measures	Smets et al. 1995	Multidimensional Fatigue Inventory (MFI): 20-item 7-point scale	5 dimensions: general fatigue, physical and mental fatigue, reduced motivation, and reduced activity	'During the previous days'
	Hann et al. (1998)	Fatigue Symptom Inventory (FSI): 13-item 0–10 numeric rating scale	Intensity and duration of fatigue and interference with daily life	'In the past week'
	Piper et al. (1989)	Original Piper Fatigue Scale (PFS) includes Piper Fatigue Self-Report Scale-Baseline (PFS-B): 42-item 100 mm horizontal VAS; and Piper Fatigue Self-Report Scale-Current (PFS-C): 40 items	7 dimensions: temporal, intensity/severity, affective, sensory, evaluative, associated symptom, and relief	'Usually'
	Piper et al. (1998)	Revised Piper Fatigue Scale (Revised PFS): 22-item 0–10 numerical scale and 5 open-ended questions	4 dimensions: behavioural/severity, affective meaning, sensory, and cognitive/mood	'Now'

Reliability and validity	Population	Comment
Reliability: reasonable to good ($\alpha = 0.65$–0.80) internal consistency. Construct validity: significant differences found between known groups, circumstances and/or activity levels. Convergent validity: significant correlations between VAS-Fatigue and MFI in radiotherapy patients ($0.22 < r < 0.78$)	111 cancer patients on radiotherapy, 357 chronic fatigue syndrome patients, various students and military groups ($n = 46$–481)	Strength: multidimensional measure of fatigue; no somatic items reduces the contamination with somatic illness; groups with/without cancer compared in different circumstances and activity levels. Limitation: reference period not clearly defined
Reliability: interference subscale $\alpha = 0.93$–0.95, total correlations > 0.70; test–retest $r = 0.35$–0.75 in active treatment group, 0.10–0.74 in healthy group. Convergent validity: significant positive correlations of FSI with POMS-F and negative ones of FSI with SF-36 vitality subscale. Divergent validity: FSI and MC-Social Desirability uncorrelated. Construct validity: known groups differed in fatigue; large positive correlations between intensity, duration and interference ratings	107 women undergoing breast cancer treatment, 113 women completed breast cancer treatment, and 50 women with no history of cancer	Strength: a short multidimensional fatigue measure; demonstrated divergent validity. Limitation: test–retest reliability was weak; methods of administration of the study measure to the patient group and healthy controls differed, which may affect differences in their responses
Reliability: total fatigue score $\alpha = 0.85$; subscale $\alpha = 0.69$–0.95. Content validity: items of temporal, severity, affective, and sensory dimensions met preset 78% criterion level of relevance. Convergent and discriminant validity: moderate correlations between PFS, POMS, and FSCL. Construct validity: 10 clusters solution supported PFS-B's multidimensionality	11 national fatigue experts for content validation; 42 newly diagnosed breast and lung cancer patients undergoing radiation therapy for psychometric testing	Strength: most comprehensive, multidimensional measure; specifically for CRF; uses VAS to measure subjective experience. Limitation: length of PFS-B may burden patients; not designed to be used clinically; questions presume presence of fatigue experience; reference period not specified
Reliability: total scale $\alpha = 0.97$; $\alpha = 0.92$–0.96 for 4 subscales. Construct validity: 4 factor solutions	382 women breast cancer survivors	Strength: shorter and easier to use than PFS; multidimensional measure. Limitation: underlying constructs may not be genuinely bipolar; wording of all responses to items in the same direction may invite response sets

Table 9.1 (continued) Measurement of cancer-related fatigue by self-report instruments

Type of measure	Study	Instrument	Characteristics of measure	Reference period
	Stein *et al.* (1998)	Multidimensional Fatigue Symptom Inventory (MFSI): 83 items 0–4 scale (rationally derived scales); MFSI-SF: 30 items 0–4 scale (empirically derived scales)	5 dimensions: general, emotional, physical, mental fatigue, and vigour	'In the past 7 days
	Schwartz (1998)	Schwartz Cancer Fatigue Scale (SCFS): 28-item, 1–5 rating scale	4 dimensions: physical, emotional, cognitive, and temporal	'In the prior 2 to 3 days'
	Schwartz and Meek (1999)	Revised Schwartz Cancer Fatigue Scale (SCFS-6): 6-item 1–5 scale	2 dimensions: physical and perceptual	'In the past 2 to 3 days'

Reliability and validity	Population	Comment
Reliability: MFSI subscale $\alpha = 0.87$–0.92; MFSI-SF subscale $\alpha = 0.85$–0.96; moderate 6–8 week test–retest reliability coefficients for MFSI (0.54–0.68) and MFSI-SF (0.51–0.70). Concurrent validity: both showed moderate to high correlations with POMS-F and SF-36. Convergent validity: both had significant positive correlations with STAI and CES-D. Divergent validity: both showed low but significant correlations with MC-20. Construct validity: known groups differed in MFSI and MFSI-SF fatigue levels	Preliminary MFSI (informal content validation): 15 breast cancer patients, 10 women with no history of cancer, and 8 oncology care providers; MFSI: 146 women in breast cancer treatment, 92 women > 3 months past treatment, and disease, and 54 women with no cancer history	Strength: was validated by cancer patients; good psychometric properties; rationally and empirically derived scales provide options to choose; can be used at frequent intervals; does not assume the presence of fatigue or chronic disease. Limitation: length of rationally derived scales can burden patients
Reliability: α internal consistency was 0.96 for total scale, 0.82–0.93 for subscales. Content validity: supported by item evaluation by both cancer patients and oncology nurse experts. Construct validity: factor analysis resulted in 4-factor solution for 70% of variance; construct validity was supported by differences in fatigue between those in and post treatment and by VAS fatigue scores	Informal content validity: 10 healthy people and 10 ambulatory cancer patients; formal content validity: 5 expert oncology nurses and 6 cancer patients; construct validity: 166 cancer patients (20 were in treatment)	Strength: simple wording and relatively brief, multidimensional measure of CRF; content validated by cancer patients and has strong content validity. Limitation: majority of validation sample had completed cancer treatment; confirmatory analysis did not support 4-factor structure
Reliability: good internal consistency of $\alpha = 0.90$ for total scale, $\alpha = 0.88$ for physical subscale and $\alpha = 0.81$ for perceptual subscale. Construct validity: was supported by GFI > 0.98 and AGFI > 0.94; subjects in treatment scored higher on all items, both subscales and total scale, than those who had completed treatment; there were significant differences by time since treatment	303 adult cancer patients with various cancers, treatments, and time since treatment (157 were in treatment)	Strength: brief, simple, easy to use; strong evidence of construct validity; the shortest multidimensional measure specifically for CRF and first measuring perceptual aspect of CRF; electronic version (computer-touch screen) is available. Limitation: test–retest reliability and sensitivity to change over time need further examination

Table 9.1 (continued) Measurement of cancer-related fatigue by self-report instruments

Type of measure	Study	Instrument	Characteristics of measure	Reference period
	Okuyama *et al.* (2000a)	Cancer Fatigue Scale (CFS): 15-item 1–5 numeric rating scale	3 dimensions: physical, affective, and cognitive	'Right now'
	Passik *et al.* (2002)	Fatigue Management Barriers Questionnaire (FMBQ): 28-item, 1–5 Likert scale	10 concerns of patients thought to be barriers to fatigue management	Not Specified

Reliability and validity	Population	Comment
Reliability: good internal consistency, $\alpha = 0.79$–0.89 for subscales and total scale; test–retest $r > 0.50$ for subscales and total scale. Construct validity: 3-factor solution was confirmed by repeating factor analysis. Convergent validity: large correlations between CFS and VAS for fatigue, and between VAS and each subscale (average $r = 0.49$)	Scale development: 89 oncology nurses; scale validation phases: 307 adult cancer patients	Strength: items pool was generated based on interviews with cancer patients; simple, easily completed in 2 minutes even by advanced cancer patients; multidimensional measure of CRF; comprehensive psychometric tests showed good validity and reliability. Limitation: was done in Japanese patient populations; did not investigate the cross-cultural validity, although an English version is available
Reliability: acceptable internal consistency, $\alpha = 0.88$ for total scale; $\alpha = 0.34$–0.77 for subscales	200 oncology patients (lung, breast, colon, and lymphoma) with various stages of cancer	Strength: first instrument attempting to assess communication barriers in CRF management. Limitation: not validated; requires further psychometric testing before drawing inferences from the results of assessment

multidimensional: the Multidimensional Fatigue Inventory (MFI) (Smets *et al.* 1995; Gentile 2003; Fillion *et al.* 2003; Schwartz *et al.* 2003), the Fatigue Symptom Inventory (FSI) (Hann *et al.* 1998), the Piper Fatigue Scale (PFS and revised PFS) (Piper *et al.* 1989, 1998), the Multidimensional Fatigue Symptom Inventory (MFSI and MFSI-SF) (Stein *et al.* 1998), the Schwartz Cancer Fatigue Scale (SCFS and revised SCFS-6) (Schwartz 1998; Schwartz and Meek 1999), the Cancer Fatigue Scale (CFS) (Okuyama *et al.* 2000*a*), and the Fatigue Management Barriers Questionnaire (FMBQ) (Passik *et al.* 2002). Six of the 19 instruments (RFS, ZSDS, POMS, SF-36, FACT, and MFI) were not specifically developed to measure CRF.

Most of the multi-item instruments and some of the fatigue subscales incorporated in larger instruments report good internal consistency reliability. Evidence of test–retest reliability is largely absent or relatively modest in the case of the FSI, MFSI, MFSI-SF, and CFS. Known groups and factor analytic approaches to construct validity and convergent and divergent validity are frequently reported, with good results. The psychometric properties of a few of the subscales are not reported although the properties of their parent instruments have been studied thoroughly.

Psychometric testing is a sample-dependent and on-going process (Nunnally and Bernstein 1994). Although the psychometric properties reported from past studies may support the reliability and validity of an instrument, users still need to test and revalidate the instrument when employing it with different populations or modifying the instrument or its mode of use.

Subjective indicators are essential to understanding the fatigue experience (Piper *et al.* 1989). However, few of the instruments to measure CRF have been developed from qualitative studies of patients' experiences, although some have been content validated by cancer patients or cancer survivors. Patients and healthcare providers often perceive cancer-related symptoms differently (Fernsler 1986; Greene *et al.* 1994; Beisecker *et al.* 1997; Macquart-Moulin *et al.* 1997; Magnusson *et al.* 1997; Newell *et al.* 1998; Knowles *et al.* 2000; Schwartz 1998; Rustoen *et al.* 2003). Consequently, instruments generated by investigators without being validated by persons who have experienced CRF should be viewed cautiously.

Although a number of multidimensional measures are currently available, some focus on the physical sensations and the impact of fatigue (MFI, FSI). Others include the mental and emotional components of fatigue as well (PFS, revised PFS, MFSI, SCFS, SCFS-6, CFS). The CRFDS assesses the distress caused by CRF in multiple domains of the person's life. The FMBQ identifies the barriers that limit the communication between patients and their oncologists about CRF management. The PFS includes items measuring causes of fatigue and strategies to relieve it while the SCFS-6 includes perceptual aspects of CRF. None of the currently available instruments evaluates patients' expectations of fatigue that were often noted by participants in qualitative studies of CRF.

Four major characteristics of CRF can be identified by focusing on the attributes of CRF revealed in qualitative studies and inferred from the dimensions of CRF in currently available instruments. They are:

◆ the physical sensation of fatigue, including severity and intensity of its indicators;

◆ mood, emotion, or affective feelings;

◆ the cognitive or mental dimension of fatigue; and

◆ temporal components, including frequency and duration of the fatigue.

These four aspects of CRF should all be considered when assessing CRF symptomatology.

A critique of the methodology of fatigue research

Design issues in fatigue research

Diversity in study methods

Quantitative fatigue research is characterized by great diversity in the populations under study, the definitions of fatigue, the instruments used, and the time frame under measurement. This variation is reflected in Table 9.1 under the entries for population, instrument, and reference period. It can be seen more comprehensively in the fatigue tables of the *AHRQ Evidence Report No 61 Management of Cancer Symptoms: Pain, Depression, and Fatigue* (Carr *et al.* 2002). So much variation across studies makes it difficult to establish an unequivocal body of evidence based on replicated studies. It also leaves unresolved whether the differences in outcomes between studies reflect methodological or substantive differences or both.

Results attributable to chance

There have been few large, randomized controlled trials (RCTs) of interventions to treat CRF. Of the 10 RCTs identified by Carr *et al.* (2002), most had relatively small sample sizes and multiple outcome measures, none of which were defined prospectively as primary. Thus the scattering of significant findings obtained across various outcomes may be an artefact of chance.

Distinguishing fatigue from its correlates

The correlation of fatigue with other symptoms such as pain and depression (Piper *et al.* 1987; Blesch *et al.* 1991; Irvine *et al.* 1991; Visser and Smets 1998; Curt 2000; Okuyama *et al.* 2000b; Redeker *et al.* 2000; Stone *et al.* 2000; Ancoli-Israel *et al.* 2001; Bender *et al.* 2002; Langeveld *et al.* 2003) raises the question of whether fatigue should be treated as an individual symptom, as a syndrome, or as part of a symptom cluster for design and analysis. Earlier studies focused more on fatigue as an individual symptom, correlated with others; more recent studies have begun to emphasize its role as part of a symptom cluster. The increased focus on symptom clusters may lessen attention to differentiating between closely related symptoms such as fatigue, anxiety, and depression.

Assessing change in CRF

Selection of the reference period for measuring CRF and the number and spacing of discrete measurements are important in assessing change in CRF. CRF fluctuates over time with changes in severity happening even within hours (Richardson 1995). Multiple, very short reference periods may detect change but be unable to distinguish between random and clinically significant effects. Longer reference periods, such as in the preceding week, may be less sensitive to chance variations but more difficult to retrieve from memory and less accurate. The trajectory of CRF appears to vary depending on the type and stage of the cancer and of its treatments (Pickard-Holley 1991; Irvine *et al.* 1994; Schwartz 2000). These concerns may determine whether the spacing of discrete measurements is done in relation to chronological time or treatment times and whether subjects are blocked with respect to their diagnosis or treatment. The heterogeneity of existing studies and their limited discussion of the selection of time intervals suggest that these are somewhat neglected areas in assessing change in CRF. Understanding the trajectory of CRF and how temporal factors function in CRF measurement are fundamental in determining change in CRF (Camarillo 1992; Richardson 1995).

CRF as a subjective experience

One of the major changes in recent years is the increased emphasis on the individual's subjective point of view when assessing fatigue in persons with cancer (Rieger 2001; Mock *et al.* 2003). Coupled with this is abundant evidence of the discordance between patients' and healthcare providers' perceptions of cancer-related symptoms (Fernsler 1986; Greene *et al.* 1994; Beisecker *et al.* 1997; Macquart-Moulin *et al.* 1997; Magnusson *et al.* 1997; Newell *et al.* 1998; Schwartz 1998; Knowles *et al.* 2000; Velikova *et al.* 2001; Rustoen *et al.* 2003). Despite this, there are still relatively few qualitative studies of patients' fatigue experience and fewer that examine the perceptions of patients together with those of their family members and healthcare providers (Krishnasamy 2000). As noted earlier, there is also relatively little reliance on a base of qualitative research in development of CRF instruments. Qualitative approaches have not yet been fully integrated in fatigue assessment in cancer research.

Data collection and measurement issues in fatigue research

Self-selection bias in data collection

Many of the most fatigued patients are probably excluded from participation in studies of CRF with lengthy or demanding data collection tasks (for example diaries, repeated interviews, complex questionnaires). This may be on the basis of self-selection or recommendation of the healthcare provider. Consequently, the more extreme manifestations of fatigue are probably under-reported or described in terms of their impact on functioning by proxy respondents. This is particularly problematic in describing fatigue in severely ill patients.

Use of cognitive psychology and technology in facilitating data collection

Little attention is given to the cognitive aspects of questionnaire response in facilitating the collection of self-report data on CRF (Mullin *et al.* 2000; Tourangeau *et al.* 2000). This is an overlooked opportunity to ease the data collection burden for respondents and improve the quality of the data generated. When coupled with the use of benchmarks, cognitive psychology techniques may be useful in counteracting the phenomenon of 'response shift' (Sprangers *et al.* 1999) in assessing change in fatigue over the course of treatment. Patients whose fatigue has increased over treatment are likely to view their early fatigue as 'mild' or 'absent' when assessed retrospectively in comparison with their current more severe fatigue. A contemporaneous assessment of their earlier fatigue might have found it 'moderate'.

Technological innovations such as computer touch-screen questioning or use of handheld computers in screening for fatigue, interactive voice responding for routine assessment of ongoing fatigue, and computer-adaptive testing to individualize testing are not widely implemented. Recent work by Velikova *et al.* (1999a, 2002), Cleeland *et al.* (2000), and Cull *et al.* (2001) suggests their value in easy, more comprehensive screening and rapid reporting of probable symptomatology to the healthcare provider.

Confounding fatigue symptoms with outcomes

Winningham *et al.* (1994) criticised some instruments used to evaluate CRF for combining the symptoms of fatigue (physical, emotional, and cognitive manifestations of fatigue) with the consequences of fatigue (for example impairment of functional performance and quality of life) in a single composite score to indicate fatigue status. This problem persists in more recent instruments. As a result, various combinations of high/low symptom scores and impairment scores can yield similar composite scores but very different fatigue experience. Measures of symptoms of fatigue should be distinguished from measures of consequences of fatigue, at least through the use of separate subscale scores or separate instruments.

Equating findings across different measurements of fatigue

Carr *et al.* (2002) found that in 27 studies of the prevalence of CRF, 26 of them from 1993–2001, only one instrument (the fatigue subscale of EORTC QLQ-C30) was used in four studies; all other instruments were used in either one or two studies. No nomograms or algorithms are available for equating the findings across dissimilar measurements of fatigue. Some attempts have been made to define cutting points for 'moderate', and 'severe' fatigue, but these gradations are not defined uniformly across instruments (Mendoza *et al.* 1999; Cleeland *et al.* 2000; Cella *et al.* 2002). Somewhat more promising are the attempts to define what constitutes a clinically significant difference by comparing multiple instruments on the same study population (Schwartz *et al.* 2002).

Implications for practice and research

Recommendations for assessing and measuring fatigue in people in cancer

Frequent and accurate symptom assessment and communication between patients and healthcare providers foster optimal management of cancer-related symptoms (Cleeland *et al.* 2000). Regular use of standardized instruments for fatigue assessment can improve patient–provider communication by stimulating providers to initiate discussion of specific aspects of cancer patients' fatigue and by increasing both patients' and providers' awareness of the issues.

Single-item instruments, such as RFS and VAFS, and the three-item fatigue subscale of the EORTC QLQ-C30 are easy approaches for fatigue screening. All measure the current level of fatigue intensity, and each can serve as a simple indicator for comparing changes over time. The EORTC QLQ-C30 measures fatigue in the context of other cancer symptoms in a widely used 30-item instrument that has been validated in many languages (www.eortc.be/home/qol). More complex instruments, such as MFSI-SF, SCFS, SCFS-6, and CFS, are multidimensional instruments with strong psychometric properties developed specifically for measuring CRF and validated by cancer patients. They are best suited for more in-depth assessment of fatigue and for research settings.

The standardized ICD-10 criteria will help to clarify the conceptualization of CRF, improve its detection in clinical practice, and promote consistency and accuracy of the estimation of prevalence in CRF research. The finalized ICD-10 CRF criteria may serve as a 'gold standard' for fatigue diagnosis in clinical and research practice (see Box 9.1).

Box 9.1 Areas for future research

- Continue to validate and disseminate standardized criteria for CRF assessment.
- Compare the effectiveness of simple assessment strategies with more complex screening and diagnostic approaches in clinical practice.
- Explore the temporal issues of recency, episodicity, and duration of CRF in the measurement of CRF.
- Continue to examine CRF in the context of symptom clusters.
- Investigate strategies to address special issues in the measurement of CRF in elderly patients and in advanced cancer patients.
- Document cancer aetiology, stage, and treatment regimen; instruments used to assess CRF and time intervals for reference, its characteristics, and its consequences in reports of research on CRF, to contribute to a less equivocal body of evidence about CRF.

Computerized assessments

Advances in computer technology provide an opportunity for innovative symptom assessment in clinical practice using computer touch-screen assessment, interactive voice-response systems, or computer-adaptive testing. Using technology-based assessments may reduce the time required to collect, record, and retrieve the data in clinical and research settings.

Computer touch-screen assessment uses a computer program to administer an assessment instrument. The application of computer technology to quality of life assessment has been shown to be feasible and equivalent in psychometric properties to the traditional paper-and-pencil format (Velikova *et al.* 1999*a*,*b*, 2002; Cull *et al.* 2001; Wilkie *et al.* 2001). Compared with the paper format, computer touch-screens were acceptable to participants, quicker to use, facilitated the communication of symptoms, and provided better-quality data in oncology practice (Cull *et al.* 2001; Wilkie *et al.* 2001). Use of a handheld computer can facilitate rapid screening and transmission of patient information to the clinician without the active hands-on involvement of the patient that is possible with touch-screen assessment.

An interactive voice-response (IVR) system was incorporated in the development of MDASI (Cleeland *et al.* 2000; Naughton and Homsi 2002). The IVR system automatically calls patients at a designated time and invites them to respond to voiced questions by pressing the keypad of their telephone. For research purposes, the information can be delivered immediately to the investigators. For clinical purposes, thresholds can be set for each assessed symptom. If the response is above the threshold value, the system will automatically notify the healthcare providers and direct their immediate attention to the symptom.

CRF assessment for the future is moving towards computer-adaptive testing (CAT). CAT employs item response theory and an item bank with a large number of items within different domains of interest (Revicki and Cella 1997; Velikova *et al.* 1999*b*; Cull *et al.* 2001) to tailor the assessment to the specific person. Each individual is asked only those questions that are most relevant to his/her condition and thus is assessed very efficiently. The advantages of using computer-adaptive testing in measuring CRF are numerous: individually tailored assessment, reduced testing time and respondent burden, and immediate scoring and feedback of data.

Each of these technology-based approaches requires a substantial initial commitment to programming and/or item generation in order to realize the gains in data quality, data feedback, and reduced respondent burden.

Conclusion

Recent growth in the area of assessment and measurement of CRF has been fruitful. Clinicians show a greater receptivity to assessing CRF, and they have more assistance in doing so—the ICD-10 diagnostic criteria, the NCCN fatigue assessment algorithm,

Box 9.2 Summary points

♦ The choice of assessment instrument for measuring CRF should be based on the purpose of measurement and the characteristics of the particular tool.

♦ Using uniform CRF diagnostic criteria will better define CRF, contribute to greater consistency in assessing its prevalence, facilitate understanding its persistence and severity, and support clinical management of CRF.

♦ Instruments generated by investigators without being validated by persons who have experienced CRF should be viewed cautiously.

♦ Measures of fatigue symptoms should be distinguished from measures of fatigue consequences.

♦ Psychometric testing is a sample-dependent, on-going process. Users should test and revalidate an instrument when employing it with different populations or modifying the instrument or its mode of use.

a wide range of screening instruments, and more complex assessment instruments. Clinicians need more information about the availability, use, and interpretation of these criteria, algorithms, and instruments so that the gap between availability and use is reduced.

Researchers have identified and tackled some of the persistent problems in the measurement of CRF. These include the fundamental problem of how to conceptualize CRF, the inclusion of the patients' perspective in the development and/or validation of measures of CRF, and the linking of scores on the various instruments with clinically significant change in CRF. Study of the psychometric properties of instruments to measure CRF has become more thorough, often incorporating attention to internal consistency reliability, content validity, and either construct or criterion-related validity (Norbeck 1985). However, temporal issues in measurement of CRF need far more attention. Test–retest reliability is infrequently reported; measures differ greatly in their time frames; and longitudinal studies of fatigue across the trajectory of cancer diagnosis, treatment, and survivorship or palliative care are rare. Cognitive psychology and technology offer advantages in data collection and retrieval that need to be exploited. As is true of other cancer-related symptoms, assessing and measuring fatigue in people with cancer requires serious and sustained efforts by clinicians and researchers (see Box 9.2).

References

Aaronson, N.K., Ahmedzai, S., Bergman, B., Bullinger, M., Cull, A., Duez, N.J. *et al.* (1993) The European Organization for Research and Treatment of Cancer QLQ-C30: a quality-of-life instrument for use in international clinical trials in oncology. *Journal of the National Cancer Institute*, **85**(5), 365–76. (See also http://www.eortc.be/home/qol/)

Ancoli-Israel, S., Moore, P.J., and Jones, V. (2001) The relationship between fatigue and sleep in cancer patients: a review. *European Journal of Cancer Care*, **10**(4), 245–55.

Beisecker, A., Cook, M.R., Ashworth, J., Hayes, J., Brecheisen, M., Helmig, L. *et al.* (1997) Side effects of adjuvant chemotherapy: perceptions of node-negative breast cancer patients. *Psycho-oncology*, **6**(2), 85–93.

Bender, C., Kramer, P., and Miaskowski, C. (2002) *New Directions in the Management of Cancer-Related Cognitive Impairement, Fatigue, and Pain.* Oncology Nursing Society, Pittsburgh, PA.

Berger, A.M., Von Essen, S., Kuhn, B.R., Piper, B.F., Agrawal, S., Lynch, J.C. *et al.* (2003) Adherence, sleep, and fatigue outcomes after adjuvant breast cancer chemotherapy: results of a feasibility intervention study. *Oncology Nursing Forum*, **30**(3), 513–22.

Blesch, K.S., Paice, J.A., Wickham, R., Harte, N., Schnoor, D.K., Purl, S. *et al.* (1991) Correlates of fatigue in people with breast or lung cancer. *Oncology Nursing Forum*, **18**(1), 81–7.

Camarillo, M. (1992).The oncology patient's experience of fatigue. *Quality of Life*, **1**(1), 39–44.

Carr, D., Goudas, L., and Lawrence, D. (2002) *Management of Cancer Symptoms: Pain, Depression, and Fatigue.* Evidence report/technology assessment number 61. AHRQ Publication No 02-E032, July. Rockville, MD: Agency for Healthcare Research and Quality. (Available at: http://www.ahrq.gov/clinic/evrptfiles.htm (see Cancer symptoms: pain, depression, and fatigue, management).)

Cella, D., Davis, K., Breitbart, W., Curt, G., and Fatigue Coalition (2001) Cancer-related fatigue: prevalence of proposed diagnostic criteria in a United States sample of cancer survivors. *Journal of Clinical Oncoogy*, **19**(14), 3385–91.

Cella, D., Lai, J.S., Chang, C.H., Peterman, A., and Slavin M. (2002) Fatigue in cancer patients compared with fatigue in the general United States population. *Cancer*, **94**(2), 528–38.

Cleeland, C.S., Mendoza, T.R., Wang, X.S., Chou, C., Harle, M.T., Morrissey, M. *et al.* (2000) Assessing symptom distress in cancer patients: the M.D. Anderson Symptom Inventory. *Cancer*, **89**(7), 1634–46.

Cull, A., Gould, A., House, A., Smith, A., Strong, V., Velikova, G. *et al.* (2001) Validating automated screening for psychological distress by means of computer touchscreens for use in routine oncology practice. *British Journal of Cancer*, **85**(12), 1842–9.

Curt, G.A. (2000) The impact of fatigue on patients with cancer: overview of FATIGUE 1 and 2. *Oncologist*, **5** (Supplement 2), 9–12.

Curt, G. and Johnston, P.G. (2003) Cancer fatigue: the way forward. *Oncologist*, **8**(Supplement 1), 27–30.

Daly, P.A. (2003) Introduction: All-Ireland Fatigue Coalition. *Oncologist*, **8**(Supplement 1), 1–2.

Fernsler, J.A. (1986) Comparison of patient and nurse perceptions of patients' self-care deficits associated with cancer chemotherapy. *Cancer Nursing*, **9**(2), 50–7.

Fillion, L., Gelinas, C., Simard, S., Savard, J., and Gagnon, P. (2003) Validation evidence for the French Canadian adaptation of the Multidimensional Fatigue Inventory as a measure of cancer-related fatigue. *Cancer Nursing*, **26**(2), 143–54.

Flechtner, H. and Bottomley, A. (2003) Fatigue and quality of life: lessons from the real world. *Oncologist*, **8**(Supplement 1), 5–9.

Furst, C.J. and Ahsberg, E. (2001) Dimensions of fatigue during radiotherapy. An application of the Multidimensional Fatigue Inventory. *Supportive Care in Cancer*, **9**(5), 355–60.

Gentile, S. (2003) Validation of the French Multidimensional Fatigue Inventory (MFI 20) *European Journal of Cancer Care*, **12**, 58–64.

Glaus, A. (1993) Assessment of fatigue in cancer and non-cancer patients and in healthy individuals. *Supportive Care in Cancer*, **1**(6), 305–15.

Glaus, A., Crow, R., and Hammond, S. (1996) A qualitative study to explore the concept of fatigue/tiredness in cancer patients and in healthy individuals. *European Journal of Cancer Care,* 5(Supplement 12), 8–23.

Greene, D., Nail, L.M., and Fieler, V.K. (1994) A comparison of patient-reported side effects among three chemotherapy regimens for breast cancer. *Cancer Practice,* 2(1), 57–62.

Hann, D. M., Jacobsen, P.B., Azzarello, L.M., Martin, S.C., Curran, S.L., Fields, K.K. *et al.* (1998) Measurement of fatigue in cancer patients: development and validation of the Fatigue Symptom Inventory. *Quality of Life Research,* 7(4), 301–10.

Hockenberry-Eaton, M. and Hinds, P.S. (2000) Fatigue in children and adolescents with cancer: evolution of a program of study. *Seminars in Oncology Nursing,* 16(4), 261–72 [discussion 272–8].

Hockenberry, M., Hinds, P., Barrera, P., Bryant, R., Adams-McNeill, J., Hooke, C., *et al.* (2003) Three instruments to assess fatigue in children with cancer: the child, parent and staff perspectives. *Journal of Pain and Symptom Management,* 25(4), 319–28.

Holley, S. (2000*a*) Cancer-related fatigue: suffering a different fatigue. *Cancer Practice,* 8(2), 87–95.

Holley, S.K. (2000*b*) Evaluating patient distress from cancer-related fatigue: an instrument development study. *Oncology Nursing Forum,* 27(9), 1425–31.

Irvine, D.M., Vincent, L., Bubela, N., Thompson, L., and Graydon, J. (1991) A critical appraisal of the research literature investigating fatigue in the individual with cancer. *Cancer Nursing,* 14(4),188–99.

Irvine, D., Vincent, L., Graydon, J.E., Bubela, N., and Thompson, L. (1994) The prevalence and correlates of fatigue in patients receiving treatment with chemotherapy and radiotherapy. A comparison with the fatigue experienced by healthy individuals. *Cancer Nursing,* 17(5), 367–78.

Kasper, C.E. and Sarna, L.P. (2000) Influence of adjuvant chemotherapy on skeletal muscle and fatigue in women with breast cancer. *Biological Research for Nursing,* 2(2),133–9.

Kirsh, K.L., Passik, S., Holtsclaw, E., Donaghy, K., and Theobald, D. (2001) I get tired for no reason: a single item screening for cancer-related fatigue. *Journal of Pain and Symptom Management,* 22(5), 931–7.

Knowles, G., Borthwick, D., McNamara, S., Miller, M., and Leggot, L. (2000) Survey of nurses' assessment of cancer-related fatigue. *European Journal of Cancer Care,* 9(2), 105–13.

Krishnasamy, M. (2000) Fatigue in advanced cancer: meaning before measurement? *International Journal of Nursing Studies,* 37(5), 401–14.

Kroenke, K. (2001) Studying symptoms: sampling and measurement issues. *Annals of Internal Medicine,* 134(9, Part 2), 844–53.

Krzys, T.M. (1995) Journal writing in rehabilitation: a tool to help patients and families face challenges and adapt. *Rehabilitation Nursing,* 20(4), 226–8.

Langeveld, N.E., Grootenhuis, M.A., Voute, P.A., de Haan, R.J., and van den Bos, C. (2003) No excess fatigue in young adult survivors of childhood cancer. *European Journal of Cancer,* 39, 204–14.

Lissitz, R. and Green, S. (1975) Effect of the number of scale points on reliability: a Monte Carlo approach. *Journal of Applied Psychology,* 60(1), 10–13.

Macquart-Moulin, G., Viens, P., Bouscary, M.L., Genre, D., Resbeut, M., Gravis, G. *et al.* (1997) Discordance between physicians' estimations and breast cancer patients' self-assessment of side-effects of chemotherapy: an issue for quality of care. *British Journal of Cancer,* 76(12), 1640–5.

Magnusson, K., Karlsson, E., Palmblad, C., Leitner, C., and Paulson, A. (1997) Swedish nurses' estimation of fatigue as a symptom in cancer patients—report of a questionnaire. *European Journal of Cancer Care,* 6(3), 186–91.

McNair, D., Lorr, M., and Droppleman, L. (1992) *Profile of Mood States Manual, Revised.* Education and Industrial Testing Service, San Diego, CA.

Meek, P.M., Nail, L.M., Barsevick, A., Schwartz, A.L., Stephen, S., Whitmer, K. *et al.* (2000) Psychometric testing of fatigue instruments for use with cancer patients. *Nursing Research,* **49**(4), 181–90.

Mendoza, T.R., Wang, X.S., Cleeland, C.S., Morrissey, M., Johnson, B.A., Wendt, J.K. *et al.* (1999) The rapid assessment of fatigue severity in cancer patients: use of the Brief Fatigue Inventory. *Cancer,* **85**(5), 1186–96.

Miller, G. (1956) The magical number seven, plus or minus two: some limits on our capacity for processing information. *Psychological Review,* **63**(2), 81–97.

Mock, V. (2001) Fatigue management: evidence and guidelines for practice. *Cancer,* **92**(6, Supplement S), 1699–707.

Mock, V., Atkinson, A., Barsevick, A., Cella, D., Cimprich, B., Cleeland, C. *et al.* for the National Comprehensive Cancer Network Cancer-Related Fatigue Panel. (2003) *NCCN Practice Guidelines for Cancer-Related Fatigue,* Version 1. National Comprehensive Cancer Network. (Available at: http://www.nccn.org/physician_gls/f_guidelines.html)

Mullin, P., Lohr, K., Bresnahan, B., and McNulty, P. (2000) Applying cognitive design principles to formatting HRQOL instruments. *Quality of Life Research,* **9**,13–27.

Nail, L.M. and Winningham, M.L. (1995) Fatigue and weakness in cancer patients: the symptom experience. *Seminars in Oncology Nursing,* **11**(4), 272–8.

Naughton, M. and Homsi, J. (2002) Symptom assessment in cancer patients. *Current Oncology Reports,* **4**(3), 256–63.

Newell, S., Sanson-Fisher, R.W., Girgis, A., and Bonaventura, A. (1998) How well do medical oncologists' perceptions reflect their patients' reported physical and psychosocial problems? Data from a survey of five oncologists. *Cancer,* **83**(8), 1640–51.

Norbeck, J.S. (1985) What constitutes a publishable report of instrument development? *Nursing Research,* **34**(6), 380–2.

Nunnally, J. and Bernstein, I. (1994) *Psychometric Theory.* McGraw-Hill, New York.

Okuyama, T., Akechi, T., Kugaya, A., Okamura, H., Shima, Y., Maruguchi, M. *et al.* (2000*a*) Development and validation of the Cancer Fatigue Scale: a brief, three-dimensional, self-rating scale for assessment of fatigue in cancer patients. *Journal of Pain and Symptom Management,* **19**(1), 5–14.

Okuyama, T., Akechi, T., Kugaya, A., Okamura, H., Imoto, S., Nakano, T. *et al.* (2000*b*) Factors correlated with fatigue in disease-free breast cancer patients: application of the Cancer Fatigue Scale. *Supportive Care in Cancer,* **8**(3), 215–22.

Okuyama, T., Wang, X.S., Akechi, T., Mendoza, T.R., Hosaka, T., Cleeland, C.S. *et al.* (2003) Validation study of the Japanese version of the Brief Fatigue Inventory. *Journal of Pain and Symptom Management,* **25**(2), 106–17.

Passik, S., Kirsh, K.L., Donaghy, K., Holtsclaw, E., Theobald, D., Cella, D. *et al.* and the Fatigue Coalition (2002) Patient-related barriers to fatigue communication: initial validation of the Fatigue Management Barriers Questionnaire. *Journal of Pain and Symptom Management,* **24**(5), 481–93.

Patrick, D., Ferketich, S., and Frame, P. (2002) *Symptom Management in Cancer: Pain, Depression, and Fatigue.* National Institutes of Health State-of-the-Science Conference, 15–17 July 2002. Final Statement 26 October 2002. (Available at: http://consensus.nih.gov/ta/022/cancer_mgmt_consensus.pdf)

Pearce, S. and Richardson, A. (1996) Fatigue in cancer: a phenomenological perspective. *European Journal of Cancer Care,* **5**(2), 111–15.

Pickard-Holley, S. (1991) Fatigue in cancer patients: a descriptive study. *Cancer Nursing,* **14**(1), 13–19.

Piper, B.F., Lindsey, A.M., and Dodd, M.J. (1987) Fatigue mechanisms in cancer patients: developing nursing theory. *Oncology Nursing Forum*, **14**(6), 17–23.

Piper, B., Lindsey, A.M., and Dodd, M. (1989) The development of an instrument to measure the subjective dimension of fatigue. In: *Key Aspects of Comfort: Management of Pain, Fatigue, and Nausea*, (ed. S. Funk, E. Tornquist, and M. Champagne), pp. 199–208. Springer, New York.

Piper, B.F., Dibble, S.L., Dodd, M.J., Weiss, M.C., Slaughter, R.E., and Paul, S.M. (1998) The revised Piper Fatigue Scale: psychometric evaluation in women with breast cancer. *Oncology Nursing Forum*, **25**(4), 677–84.

Portenoy, R.K. and Itri, L.M. (1999) Cancer-related fatigue: guidelines for evaluation and management. *Oncologist*, **4**(1), 1–10.

Radbruch, L., Sabatowski, R., Elsner, F., Everts, J., Mendoza, T., and Cleeland, C. (2003) Validation of the German version of the Brief Fatigue Inventory. *Journal of Pain and Symptom Management*, **25**(5), 449–58.

Ream, E. and Richardson, A. (1997) Fatigue in patients with cancer and chronic obstructive airways disease—a phenomenological enquiry. *International Journal of Nursing Studies*, **34**(1), 44–53.

Redeker, N.S., Lev, E.L., and Ruggiero, J. (2000) Insomnia, fatigue, anxiety, depression, and quality of life of cancer patients undergoing chemotherapy. *Scholarly Inquiry into Nursing Practice*, **14**(4), 275–90 [discussion 291–8].

Ressel, G.W. (2003) NIH releases statement on managing pain, depression, and fatigue in cancer. *American Family Physician*, **67**(2), 423–4.

Revicki, D.A. and Cella, D.F. (1997) Health status assessment for the twenty-first century: item response theory, item banking and computer adaptive testing. *Quality of Life Research*, **6**(6), 595–600.

Rhoten, D. (1982) Fatigue and the post-surgical patient. In: *Concept Clarification in Nursing* (ed C. Norris), pp. 277–300. Aspen Publishers, Rockville, MD.

Richardson, A. (1995) The pattern of fatigue in patients receiving chemotherapy. In: *Nursing Research in Cancer Care* (ed. A. Richardson and J. Wilson-Barnett), pp. 225–45. Scutari Press, London.

Rieger, P.T. (2001) Assessment and epidemiologic issues related to fatigue. *Cancer*, **92**(6, Supplement), 1733–6.

Rustoen, T., Schjolberg, T.K., and Wahl, A.K. (2003) What areas of cancer care do Norwegian nurses experience as problems? *Journal of Advanced Nursing*, **41**(4), 342–50.

Sadler, I.J., Jacobsen, P.B., Booth-Jones, M., Belanger, H., Weitzner, M.A., and Fields, K.K. (2002) Preliminary evaluation of a clinical syndrome approach to assessing cancer-related fatigue. *Journal of Pain and Symptom Management*, **23**(5), 406–16.

Schwartz, A.H. (2002) Validity of cancer-related fatigue instruments. *Pharmacotherapy*, **22**(11), 1433–41.

Schwartz, A.L. (1998) The Schwartz Cancer Fatigue Scale: testing reliability and validity. *Oncology Nursing Forum*, **25**(4), 711–17.

Schwartz, A.L. (2000) Daily fatigue patterns and effect of exercise in women with breast cancer. *Cancer Practice*, **8**(1), 16–24.

Schwartz, A. and Meek, P. (1999) Additional construct validity of the Schwartz Cancer Fatigue Scale. *Journal of Nursing Measurement*, **7**(1), 35–45.

Schwartz, A., Meek, P., Nail, L., Fargo, J., Lundquist, M., Donofrio, M. *et al.* (2002) Measurement of fatigue: determining minimally important clinical differences. *Journal of Clinical Epidemiology*, **55**, 239–44.

Schwartz, R., Krauss, O., and Hinz, A. (2003) Fatigue in the general population. *Onkologie*, **26**, 140–4.

Smets, E.M., Garssen, B., Bonke, B., and De Haes, J.C. (1995) The Multidimensional Fatigue Inventory (MFI) psychometric qualities of an instrument to assess fatigue. *Journal of Psychosomatic Research*, **39**(3), 315–25.

Sprangers, M.A., Van Dam, F.S., Broersen, J., Lodder, L., Wever, L., Visser, M.R. *et al.* (1999) Revealing response shift in longitudinal research on fatigue—the use of the Thentest approach. *Acta Oncologica*, **38**(6), 709–18.

Stein, K.D., Martin, S.C., Hann, D.M., and Jacobsen, P.B. (1998) A multidimensional measure of fatigue for use with cancer patients. *Cancer Practice*, **6**(3), 143–52.

Stone, P. (2002) The measurement, causes and effective management of cancer-related fatigue. *International Journal of Palliative Nursing*, **8**(3), 120–8.

Stone, P., Richards, M., A'Hern, R., and Hardy, J. (2000) A study to investigate the prevalence, severity and correlates of fatigue among patients with cancer in comparison with a control group of volunteers without cancer. *Annals of Oncology*, **11**(5), 561–7.

Tourangeau, R., Rips, L., and Rasinski, K. (2000) *The Psychology of Survey Response*. Cambridge University Press, New York.

Velikova, G., Wright, E.P., Smith. A.B., Cull, A., Gould, A., Forman, D. *et al.* (1999*a*) Automated collection of quality-of-life data: a comparison of paper and computer touch-screen questionnaires. *Journal of Clinical Oncology*, **17**(3), 998–1007.

Velikova, G., Stark, D., and Selby, P. (1999*b*) Quality of life instruments in oncology. *European Journal of Cancer*, **35**(11), 1571–80.

Velikova, G., Wright, P., Smith, A.B., Stark, D., Perren, T., Brown, J. *et al.* (2001) Self-reported quality of life of individual cancer patients: concordance of results with disease course and medical records. *Journal of Clinical Oncology*, **19**(7), 2064–73. [Erratum *Journal of Clinical Oncology*, **19**(20), 4091.]

Velikova, G., Brown, J.M., Smith, A.B., and Selby, P.J. (2002) Computer-based quality of life questionnaires may contribute to doctor-patient interactions in oncology. *British Journal of Cancer*, **86**(1), 51–9.

Visser, M.R.M. and Smets, E.M.A. (1998) Fatigue, depression and quality of life in cancer patients—how are they related? *Supportive Care in Cancer*, **6**(2), 101–8.

Wang, L. (2002) Cancer care should include symptom management, panel says. *Journal of the National Cancer Institute*, **94**(15), 1123–4.

Ware, J.E, Jr. and Sherbourne, C.D. (1992) The MOS 36-item short-form health survey (SF-36). I. Conceptual framework and item selection. *Medical Care*, **30**(6), 473–83.

Ware, J.E., Jr., Snow, K., Kosinski, M., and Gandek, B. (1993) *SF-36 Health Survey: Manual and Interpretation Guide*. Boston, MA: The Health Institute, New England Medical Center.

Wilkie, D.J., Huang, H.Y., Berry, D.L. Schwartz, A., Lin, Y.C., Ko, N.Y. *et al.* (2001) Cancer symptom control: feasibility of a tailored, interactive computerized program for patients. *Family and Community Health*, **24**(3), 48–62.

Winningham, M.L. (2001) Strategies for managing cancer-related fatigue syndrome: a rehabilitation approach. *Cancer*, **92**(4, Supplement), 988–97.

Winningham, M.L., Nail, L.M., Burke, M.B., Brophy, L., Cimprich, B., Jones, L.S. *et al.* (1994) Fatigue and the cancer experience: the state of the knowledge. *Oncology Nursing Forum*, **21**(1), 23–36.

Wu, H.S. and McSweeney, M. (2001) Measurement of fatigue in people with cancer. *Oncology Nursing Forum*, **28**(9), 1371–86.

Yellen, S.B., Cella, D.F., Webster, K., Blendowski, C., and Kaplan, E. (1997) Measuring fatigue and other anaemia-related symptoms with the Functional Assessment of Cancer Therapy (FACT) measurement system. *Journal of Pain and Symptom Management*, **13**(2), 63–74.

Chapter 10

Fatigue and depression in cancer patients: Conceptual and clinical issues

Paul Jacobsen and Michael Weitzner

Introduction

There is a growing recognition among oncology professionals that fatigue is one of the most common and distressing symptoms experienced by cancer patients (Winningham *et al.* 1994; Richardson 1995). In seeking to learn more about the aetiology and treatment of fatigue, clinicians and researchers alike have been challenged to understand how fatigue and depression may be related in patients with cancer. The need to understand this relationship stems from two basic facts: (1) fatigue, in addition to being a symptom of cancer and its treatment, is a symptom of depression (American Psychiatric Association 1994) and (2) depression, like fatigue, is relatively common among cancer patients (Bottomley 1998). In our attempt to clarify the fatigue–depression relationship in cancer patients, we have identified four questions that are of particular importance and will serve to organize this chapter. What are the conceptual similarities and differences between fatigue and depression? To what extent are fatigue and depression related and how might they be distinguished? What are the causal relationships between fatigue and depression? And what are the treatment implications of relationships between fatigue and depression?

Any attempt to answer these questions should be based on empirical findings and, whenever possible, we have done so. However, given the limited amount of research on fatigue in cancer patients, there is relatively little empirical evidence currently available to answer several of our questions. We hope that, by identifying areas where evidence is lacking, this chapter will stimulate additional and much needed research into the relationship between fatigue and depression in patients with cancer.

What are the conceptual similarities and differences between fatigue and depression?

In order to understand the conceptual similarities and differences between depression and fatigue, it is necessary to consider how these two concepts have been defined.

Our approach to this issue focuses on the different ways in which fatigue and depression have been assessed in cancer patients.

Three distinct approaches to the measurement of depression can be identified: the single-symptom approach, the symptom cluster approach, and the clinical syndrome approach. The single-symptom approach refers to assessment methods that focus specifically on measuring depressed mood. This symptom can be measured as a continuous variable (for example visual analogue scales measuring severity of depressed mood) or a categorical variable (for example clinical interview items measuring presence/absence of depressed mood).

The symptom cluster approach refers to assessment methods that focus on measuring depressive symptomatology. A common approach to measuring depressive symptomatology in cancer patients has been to administer a multi-item self-report scale, such as the Beck Depression Inventory (BDI) (Beck *et al.* 1961) or the Center for Epidemiologic Studies Depression Scale (CES-D) (Radloff 1977). Both instruments assess a constellation of symptoms (for example depressed mood, loss of appetite, and difficulty concentrating) that are theorized to reflect the construct of depression. Higher scores on these measures suggest the presence of more depressive symptoms as well as the increased severity of those symptoms. Since fatigue is generally regarded as one of the core symptoms of depression (American Psychiatric Association 1994), it is not surprising to find that many depressive symptomatology measures include at least one item assessing fatigue-related phenomena. For example, the BDI asks respondents to chose among alternatives ranging from 'I don't get more tired than usual' to 'I am too tired to do anything'. Similarly, on the CES-D respondents are asked to rate the extent to which they 'could not get "going"' from 'rarely or none of the time' to 'most or all of the time'.

The clinical syndrome approach refers to assessment methods that focus on detecting the presence of a mood disorder, such as major depressive disorder. As defined in the fourth edition of the American Psychiatric Association's *Diagnostic and Statistical Manual of Mental Disorders* (DSM-IV) (American Psychiatric Association 1994), a diagnosis of major depressive disorder requires, in part, the presence of five or more depressive symptoms during the same 2-week period. Depressed mood or loss of interest or pleasure in usual activities must be present for the diagnosis to be made. Among the other symptoms whose presence counts toward the criterion of five or more symptoms is 'fatigue or loss of energy'. Accordingly, items assessing fatigue are a standard feature of structured interviews designed to diagnose major depressive disorder (First *et al.* 1996).

Fatigue can also be assessed as a single symptom, a cluster of symptoms, and a clinical syndrome. The single-symptom approach refers to assessment methods in which fatigue is conceptualized as a unidimensional phenomenon. Measures of fatigue severity, such as the Profile of Mood States Fatigue Scale (POMS-F) (McNair *et al.* 1971), exemplify this approach. Overlap can be identified between the single-symptom approach to measuring fatigue and both the symptom cluster and clinical syndrome approaches to measuring depression. As described above, instruments used to measure depressive symptomatology and diagnose major depressive disorder typically include one or more items assessing the presence or severity of fatigue-related phenomena.

The symptom cluster approach refers to assessment methods in which fatigue has been conceptualized as a multidimensional phenomenon. Although the specific dimensions that characterize fatigue in cancer patients remain a topic of debate (Winningham *et al.* 1994; Richardson 1995), at least two independent teams of investigators (Smets *et al.* 1996; Stein *et al.* 1998) have identified similar clusters of symptoms. These clusters include: general symptoms (for example tiredness), physical symptoms (for example feelings of weakness or heaviness), and mental symptoms (for example difficulty concentrating). Self-report measures reflecting this conceptualization of fatigue include the Multidimensional Fatigue Inventory (MFI) (Smets *et al.* 1996) and the Multidimensional Fatigue Symptom Inventory (MFSI) (Stein *et al.* 1998). Overlap can be identified between this approach to measuring fatigue and both the symptom cluster and clinical syndrome approaches to measuring depression. For example, both multidimensional fatigue measures referred to above assess a general symptom of fatigue (that is, tiredness) and a mental symptom of fatigue (that is, difficulty concentrating) that are also included in instruments used to measure depressive symptomatology and diagnose major depressive disorder.

The clinical syndrome approach represents a relatively new method of assessing fatigue in cancer patients. Recognizing the need for a standard case definition, a group of investigators (Cella *et al.* 1998) recently proposed a set of criteria for the diagnosis of 'cancer-related fatigue'. These diagnostic criteria (Table 10.1) have been submitted for inclusion in the 10th edition of the International Classification of Diseases (ICD-10). Examination of the criteria indicates that overlap exists between this approach to measuring fatigue and both the symptom cluster and clinical syndrome approaches to measuring depression.

As shown in Table 10.1, a diagnosis of cancer-related fatigue requires the presence of six or more symptoms listed in Criterion A. Several of the symptoms listed (for example fatigue, sleep disturbance, diminished concentration, and decreased interest in usual activities) are also present in measures of depressive symptomatology and are included in diagnostic criteria for major depressive disorder.

Although similarities are present in approaches to measuring fatigue and depression, important differences can also be identified. Symptom cluster and clinical syndrome conceptualizations of depression generally include a number of symptoms that are not consistent with symptom cluster and clinical syndrome conceptualizations of fatigue. These include changes in appetite or weight, recurrent thoughts of death, feelings of worthlessness or excessive guilt, and psychomotor agitation or retardation. Likewise, symptom cluster and clinical syndrome conceptualizations of fatigue include a number of symptoms that are not consistent with symptom cluster and clinical syndrome

Table 10.1 ICD-10 criteria for cancer-related fatigue

A. Six (or more) of the following symptoms have been present every day or nearly every day during the same 2-week period in the past month, and at least one of the symptoms is (1) significant fatigue:

1. Significant fatigue, diminished energy, or increased need to rest, disproportionate to any recent change in activity level

2. Complaints of generalized weakness or limb heaviness

3. Diminished concentration or attention

4. Decreased motivation or interest to engage in usual activities

5. Insomnia or hypersomnia

6. Experience of sleep as unrefreshing or non-restorative

7. Perceived need to struggle to overcome inactivity

8. Marked emotional reactivity (e.g. sadness, frustration, or irritability) to feeling fatigued

9. Difficulty completing daily tasks attributed to feeling fatigued

10. Perceived problems with short-term memory

11. Postexertional malaise lasting several hours

B. The symptoms cause clinically significant distress or impairment in social, occupational, or other important areas of functioning

C. There is evidence from the history, physical examination, or laboratory findings that the symptoms are a consequence of cancer or cancer therapy

D. The symptoms are not primarily a consequence of co-morbid psychiatric disorders such as major depression, somatization disorder, somatoform disorder, or delirium

conceptualizations of depression. These symptoms include generalized feelings of weakness or heaviness, postexertional malaise, and difficulty completing daily tasks due to fatigue. Moreover, clinical syndrome approaches to measuring both fatigue and depression include criteria that seek to differentiate cancer-related fatigue and major depressive disorder. Criterion D for cancer-related fatigue (Table 10.1) states that this syndrome is not diagnosed if symptoms of fatigue are considered to be the primary consequence of a co-morbid psychiatric disorder. Similarly, DSM-IV criteria (American Psychiatric Association 1994) specify that major depressive disorder is not diagnosed if depressive symptoms (including fatigue) are considered to be the direct physiological effects of substance use or a general medical condition such as cancer.

In summary, a review of measurement approaches indicates that overlap is present between all three approaches to measuring fatigue and both the symptom cluster and clinical syndrome approaches to measuring depression. This overlap is consistent with the fact that the symptom of fatigue is encompassed within current conceptualizations of depressive symptomatology and major depressive disorder. Overlap also reflects the fact that several symptoms commonly associated with depression (for example tiredness, diminished attention, and sleep disturbance) are encompassed within symptom cluster and clinical syndrome approaches to measuring fatigue in cancer patients. Based on these considerations, one would expect empirical studies to show that fatigue and depression are related in patients with cancer.

To what extent are fatigue and depression related and how might they be distinguished?

A search of the literature yielded 14 published studies in which fatigue and depression were assessed concurrently in patients with cancer (Table 10.2).

Depression was usually assessed in these studies using measures of depressive symptomatology, such as the CES-D (Radloff 1977), the BDI (Beck *et al.* 1961), or the depression subscale of the Hospital Anxiety and Depression Scale (HADS) (Zigmond and Snaith 1983). Exceptions include two studies (Blesch *et al.* 1991; Dimeo *et al.* 1997) that used the POMS Depression Scale, a measure that reflects primarily depressed mood, and one study (Visser and Smets 1998) that included only mood items from the CES-D. No studies were identified that assessed fatigue and the presence/absence of a mood disorder syndrome (for example major depressive disorder) concurrently in cancer patients. Fatigue was usually assessed in these studies using measures of general fatigue severity, such as the POMS Fatigue Scale or the MFI General Scale. Three studies were identified (Smets *et al.* 1996; Schneider 1998; Stein *et al.* 1998) in which general, mental, and physical symptoms of fatigue were assessed as part of a multidimensional approach. No studies were identified that assessed the clinical syndrome of cancer-related fatigue concurrent with depression.

Correlations between measures of fatigue and depression reported in these studies were all positive and ranged from a low of $r = 0.16$ to a high of $r = 0.80$. The average correlation between fatigue and depression across studies (weighted for sample size) was $r = 0.54$. Thus, on average, measures of fatigue and depression administered concurrently to cancer patients share approximately 29% of their variance. There was little evidence that the individual dimensions of fatigue were differentially related to depression. Specifically, in those studies that used a multidimensional approach (Smets *et al.* 1996; Schneider 1998; Stein *et al.* 1998), the average weighted correlations between depression and general fatigue ($r = 0.68$), mental fatigue ($r = 0.62$), and physical fatigue ($r = 0.61$) were all quite similar. In contrast, there was evidence that depressed mood and depressive symptomatology were differentially related to fatigue. The average weighted correlation between measures of fatigue and depressed mood ($r = 0.44$) was found to be considerably less than the average weighted correlation between measures of fatigue and depressive symptomatology ($r = 0.60$). This pattern of results is consistent with the view that measures assessing depressive

Table 10.2 Studies assessing fatigue and depression concurrently in cancer patients

Study	Cancer diagnoses	n	Treatment modalities	Depression measure	Fatigue measure	r
Andrykowski et al. (1998)	Breast	88	Radiation, chemotherapy	CES-D	CFS (total)	0.68
				CES-D	PFS (total)	0.68
				CES-D	Weakness rating	0.47
				CES-D	Tiredness rating	0.63
Blesch et al. (1991)	Breast, lung	77	Radiation, chemotherapy	POMS Depression	VAS Fatigue	0.46
Dimeo et al. (1997)	Mixed	78	Transplantation	POMS Depression	POMS Fatigue	0.61
				SCL-90 Depression	POMS Fatigue	0.68
Hann et al. (1997)	Breast	43	Transplantation	CES-D	POMS Fatigue	0.80
Hann et al. (1998)	Breast	45	Radiation	CES-D	FSI (severity)	0.68
				CES-D	FSI (interference)	0.73
Hann et al. (1999)	Breast	31	Transplantation	CES-D	POMS Fatigue	.77
Pickard-Holley, 1991	Ovarian	12	Chemotherapy	BDI	RFS	.20
Schneider (1998)	Mixed	54	Radiation, chemotherapy	BDI	MFI General	0.56
				BDI	MFI Mental	0.55
				BDI	MFI Physical	0.61
Smets et al. (1996)	Mixed	116	Radiation	HADS-D	MFI General	0.77
				HADS-D	MFI Mental	0.61
				HADS-D	MFI Physical	0.67
				HADS-D (minus item 8)	MFI General	0.67
				HADS-D (minus item 8)	MFI Mental	0.58
				HADS-D (minus item 8)	MFI Physical	0.56

Smets et al. (1998a)	250	Mixed	Radiation	CES-D	MFI General	0.43
Smets et al. (1998b)	154	Mixed	Radiation	CES-D	MFI General	0.49
Stein et al. (1998)	326	Breast	Radiation, chemotherapy, transplantation	CES-D	MFSI General	0.68
				CES-D	MFSI Mental	0.64
				CES-D	MFSI Physical	0.61
Stone et al. (1999)	95	Mixed	Unknown	HADS-D (minus item 8)	FSS	0.16
Visser and Smets (1998)	250	Mixed	Radiation	CES-D (mood only) time 1	MFI General	0.35
				CES-D (mood only) time 2	MFI General	0.43
				CES-D (mood only) time 3	MFI General	0.48
				CES-D (mood only) time 1	MFI Physical	0.37
				CES-D (mood only) time 2	MFI Physical	0.50
				CES-D (mood only) time 3	MFI Physical	0.46

r = correlation coefficient; BDI = Beck Depression Inventory; CES-D = Center for Epidemiologic Studies Depression Scale; CFS = Chalder Fatigue Scale; FSI = Fatigue Symptom Inventory; FSS = Fatigue Severity Scale; HADS-D = Hospital Anxiety and Depression Scale—Depression Subscale; MFI = Multidimesional Fatigue Inventory; MFSI = Multidimensional Fatigue Symptom Inventory; PFS = Piper Fatigue Scale; POMS = Profile of Mood States; RFS = Rhoten Fatigue Scale; SCL-90 = Symptom Checklist 90; VAS = Visual Analog Scale.

symptomatology, but not depressed mood, include symptoms that overlap with fatigue.

One of the studies listed in Table 10.2 included analyses designed specifically to examine the effects of overlap on correlations between measures of fatigue and depression. In this study (Smets et al. 1996), the MFI and the depression subscale of the HADS were administered concurrently to cancer patients undergoing radiotherapy. The latter measure includes one item ('I feel as if I am slowed down') that would appear to overlap with fatigue. Correlations were computed between the MFI and both the original version of the HADS depression subscale and a version that excluded this item. As shown in Table 10.2, exclusion of the item yielded decreases in the magnitude of correlations with the General, Mental and Physical subscales of the MFSI. It should be noted, however, that correlations between depression and fatigue remained relatively high ($r = 0.56$ to 0.67) even after elimination of the item.

In summary, empirical studies yield consistent evidence that levels of fatigue and depression correspond in patients with cancer. The relatively high magnitude of the correlations between measures of fatigue and depressive symptomatology are not surprising considering the overlap present in current approaches to assessing these constructs. There is evidence to suggest, however, that this correspondence is not solely a function of overlap in measurement approaches. First, correlations between fatigue and depressive symptomatology remain relatively high even when items reflecting phenomena associated with fatigue are removed from the depressive symptomatology measures (Smets et al. 1996). Second, correlations are relatively high between measures of fatigue and measures assessing only depressed mood (Blesch et al. 1991; Dimeo et al. 1997; Visser and Smets 1998).

Taken together, the findings from empirical studies suggest that the two measurement approaches currently in use (that is, the single symptom and symptom cluster approaches) are of limited usefulness in attempts to distinguish fatigue and depression. One strategy that has yet to be investigated for its ability to distinguish fatigue and depression is the clinical syndrome approach. As noted earlier, criteria have been proposed for diagnosing a clinical syndrome of cancer-related fatigue (Cella et al. 1998). With the advent of these criteria, there is a need for research in which clinical syndrome measures of depression and fatigue are administered concurrently to cancer patients. The results of this research would indicate the extent to which it is possible to distinguish fatigue associated with cancer and its treatment from fatigue associated with mood disorder. Likewise, this research would indicate the extent to which it is possible to distinguish whether certain 'depressive symptoms' (for example loss of concentration) are a reflection of an underlying mood disorder or are part of a cancer-related fatigue syndrome. The ability to distinguish clinical syndromes of fatigue and depression may be particularly important as studies are initiated that seek to determine the efficacy of antidepressant medications in relieving fatigue in cancer patients (see below).

What are the causal relationships between fatigue and depression?

As noted earlier, there is considerable evidence that levels of fatigue and depression correspond in cancer patients. At least three different causal relationships can be theorized to explain this correspondence. One possibility is that the fatigue produced by cancer and its treatment may result in patients becoming depressed. A second possibility is that fatigue may develop in cancer patients as a consequence of their being depressed. Yet a third possibility is that no causal relationship exists; instead, the correspondence may reflect the presence of a third factor that is the cause of both fatigue and depression in patients with cancer. As will be shown, there is evidence to suggest the existence of each of these mechanisms.

Two lines of research provide support for the view that cancer patients can become depressed as a consequence of experiencing disease-related or treatment-related fatigue. One line of research consists of reports indicating that patients perceive disease-related or treatment-related fatigue as having adverse effects on their mood. For example, women undergoing bone marrow transplantation for breast cancer have been found to report more severe fatigue and greater interference of fatigue with their mood than a comparison group of women with no history of cancer (Hann *et al.* 1999). Differences between groups on these measures were evident only after the breast cancer patients had started treatment. A second line of evidence consists of research examining whether, over the course of cancer treatment, fatigue predicts subsequent depression better than depression predicts subsequent fatigue. Of particular relevance is a study in which fatigue and depression were assessed before the start of radiotherapy treatment and again 2 weeks after completion of treatment (Visser and Smets 1998). Pretreatment fatigue severity was found to account for 11% of the variability in subsequent depressed mood whereas pretreatment depressed mood accounted for only 4% of the variability in subsequent fatigue severity. Additional supportive evidence comes from a study that examined relations between psychiatric disorder (that is, mood, anxiety, and adjustment disorders) and fatigue in women previously treated with adjuvant chemotherapy for breast cancer (Broeckel *et al.* 1998). The presence of a psychiatric disorder prior to cancer diagnosis was not related to fatigue severity following chemotherapy treatment; in contrast, more severe fatigue following chemotherapy treatment was related to the concurrent presence of a psychiatric disorder.

The possibility that cancer patients may develop fatigue as a consequence of being depressed is intuitively obvious. Actually demonstrating this relationship represents a methodological challenge, since most cancer patients can also develop fatigue as a consequence of their disease or its treatment. There is, however, indirect evidence to support the possibility that fatigue in cancer patients may occur as a consequence of depression. Research has shown that patients with a prior history of depression are more likely to develop mood disorders following the diagnosis of cancer (Leopold *et al.* 1998).

Evidence indicating that these patients also experience worse fatigue than patients without mood disorders would be consistent with the possibility that fatigue can occur as a consequence of depression. Another indirect piece of evidence consists of reports indicating that reliance on specific forms of coping characteristic of depressed individuals is related to fatigue severity in cancer patients. For example, among women with breast cancer previously treated with chemotherapy, greater reliance on catastrophizing (a coping strategy characterized by negative self-statements and overly negative thoughts about the future) was found to be associated with more severe fatigue (Broeckel *et al.* 1998). Greater reliance on this coping strategy has also been shown to be related to higher levels of depressive symptomatology in breast cancer patients (Jacobsen *et al.* 1999).

There is considerable evidence to suggest that the correspondence between fatigue and depression in cancer patients may be due to their causal relationship to a third factor. Along these lines, attention has focused on certain cancers that are believed to cause depressive symptoms. Pancreatic cancer is one neoplasm that appears to display these characteristics. The prevalence of depression-related disorders among patients with pancreatic cancer is estimated to be as high as 71% (Green and Austin 1993). Moreover, numerous reports have documented the presence of depressive symptoms in patients before their pancreatic cancer was diagnosed (Joffe *et al.* 1986; Holland *et al.* 1986; Kelsen *et al.* 1995). Recent physiological findings provide further evidence of a causal link between pancreatic cancer and depression. Pancreatic tumours have been shown to secrete various neuropeptides and neurohormones, such as adrenocorticotropic hormone (ACTH) and cortisol (Raddatz *et al.* 1998; Drake *et al.* 1998). These findings are consistent with a wealth of data showing that hypercortisolaemia, as evidenced by non-suppression of cortisol after dexamethasone administration, is associated with major depressive disorder (Geffken *et al.* 1998). Pancreatic tumours have also been shown to secrete calcitonin. These secretions can result in hypercalcaemia (Sugimoto *et al.* 1998; Fleury *et al.* 1998), a condition characterized by prominent symptoms of lethargy and fatigue (Hutto 1998). In addition, there is evidence that pancreatic tumours also secrete growth hormone (Kawa *et al.* 1997; Losa and von Werder 1997), another substance known to be associated with increased depressive symptoms (Geffken *et al.* 1998).

Certain forms of cancer treatment may also be a direct cause of both fatigue and depression. Along these lines, attention has focused on biological response modifiers such as the interferons and the interleukins. These agents are used increasingly to treat a variety of cancers, including renal cell cancer and melanoma, and to control chronic myelogenous leukaemia. Administration of supraphysiological doses of these substances has been shown to be associated with prominent depressive symptoms, including fatigue (Valentine *et al.* 1998; Licinio *et al.* 1998; Meyers 1999). The occurrence of these psychiatric side-effects is consistent with research showing that elevated levels of both interferons and interleukins are present in psychiatric patients with major depressive disorder (Maes *et al.* 1995*a*,*b*; Anforth *et al.* 1998; Anisman *et al.* 1999; Licinio and Wong 1999).

What are the treatment implications of relationships between fatigue and depression?

In the previous section, we reviewed evidence suggesting the existence of three different causal relationships between fatigue and depression in cancer patients. One possibility suggested by prior research is that patients experience fatigue as part of an underlying mood disorder. A second possibility is that patients develop symptoms of depression (for example depressed mood) as a result of experiencing disease-related or treatment-related fatigue. Yet a third possibility is that the correspondence between fatigue and depression in cancer patients is due a third factor, such as administration of high-dose interferon therapy. In this section, we examine how consideration of these causal mechanisms may have implications for the management of fatigue.

The situation in which fatigue is part of a mood disorder is perhaps the easiest to manage, since therapy will revolve around treatment of the underlying mood disorder. The treatment of major depressive disorder in cancer patients typically involves the use of both pharmacological and non-pharmacological therapies (Pirl and Roth 1999). The selection of a specific antidepressant is likely to be guided by the symptom presentation. For example, if sleep disturbance is one of the chief presenting symptoms of depression, an antidepressant with sedating properties (for example amitriptyline) would be preferred. If, on the other hand, the patient's depression is accompanied by problems with diarrhoea, as with several gastrointestinal cancers, then an antidepressant with constipating properties (for example paroxetine) would be preferred. By and large, research indicates that serotonin selective re-uptake inhibitors (SSRIs) (for example paroxetine, sertraline, and citalopram) and medications that inhibit primarily norepinephrine re-uptake (for example venlafaxine, amfebutamone, and the tricyclic antidepressants) are equally efficacious in the treatment of major depressive disorder (Feighner *et al.* 1993; Moller *et al.* 1993; Stuppaeck *et al.* 1994). As depressed mood improves, the associated fatigue can also be expected to resolve.

The management of disease-related or treatment-related fatigue that is accompanied by depressive symptoms is more complex. This situation reflects, in part, the relative lack of empirically supported interventions for fatigue in cancer patients. In the absence of a strong body of empirical evidence, several authors (Cella *et al.* 1998; Portenoy and Itri 1999) have proposed preliminary guidelines for the management of fatigue based largely on clinical experience with cancer patients and research with other patient populations (Fig. 10.1). According to these guidelines, efforts to manage fatigue should focus on correcting potential aetiologies as well as relieving symptoms. Potentially correctable aetiologies, besides depression, include anaemia, infection, other symptoms (for example pain), and centrally acting medications (for example opioids).

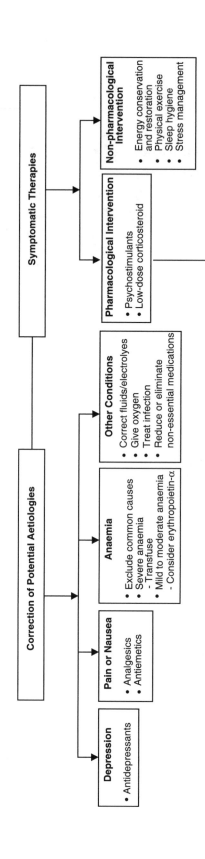

Fig. 10.1 Algorithm for management of cancer-related fatigue. (Adapted from Portenoy and Itri (1999) and Cella et al. (1998).)

Symptomatic therapies may include pharmacological as well as non-pharmacological interventions. It is worth noting that several of the proposed symptomatic therapies for fatigue (for example physical exercise, psychostimulant medications, and antidepressant medications) also have antidepressant properties.

A growing body of evidence indicates that exercise may be effective in relieving fatigue in patients who are undergoing or recovering from cancer treatment (Courneya and Friedenreich 1999). Positive changes in mood are a likely consequence of regular practice of exercise. However, at least one study (Mock *et al.* 1997) has documented that reductions in treatment-related fatigue among regular exercisers were not accompanied by corresponding reductions in depressed mood. These findings suggest that the beneficial effects of exercise on fatigue in cancer patients are not due solely to the mood-enhancing properties of exercise.

With regard to psychostimulants (for example methylphenidate, dextroamphetamine, and pemoline), there is evidence that this class of medications may be useful in relieving fatigue related to opioid-induced somnolence (Bruera *et al.* 1989), neurobehavioural slowing (Weitzner *et al.* 1995; Meyers *et al.* 1998), and depression (Breitbart and Mermelstein 1992) in cancer patients. Clinical experience suggests that these agents are also useful in relieving disease-related or treatment-related fatigue in cancer patients. The mechanisms by which psychostimulants may relieve disease-related or treatment-related fatigue have yet to be identified. In particular, it is unclear whether the effects of psychostimulants on fatigue are related to or distinct from their mood-enhancing properties.

Recommendations regarding the use of antidepressant medications to relieve fatigue in cancer patients are based largely on clinical observations that these agents can produce increases in energy disproportionate to any changes in mood (Portenoy and Itri 1999). Accordingly, administration of these agents may be indicated for non-depressed patients experiencing disease-related or treatment-related fatigue in cancer. Controlled trials are needed to identify the specific antidepressant agents that are effective in relieving fatigue. Two agents that appear to merit study are venlafaxine and amfebutamone. This suggestion is based on clinical observations that these two agents have particularly energizing effects (Marin 1996). Both agents appear to function similarly to psychostimulants, in that their use is associated with increased synaptic levels of norepinephrine (Hyman *et al.* 1995). These findings are consistent with animal and human studies suggesting that increased levels of norepinephrine and/or dopamine are associated with increased levels of cortical arousal (Duffy 1997). As with the psychostimulants, it will be important to clarify whether any observed effects of these agents on fatigue are related to or distinct from their mood-enhancing effects.

The guidelines described above (Cella *et al.* 1998; Portenoy and Itri 1999) are also applicable to the management of fatigue and depression that is related to a third factor. To the extent that the aetiology of these symptoms is identifiable and correctable, efforts should focus on correcting the underlying cause(s). Often, correction of the underlying aetiology is not practical or feasible. For example, it may be inadvisable to discontinue interferon even though a patient has become severely fatigued and depressed during the course of therapy. Under these circumstances, management efforts should focus on symptomatic relief. In the absence of a strong body of empirical evidence, clinical experience would suggest the use of agents that are likely to have beneficial effects on both fatigue and depression (for example, 'activating' antidepressants or psychostimulants). Clearly, this is an area in which controlled outcomes studies are needed (see Box 10.1).

Conclusions

In this chapter we have sought to address four issues regarding the relationship between fatigue and depression in cancer patients (Box 10.2). First, we have identified conceptual similarities and differences between fatigue and depression. As noted previously, fatigue and depression have both been assessed as a single symptom, a cluster of symptoms, and a clinical syndrome. Overlap was found to be present between all three of these approaches to measuring fatigue and both the symptom cluster and clinical syndrome approaches to measuring depression. This overlap reflects the inclusion of the symptom of fatigue within symptom cluster and clinical syndrome approaches to measuring depression and the inclusion of certain symptoms of depression (for example difficulty concentrating) within symptom cluster and clinical syndrome approaches to measuring fatigue. Important conceptual differences were also identified. Certain symptoms (for example recurrent thoughts of death) generally appear only in measures of depression, whereas other symptoms (for example postexertional malaise) generally appear only in measures of fatigue. Moreover, it was noted that the clinical syndrome measurement approaches include criteria intended to differentiate cancer-related fatigue and major depressive disorder.

Box 10.1 Future areas for research

- Studies promoting understanding of the similarities and differences between cancer-related fatigue and depression are needed.
- Studies to assess both mood disorder and fatigue concurrently in patients with cancer should be undertaken.
- Studies to evaluate the efficacy of therapies targeted at the management of cancer-related fatigue and depression represent high priorities for research in this area.
- Studies that contribute to understanding the mechanisms of action of therapies targeted at cancer-related fatigue and depression are urgently needed.

A second aim of this chapter was to determine the extent to which fatigue and depression are related in cancer patients. A review of the literature indicated that research on this topic has been limited to the use of either single-symptom or symptom cluster approaches to measuring fatigue and depression. The average correlation between fatigue and depression across studies was found to be relatively high ($r = 0.54$). The magnitude of this correlation is consistent with the previously noted overlap between measures of fatigue and measures of depressive symptomatology. There is evidence, however, that this correspondence is not solely a function of overlap in measurement approaches. For example, correlations between measures of fatigue and depression were found to remain relatively high even when items reflecting phenomena associated with fatigue were removed from measures of depressive symptomatology. These findings suggest that the two measurement approaches currently in use (that is, the single-symptom and the symptom cluster approaches) are of limited usefulness in attempts to distinguish fatigue and depression. Clinical syndrome approaches to measuring fatigue and depression may be better suited to this task and merit further study.

A third aim of the chapter was to explore the causal relationships between fatigue and depression in cancer patients. A review of the literature suggested the existence of three different causal mechanisms. First, there is evidence consistent with the view that cancer patients may become depressed as a consequence of experiencing disease-related or treatment-related fatigue. Second, there is evidence suggesting that fatigue may develop in cancer patients as a consequence of their becoming depressed. Third, there is evidence indicating that the correspondence between fatigue and depression in cancer patients may be due to the presence of a third factor. Examples of such a third factor include certain neoplasms (for example pancreatic cancer) and certain forms of cancer treatment (for example interferon therapy) that appear to be a direct cause of both fatigue and depression. The specific mechanisms by which these neoplasms and treatments give rise to both fatigue and depression are not well understood and need to be investigated further.

The fourth and final aim was to consider the treatment implications of relationships between fatigue and depression in cancer patients. When evidence suggests that fatigue is the consequence of a mood disorder, then efforts to manage fatigue typically focus on treatment of the underlying mood disorder. The management of fatigue that is disease-related or treatment-related and accompanied by depressive symptoms is more complex owing, in part, to the relative lack of empirically validated interventions. Current guidelines (Cella *et al.* 1998; Portenoy and Itri 1999), based largely on clinical experience and research with other patient populations, suggest that efforts to manage fatigue under these circumstances should focus on correcting potential aetiologies and relieving symptoms. Several of the proposed symptomatic therapies (for example physical exercise, psychostimulant medications, and antidepressant medications) are known to have antidepressant properties. These therapies may be particularly useful in

Box 10. 2 Summary points

1. A review of measurement approaches indicates that overlap is present between measurement of fatigue and depression as single symptoms, as clusters, and as clinical syndromes.

2. Epidemiological studies yield consistent evidence that levels of fatigue and depression correspond in patients with cancer.

3. At least three different causal relationships can be theorized to echo the correspondence between fatigue and depression:

  ◆ That fatigue produced by cancer and its treatment may result in depression.

  ◆ That fatigue may develop in patients with cancer as a consequence of depression.

  ◆ The correspondence may reflect the presence of a third factor that results in both fatigue and depression in patients with cancer, for example high-dose interferon therapy.

managing fatigue accompanied by depressive symptoms as well as fatigue and depression that are attributable to a common third factor. Evaluating the efficacy of these therapies and understanding their mechanisms of action in relieving fatigue should be considered high priorities for future research.

References

American Psychiatric Association (1994) *Diagnostic and Statistical Manual of Mental Disorders*, 4th edn. American Psychiatric Press, Washington, DC.

Andrykowski, M.A., Curran, S.L., and Lightner, R. (1998) Off-treatment fatigue in breast cancer survivors: a controlled comparison. *Journal of Behavioral Medicine*, **21**, 1–18.

Anforth, H.R., Bluthe, R.M., Bristow, A., Hopkins, S., Lenczowski, M.J., Luheshi, G. *et al.* (1998) Biological activity and brain actions of recombinant rat interleukin-1-alpha and interleukin-1-beta. *European Cytokine Network*, **9**, 279–88.

Anisman, H., Ravindran, A.V., Griffiths, J., and Merali, Z. (1999) Endocrine and cytokine correlates of major depression and dysthymia with typical or atypical features. *Molecular Psychiatry*, **4**, 182–8.

Beck, A.T., Ward, C.H., Mendelson, M., Mock, J., and J, Erbaugh, J. (1961) An inventory for measuring depression. *Archives of General Psychiatry*, **4**, 53–63.

Blesch, K.S., Paice, J.A., Wickham, R., Harte, N., Schnoor, D.K., Purl, S. *et al.* (1991) Correlates of fatigue in people with breast or lung cancer. *Oncology Nursing Forum*, **18**, 81–7.

Bottomley, A. (1998) Depression in cancer patients: a literature review. *European Journal of Cancer Care*, **7**, 181–91.

Breitbart, W. and Mermelstein, H. (1992) An alternative psychostimulant for the management of depressive disorders in cancer patients. *Psychosomatics*, **33**, 352–6.

Broeckel, J.A., Jacobsen, P.B., Horton, J., Balducci, L., and Lyman, G.H. (1998) Characteristics and correlates of fatigue after adjuvant chemotherapy for breast cancer. *Journal of Clinical Oncology*, **16**, 1689–96.

Bruera, E., Brenneis, C., Paterson, A.H., and MacDonald, R.N. (1989) Use of methylphenidate as an adjuvant to narcotic analgesics in patients with advanced cancer. *Journal of Pain and Symptom Management*, **4**, 3–6.

Cella, D., Peterman, A., Passik, S., Jacobsen, P.B., and Breitbart, W. (1998) Progress toward guidelines for the management of fatigue. *Oncology*, **12**, 369–77.

Courneya, K.S. and Friedenreich, C.M. (1999) Physical exercise and quality of life following cancer diagnosis: a literature review. *Annals of Behavioral Medicine*, **21**, 171–9.

Dimeo, F., Stieglitz, R.D., Novelli-Fischer, U., Fetscher, S., Mertelsmann, R., and Keul, J. (1997) Correlation between physical performance and fatigue in cancer patients. *Annals of Oncology*, **8**, 1251–5.

Drake, W.M., Perry, L.A., Hinds, C.J., Lowe, D.G., Reznek, R.H., and Besser, G.M. (1998) Emergency and prolonged use of intravenous etomidate to control hypercortisolemia in a patient with Cushing's syndrome and peritonitis. *Journal of Clinical Endocrinology and Metabolism*, **83**, 3542–4.

Duffy, J.D. (1997) The neural substrates of motivation. *Psychiatric Annals*, **27**, 24–9.

Feighner, J., Cohn, J., Fabre, L., Fieve, R.R., Mendels, J., Shrivastava, R.K. *et al.* (1993) A study comparing paroxetine, placebo, and imipramine in depressed patients. *Journal of Affective Disorders*, **28**, 71–9.

First, M.B., Gibbon, M., Spitzer, R.L., and Williams, J.B. (1996) *User's Guide for the Structured Clinical Interview for DSM-IV Disorders*. Biometrics Research, New York.

Fleury, A., Flejou, J.F., Sauvanet, A., Molas, G. Vissuzaine, C., Hammel, P. *et al.* (1998) Calcitonin-secreting tumors of the pancreas: about six cases. *Pancreas*, **16**, 545–50.

Geffken, G.R., Ward, H.E., Staab, J.P., Carmichael, S.L.K., and Evans, D.L. (1998) Psychiatric morbidity in endocrine disorders. *Psychiatric Clinics of North America*, **21**, 473–89.

Green, A.I. and Austin, C.P. (1993) Psychopathology of pancreatic cancer: a psychobiologic probe. *Psychosomatics*, **34**, 208–21.

Hann, D.M., Jacobsen, P.B., Martin, S.C., Kronish, L.E., Azzarello, L.M., and Fields, K.K. (1997) Fatigue in women treated with bone marrow transplantation for breast cancer: a comparison with women with no history of cancer. *Supportive Care in Cancer*, **5**, 44–52.

Hann, D.M., Jacobsen, P.B., Martin, S., Azzarello, L.M., and Greenberg, H. (1998) Fatigue and quality of life following radiotherapy for breast cancer: a comparative study. *Journal of Clinical Psychology in Medical Settings*, **5**, 19–33.

Hann, D.M., Garovoy, N., Finkelstein, B., Jacobsen, P.B., Azzarello, L.M., and Fields, K.K. (1999) Fatigue and quality of life in breast cancer patients undergoing autologous stem cell transplantation: a longitudinal comparative study. *Journal of Pain and Symptom Management*, **17**, 311–19.

Holland, J.C., Korzun, A., Tross, S., Silberfarb, P., Perry, M., Comis, R. *et al.* (1986) Comparative psychological disturbance in patients with pancreatic and gastric cancer. *American Journal of Psychiatry*, **143**, 982–6.

Hutto, B. (1998) Subtle psychiatric presentations of endocrine diseases. *Psychiatric Clinics of North America*, **21**, 905–16.

Hyman, S.E., Arana, G.W., and Rosenbaum, J.F. (1995) *Handbook of Psychiatric Drug Therapy*, 3rd edn. New York: Little, Brown and Company.

Jacobsen, P.B., Azzarello, L.M., and Hann, D.M. (1999) Relation of catastrophizing to fatigue severity in women with breast cancer. *Cancer Research Therapy and Control*, **8**, 155–64.

Joffe, R., Rubinow, D., Demicoff, K., Maher, M., and Sindelar, W.F. (1986) Depression and carcinoma of the pancreas. *General Hospital Psychiatry*, **8**, 241–5.

Kawa, S. Ueno, T., Iijima, A., Midorikawa, T., Fujimori, Y., Tokoo, M. *et al.* (1997) Growth hormone-releasing hormone (GRH)-producing pancreatic tumor with no evidence of multiple endocrine neoplasia type 1. *Digestive Diseases and Sciences,* **42**, 1480–5.

Kelsen, D., Portenoy, R., Thaler, H., Niedzwiecki, D., Passik, S., Tao, Y. *et al.* (1995) Pain and depression in patients with newly diagnosed pancreas cancer. *Journal of Clinical Oncology,* **13**, 748–55.

Leopold, K.A., Ahles, T.A., Walch, S., Amdur, R.J., Mott, L.A., Wiegand-Packard, L. *et al.* (1998) Prevalence of mood disorders and utility of the prime-MD in patients undergoing radiation therapy. *International Journal of Radiation Oncology Biology Physics,* **42**, 1105–12.

Licinio, J. and Wong, M.L. (1999) The role of inflammatory mediators in the biology of major depression: central nervous system cytokines modulate the biological substrate of depressive symptoms, regulate stress-responsive systems, and contribute to neurotoxicity and neuroprotection. *Molecular Psychiatry,* **4**, 317–27.

Licinio, J., Kling, M.A., and Hauser, P. (1998) Cytokines and brain function: relevance to interferon-alpha-induced mood and cognitive changes. *Seminars in Oncology,* **25**(Supplement 1), 30–8.

Losa, M. and von Werder, K. (1997) Pathophysiology and clinical aspects of the ectopic GH-releasing hormone syndrome. *Clinical Endocrinology,* **47**, 123–35.

Maes, M., Bosmans, E., and Meltzer, H.Y. (1995*a*) Immunoendocrine aspects of major depression. Relationships between plasma interleukin-6 and soluble interleukin-2 receptor, prolactin and cortisol. *European Archives of Psychiatry and Clinical Neuroscience,* **245**, 172–8.

Maes, M., Meltzer, H.Y., Bosmans, E., Bergmans, R., Vandoolaeghe, E., Ranjan, R. *et al.* (1995*b*) Increased plasma concentrations of interleukin-6, soluble interleukin-6, soluble interleukin-2 and transferrin receptor in major depression. *Journal of Affective Disorders,* **34**, 301–9.

Marin, R.S. (1996) Apathy: concept, syndrome, neural mechanisms, and treatment. *Seminars in Neuropsychiatry,* **1**, 304–14.

McNair, D.M., Lorr, M., and Droppleman, L.F. (1971) *Profile of Mood States Manual.* Educational and Industrial Testing Service, San Diego, CA.

Meyers, C.A. (1999) Mood and cognitive disorders in cancer patients receiving cytokine therapy. *Advances in Experimental Medicine and Biology,* **461**, 75–81.

Meyers, C.A., Weitzner, M.A., Valentine A.D., and Levin, V.A. (1998) Methylphenidate therapy improves cognition, mood, and function in brain tumor patients. *Journal of Clinical Oncology,* **16**, 2522–7.

Mock, V., Dow, K.H., Meares, C.J., Grimm, P.M., Dienemann, J.A., Haisfield-Wolfe, M.E. *et al.* (1997) Effects of exercise on fatigue, physical functioning, and emotional distress during radiation therapy for breast cancer. *Oncology Nursing Forum,* **24**, 991–1000.

Moller, H., Berzewski, H., Eckmann, F., Gonzalves, N., Kissling, W., Knorr, W. *et al.* (1993) Double-blind multicenter study of paroxetine and amitriptyline in depressed inpatients. *Pharmacopsychiatry,* **26**, 75–8.

Pickard-Holley, S. (1991) Fatigue in cancer patients. *Cancer Nursing,* **14**, 13–19.

Pirl, W.F. and Roth, A.J. (1999) Diagnosis and treatment of depression in cancer patients. *Oncology,* **13**, 1293–1301.

Portenoy, R.K. and Itri, L.M. (1999) Cancer-related fatigue: guidelines for evaluation and management. *The Oncologist,* **4**, 1–10.

Raddatz, D., Horstmann, O., Basenau, D., Becker, H., and Ramadori, G. (1998) Cushing's syndrome due to ectopic adrenocorticotropic hormone production by a non-metastatic gastrinoma after long-term conservative treatment of Zollinger-Ellison syndrome. *Italian Journal of Gastroenterology and Hepatology,* **30**, 636–40.

Radloff, L.S. (1977) The CES-D scale: a self-report depression scale for research in the general population. *Applied Psychological Measures*, **1**, 385–401.

Richardson, A. (1995) Fatigue in cancer patients: a review of the literature. *European Journal of Cancer Care*, **4**, 20–32.

Schneider, R.A. (1998) Concurrent validity of the beck depression inventory and the multidimensional fatigue inventory-20 in assessing fatigue among cancer patients. *Psychological Reports*, **82**, 883–6.

Smets, E.M.A., Garssen, B., Cull, A., and de Haes, J.C. (1996) Application of the multidimensional fatigue inventory (MFI-20) in cancer patients receiving radiotherapy. *British Journal of Cancer*, **73**, 241–5.

Smets, E.M., Visser, M.R., Willems-Grott, A.F., Garssen B., Oldenburger, F., van Tienhoven, G. *et al.* (1998*a*) Fatigue and radiotherapy: (A) experience in patients undergoing treatment. *British Journal of Cancer*, **78**, 899–906.

Smets, E.M., Visser, M.R., Willems-Grott, A.F., Garssen B., Schuster-Uitterhoeve, A.L., and de Haes, J.C. (1998*b*) Fatigue and radiotherapy: (B) experience in patients 9 months following treatment. *British Journal of Cancer*, **78**, 907–12.

Stein, K.D., Martin, S.C., Hann, D.M., and Jacobsen, P.B., (1998) A multidimensional measure of fatigue for use with cancer patients. *Cancer Practice*, **6**, 143–52.

Stone, P., Hardy, J., Broadley, K., Tookman, A.J., Kurowska, A., and Hern, R.A. (1999) Fatigue in advanced cancer: a prospective controlled cross-sectional study. *British Journal of Cancer*, **79**, 1479–86.

Stuppaeck, C.H., Geretsegger, C., Whitwirth, A.B., Schubert, H., Platz, T., Konig, P. *et al.* (1994) A multicenter double-blind trial of paroxetine versus amitriptyline in depressed inpatients. *Journal of Clinical Psychopharmacology*, **14**, 241–6.

Sugimoto, F., Sekiya, T., Saito, M., Iiai, T., Suda, K., Nozawa, A. *et al.* (1998) Calcitonin-producing pancreatic somatostatinoma: report of a case. *Surgery Today*, **28**, 1279–82.

Valentine, A.D., Meyers, C.A., Kling, M.A., Richelson, E., and Hauser, P. (1998) Mood and cognitive side effects of interferon-alpha therapy. *Seminars in Oncology*, **25**(Supplement 1), 35–47.

Visser, M.R.M. and Smets, E.M.A. (1998) Fatigue, depression and quality of life in cancer patients: how are they related? *Supportive Care in Cancer*, **6**, 101–8.

Weitzner, M.A., Meyers, C.A., and Valentine, A.D. (1995) Methylphenidate in the treatment of neurobehavioral slowing associated with cancer and cancer treatment. *Journal of Neuropsychiatry and Clinical Neurosciences*, **7**, 347–50.

Winningham, M.L., Nail, L.M., Burke, M.B., Brophy, L., Cimprich, B., Jones, L.S. *et al.* (1994) Fatigue and the cancer experience, the state of the knowledge. *Oncology Nursing Forum*, **21**, 23–36.

Zigmond, A.S. and Snaith, R.P. (1983) The Hospital Anxiety and Depression Scale. *Acta Psychiatrica Scandinavica*, **67**, 361–70.

Chapter 11

Mental fatigue and cognitive dysfunction

Christina A. Meyers

Introduction

Fatigue is the most widespread adverse symptom related to cancer and cancer therapy (Cleeland 2000). Although there is growing awareness of the prevalence of cancer-related fatigue, there is very little scientific literature about the aetiology and natural history of this debilitating symptom, unlike other illnesses with associated fatigue such as multiple sclerosis and lupus erythematosus. Fatigue can be physical (e.g. associated with muscle weakness or lack of stamina), mental (including poor concentration and lack of motivation), or both. Fatigue can have adverse effects on cognitive function and mood. However, impaired cognitive function and mood disorders may also cause fatigue. The multidimensional nature of fatigue, and its frequent association with cognitive disorders, makes assessment and interventions challenging. However, current research into the underlying mechanisms of cancer-related symptoms is promising and will guide the development of new, targeted treatments (see Chapter 4).

Components of mental fatigue

Mental fatigue is an extremely common side-effect of cancer and cancer treatment. It occurs in the majority of patients who are in active therapy and persists in a substantial proportion of patients after treatment is discontinued. Many patients refer to the syndrome as 'chemobrain'. Mental fatigue is a manifestation of toxicity to the central nervous system. Patients who suffer from mental fatigue often report that they become exhausted from performing their normal routine, and so find it hard to put in a full day's work. They have difficulty with multitasking and become overwhelmed when more than one thing is happening at once. For instance, they have problems following several conversations at a party or working in an office where they must answer several phone lines. Patients report having difficulty sustaining focused attention that manifests itself as vulnerability to distraction. They may experience generalized slowing of cognitive processes, so that they miss points in a conversation or have difficulty meeting deadlines at work. Activities that used to be automatic now require more effort. Factors associated with mental fatigue include the person's subjective perception of burden (Smets *et al.* 1998), their overall physical condition (Smets *et al.* 1998), having multiple social roles, especially for those who work and have families (Mock 1998), and the type and pace of their daily activities.

The impact of mental fatigue will vary from individual to individual. A system for assessing the degree to which a person is disabled by mental fatigue has been developed by the World Health Organization (1980). This system was initially developed to assess the impact of a disorder of the central nervous system, such as a traumatic brain injury, on individual patients, but it is highly applicable to mental fatigue. Impairment is the assessment of mental fatigue as a disorder of the efficient function of the brain and includes the determination of aetiology and severity. This would include medical tests for underlying disturbances of thyroid function or anaemia, assessment of the patient's rating of severity and objective tests of cognitive performance. Disability is the impact of mental fatigue on the patient's ability to perform his or her usual daily activities. Handicap is the impact of mental fatigue on the patient's overall social role and ability to function within the family system, at work, and in society. This is the most individualized level of conceptualization, and is closely related to the person's particular work or leisure activities, their access to support and services, and the developmental stage they are at in life. Thus, a person may be quite handicapped by a relatively minor disability caused by mental fatigue, such as a trial lawyer experiencing mild cognitive slowing. Another person may experience little handicap from a greater disability because they are retired and can take life at their own pace. All three levels of function (impairment, disability, and handicap) need to be addressed for appropriate management of the individual.

Components of cognitive dysfunction

Symptoms of cognitive and mood disturbance are ubiquitous in cancer patients (Meyers 2000). Table 11.1 summarizes the possible contributions of cancer and cancer treatment to cognitive impairment. Advances in the successful treatment of cancer have been achieved largely by an increased aggressiveness of therapy, including surgery,

Table 11.1 Potential causes of cognitive impairment

Primary and metastatic brain cancer

Paraneoplastic disorders

Treatment neurotoxicity

Adjuvant medications

Medical complications

Coexisting medical and psychiatric conditions

Reactive mood and adjustment disorders

radiation, chemotherapy, hormonal agents, and immunotherapy. Unfortunately, cancer treatments are not highly specific and place normal tissues and organs at risk. The central nervous system (CNS) is affected in some way by most cancer treatments. In addition, many adjuvant medications necessary for the treatment of medical complications also cause adverse CNS effects, including immunosuppressive agents used in bone marrow transplantation, antibiotics, steroids, and drugs used for pain and nausea. Medical complications, such as anaemia and infection, may result in cognitive disturbance. CNS cancers, particularly malignant gliomas, cause progressive decline in mental function similar to neurodegenerative diseases. Some non-CNS cancers, including small cell lung cancer and acute leukaemia, cause brain dysfunction indirectly (paraneoplastic disorders). This can be related to an autoimmune response directed against the tumour that affects the brain, or by secretion of cytokines or other substances that cross the blood–brain barrier and are neurotoxic.

Cancer patients will typically complain of memory problems when they present for evaluation and treatment of cognitive dysfunction. However, formal neuropsychological testing often reveals a restriction of working memory capacity rather than a true impairment in the ability to retain newly learned information. For example, the person may learn fewer words than expected on a list-learning task, but retains most of the items that were initially learned over time. In essence, the person can process less information 'on-line', and information that does not get processed in working memory initially will obviously not be recalled later. In addition, patients will demonstrate variability in their ability to focus attention. For example, during a mental arithmetic test they may miss easier items and get more difficult ones correct as a result of fluctuations in attention, despite having preserved mathematical ability. Another common finding on evaluation is an impairment of divided attention. This is often assessed by having the person connect dots alternating between numbers and letters; their performance may be slower than expected when alternating between two sequences. This often correlates with subjective difficulties with multitasking. In contrast, tests of reasoning and problem solving tend not to be affected; patients will perform within expectation, given their age and education, on these tests. Individuals with mental fatigue will, therefore, often have difficulty performing their normal work even though their intellectual functions are not compromised.

The symptoms of fatigue and cognitive dysfunction frequently coexist, and both can have overlapping causes (see Table 11.2). However, the relationship between the two symptoms is not at all clear. For example, cognitive dysfunction can cause fatigue; individuals who must exert more mental effort to perform tasks because of cognitive impairment will tire easily. On the other hand, people who are exhausted report that they cannot think straight. However, these two symptoms are frequently distinguishable. For instance, Schagen et al. (1999) did not find a correlation between cognitive dysfunction and fatigue in breast cancer patients. In contrast, another study found that patients who complained of memory loss and difficulty with concentration were more

Table 11.2 Overlapping causes of fatigue and cognitive dysfunction

Cancer treatment
Medications
Anaemia
Treatment-related
Disease-related
Depression
Stress
Pain
Nausea and vomiting
Nutrition
Dyspnoea

likely to have fatigue despite unimpaired objective cognitive assessment (Cull *et al.* 1996). In addition, the severity of physical fatigue did not correlate with the severity of mental fatigue in patients with Parkinson's disease (Lou *et al.* 2001). Thus, comprehensive assessment of mental fatigue must include objective assessment of cognitive perform- ance as well as subjective patient report of symptoms.

Although there are few data exploring the relationship between mental fatigue and cognitive dysfunction in cancer patients, there is some information in other disease states. For instance, patients with chronic fatigue syndrome (CFS) have impaired cognitive function that is not highly correlated with mood disturbance (Christodoulou *et al.* 1998). Patients with multiple sclerosis (MS) manifest worsening scores on cognitive tests after a single continuous 4 h testing session, while healthy control subjects show improve- ment over the same period of time due to practice (Krupp and Elkins 2000). Both the patients with MS and the control subjects reported subjective physical and mental fatigue over the course of the testing session. Similar findings have been reported in patients with myasthenia gravis (Paul *et al.* 2000). Even healthy control subjects can develop cognitive impairments as a result of fatigue. The ability to make rapid decisions declines when people are exhausted from exercise (Féry *et al.* 1997). Sleep deprivation also causes cognitive impairment; performance on tests after 17 h without sleep is as poor as the performance of an individual who has a blood alcohol level of 0.05%, response time is 50% slower, and accuracy is much poorer (Williamson and Feyer 2000). Mental fatigue has also been found to reduce the ability to prepare for future actions in experimental paradigms (Lorist *et al.* 2000).

In addition to assessing changes in cognitive function due to mental fatigue in healthy control subjects, there have been a number of studies demonstrating physiological corre- lates of impaired cognitive function. For instance, transient cognitive impairment due to fatigue was recently assessed using neural network pattern recognition applied to electroencephalograms (EEGs) with 92% accuracy (Gevins and Smith 1999). Changes in brain energy metabolism, measured by phosphorus-31 magnetic resonance spectroscopy (31P-MRS) correlates with the degree of mental fatigue in healthy control subjects (Kato et al. 1999). Increasing mental fatigue is also associated with prolongation of the latency of the P300 peak of auditory event-related potentials (Kaseda et al. 1998), an electro-physiological measure of nerve conduction speed and the magnitude of the response.

Aetiology of mental fatigue

Research into the mechanisms of symptom development is less mature, but several lines of research have generated much interest, including the role of cytokines (Dantzer 2001; Larson and Dunn 2001; Meyers and Valentine 1995) and the impact of anaemia (Temple et al. 1995; Marsh et al. 1991). Understanding the mechanisms of cancer-related fatigue is critical for the provision of targeted interventions (see Chapter 4). The role of proinflammatory cytokines in the genesis of mental fatigue and cognitive impairment is an exciting area of research. Proinflammatory cytokines have profound effects on brain function (Meyers and Valentine 1995). For example, it is known that treatment with interferon-α increases levels of interleukin-1β (IL-1β), interleukin-6 (IL-6) and tumour necrosis factor-α (TNF-α), and that this increase is associated with the impairment of memory, motor, executive functions, and mood that are suggestive of frontal-subcortical dysfunction (Valentine et al. 1998).

Interleukin-1 (IL-1) crosses the blood–brain barrier, with the highest rate of entry occurring in the hypothalamus (Dantzer et al. 1992). The hypothalamus has rich connections with the brainstem, frontal cortex, and limbic system. IL-1 and its receptors are found in many areas of the brain. IL-1 messenger RNA is found in abundance in the hippocampus (Dantzer et al. 1992), a critical structure for memory processes. IL-1β depresses the influx of calcium into hippocampus neurons, which may explain the preponderance of memory impairment in patients with IL-1-associated toxicity (Plata-Salaman and Ffrench-Mullen 1992). TNF is also neurotoxic, and is associated with demyelination in the brain (Ellison and Merchant 1991). TNF and IL-1 are synergistically toxic (Waage and Espevik 1988) and are associated with the development of multiple sclerosis plaques and gliosis (Wollman et al. 1992). Patients with Alzheimer's disease have elevated levels of IL-6 (Huberman et al. 1995). We have found that patients who have severe neurotoxicity following administration of intraventricular IL-2, as treatment for leptomeningeal disease, also have increased IL-6 levels in the cerebrospinal fluid compared with pretreatment values (Sherman et al. 2002). In addition to their direct effects on brain function, these cytokines also provoke a stress hormone cascade that can affect mood and cognition, as well as having discrete effects on brain neurotransmitter systems (Meyers and Valentine 1995; Marsh et al. 1991). The cancer itself may also produce cytokines. Concentrations of IL-6 have been demonstrated to be higher on average in patients with large cell lymphoma and Hodgkin's disease than in normal controls. Patients with high levels are more likely to have poor performance status and B-symptoms than patients with lower levels (Preti *et al.* 1997; Seymour *et al.* 1997). IL-1, IL-6, and TNF-α appear to be elevated in patients with leukaemia and myelodysplastic syndrome (Sugiyama *et al.* 1996; Bruserud *et al.* 1995; Kurzrock *et al.* 1995).

Elevated cytokine levels are observed in other illnesses characterized by mental fatigue. For example, individuals who contract Q fever often develop a syndrome that persists after the illness remits, characterized by fatigue, pain, mood disturbance, and sleep disturbance (Pentilla *et al.* 1998). It is thought that this syndrome may be related to upregulation of certain proinflammatory cytokines, particularly IL-6. Increased IL-6 secretion has also been found in patients with CFS, although the IL-6 changes are not sufficient to explain the entire constellation of symptoms (Cannon *et al.* 1999), as well as in patients with chronic daytime sleepiness (Vgontzas *et al.* 1999). TNF is another cytokine that has been associated with CFS (Moss *et al.* 1999). These studies suggest that potential avenues for treatment may be in the development of cytokine blockers or anti-inflammatory agents.

Anaemia can also cause mental fatigue and cognitive deficits. For instance, cognitive deficits have been reported in well-dialysed patients with end-stage renal disease who are anaemic but do not have uraemia (Nissenson 1992). Cognitive deficits are also seen in patients who have anaemia due to iron deficiency (Lozoff 1988). The cognitive problems observed on neuropsychological testing include deficits in attention, perceptual–motor speed, memory, and verbal fluency (Temple *et al.* 1995; Brown *et al.* 1991; Marsh *et al.* 1991). Neurophysiological assessment of auditory evoked potentials also reveal increased latency of certain components (Brown *et al.* 1991; Marsh *et al.* 1991). These cognitive deficits and slowed evoked potentials often improve following reversal of anaemia with erythropoietin (Temple *et al.* 1995; Brown *et al.* 1991; Marsh *et al.* 1991; Nissenson 1989).

Assessment and measurement

Symptom research in cancer is well developed, with a number of validated assessment tools that measure symptoms such as fatigue, cognitive function, pain, and psychological distress (Cleeland *et al.* 2000; Mendoza *et al.* 1999; Lezak 1995). However, assessment of mental fatigue and its relationship to cognitive impairment is difficult for several reasons. Increasingly there is agreement that fatigue is a multidimensional construct and that assessment instruments, if they are to have any utility in treatment, will have to be multidimensional as well (see Chapter 9). Another factor complicating assessment is that perceptions of subjective phenomena change with time (Dimeo *et al.* 1997). This may relate to observed inconsistencies between complaints of fatigue and cognitive disturbance compared with actual tested performance, and how those inconsistencies are interpreted by clinicians. There are also issues with the ecological validity of cognitive testing in patients with mental fatigue. Usually cognitive testing occurs in a quiet setting, one-to-one with the examiner, which may bear little relationship to that person's performance after an 8 h working day.

Despite these caveats, assessment of impairment, disability, and handicap are done routinely in the clinic. Cognitive testing of impairment needs to include challenging tasks that measure sustained and divided attention, the ability to multitask, and the ability to flexibly shift mental set. In addition, the neuropsychological tests used should be reliable, validated, and provide reference values for the normal population in order to assess the patient's performance in the context of their age, education, and occupational attainments. A review of such tests can be found in Lezak (1995). In addition, there are a number of well-validated tools that measure disability and handicap, a review of which can be found in Wade (1992).

Interventions

Knowing the specific impact of mental fatigue on the individual patient allows the healthcare provider to institute proper interventions, and a multidisciplinary approach tends to be most efficacious. As with most secondary behavioural syndromes, effective intervention against mental fatigue associated with cognitive impairment begins with identification and correction, if possible, of the underlying causes. Examples of this include treatment of thyroid dysfunction or anaemia, and discontinuation or dose reduction of immunotherapy to correct the neuroendocrine or neurochemical disturbance that is a primary cause of the symptoms experienced.

Pharmacological intervention for mental fatigue at this point is symptomatic, and the most widely used class of medications is the psychostimulants. These medications (e.g. methylphenidate hydrochloride, dexamfetamine sulphate, modafinil, pemoline) have an established role in treatment of depression in the medically ill (Brown *et al.* 1998; Masand and Tesar 1996). While not studied in large controlled trials, they have been used to counter sedation associated with opioid administration in cancer patients (Bruera *et al.* 1992), fatigue and depression in AIDS (Wagner *et al.* 1997), and also against cognitive impairment and psychomotor slowing in patients with primary brain tumours (Meyers *et al.* 1996). Pharmacological interventions that could be studied, in addition to stimulant therapy, include drugs used to treat other diseases (e.g. Alzheimer's disease) and drugs that might confer protection to the nervous system to prevent the development of mental fatigue.

Behavioural interventions are often very effective and include self-hypnosis therapy or relaxation training to help focus attention when overwhelmed, energy conservation to preserve stamina, and exercise to enhance energy and fitness. Lifestyle interventions are also valuable. For instance, intervening with employers to implement reasonable accommodations can make the difference between continuing to work or applying for medical disability (e.g. establishing a more distraction-free environment for working, moving to a job that allows flexible working hours which emphasizes completing work properly and on time rather than on the number of consecutive hours spent at the job). Occasionally individuals are disabled from performing their usual work, but vocational counselling and retraining may afford them opportunities to find an area of employment that focuses on their skills and abilities and minimizes the impact of their disabilities.

Conclusion

Mental fatigue and cognitive dysfunction are very common in cancer patients. A relationship between multiple symptoms with potentially similar underlying aetiologies is not well understood at present. An understanding of mental fatigue in cancer patients may benefit by extrapolating from studies of CFS and other non-malignant diseases which show that cognitive impairment is often associated with physical and mental fatigue, and not caused by mood disturbance. Because the disability and handicap caused by mental fatigue are highly individual, it follows that interventions should be patient-specific. Different individuals would benefit from different combinations of lifestyle alterations, behavioural therapies, and pharmacological interventions. Targeted interventions against mental fatigue will benefit from a better understanding of its potential biological causes. Implications for future research are shown in Box 11.1 and a summary of the points made in this chapter in Box 11.2.

Box 11.1 Implications for future research

- Need to develop ecologically valid objective and reproducible assessments of mental fatigue.
- Need to further investigate the pathophysiological mechanisms of mental fatigue.
- Need to identify predictors of patients who are vulnerable to developing significant symptoms.

Box 11.2 Summary points

- Cognitive dysfunction and fatigue frequently overlap, but can be differentiated.
- Cognitive impairments are a result of inefficiency of brain function.
- There are multiple aetiologies of mental fatigue, and thus the requirement for multiple intervention strategies and a multidisciplinary approach to treatment.
- Knowledge of the underlying mechanisms of fatigue in other disease states will inform future research.

References

Brown, T.H., Stoudemire, A., Fogel, B.S., and Moran, M.G. (1998) Psychopharmacology in the medical patient. In: *Psychiatric Care of the Medical Patient*, (ed. A. Stoudemire, B.S. Fogel, and D.B. Greenberg) (2nd edn). Oxford University Press, New York, pp. 329–72.

Brown, W.E., Marsh, J., Wolcott, D., Takushi, R., Carr, C.R., Higa, J. *et al.* (1991) Cognitive function, mood and P3 latency: effects of the amelioration of anaemia in dialysis patients. *Neuropsychologia*, **29**, 35–45.

Bruera, E., Miller, M.J., MacMillan, K., and Kuehn, N. (1992) Neuropsychological effects of methylphenidate in patients receiving a continuous infusion of narcotics for cancer pain. *Pain*, **48**, 163–6.

Bruserud, O., Nesthus, I., Buhring, H.J., and Pawelec, G. (1995) Cytokine modulation of interleukin 1 and tumour necrosis factor-alpha secretion from acute myelogenous leukaemia blast cells *in vitro*. *Leukemia Research*, **1**, 15–22.

Cannon, J.G., Angel, J.B., Ball, R.W., Abad, L.W., Fagioli, L., and Komaroff, A.L. (1999) Acute phase responses and cytokine secretion in chronic fatigue syndrome. *Journal of Clinical Immunology*, **19**, 414–21.

Christodoulou, C., DeLuca, J., Lange, G., Johnson, S.K., Sisto, S.A., Korn, L. *et al.* (1998) Relation between neuropsychological impairment and functional disability in patients with chronic fatigue syndrome. *Journal of Neurology, Neurosurgery and Psychiatry*, **64**, 431–4.

Cleeland, C.S. (2000) Cancer-related symptoms. *Seminars in Radiation Oncology*, **10**, 175–90.

Cleeland, C.S., Mendoza, T.R., Wang, X.S., Chou, C., Harle, M.T., Morrissey, M. *et al.* (2000) Assessing symptom distress in cancer patients: the M.D. Anderson Symptom Inventory. *Cancer*, **89**, 1634–46.

Cull, A., Hay, C., Love, S.B., Mackie, M., Smets, E., and Stewart, M. (1996) What do cancer patients mean when they complain of concentration and memory problems? *British Journal of Cancer*, **74**, 1674–9.

Dantzer, R. (2001) Cytokine-induced sickness behavior: where do we stand? *Brain Behavior and Immunity*, **15**, 7–24.

Dantzer, R., Bluthe, R.M., Kent, S., and Kelley, K.W. (1992) Behavioural effects of cytokines. In: *Interleukin-1 in the Brain* (ed. N.J. Rothwell and R.D. Dantzer), Pergamon Press, New York. pp. 135–50.

Dimeo, F., Stieglitz, R.-D., Novelli-Fischer, U., Fetscher, S., Mertelsmann, R., and Keul, J. (1997) Correlation between physical performance and fatigue in cancer patients. *Annals of Oncology*, **8**, 1251–5

Ellison, M.D. and Merchant, R.E. (1991) Appearance of cytokine-associated central nervous system myelin damage coincides temporally with serum tumour necrosis factor induction after recombinant interleukin-2 infusion in rats. *Journal of Neuroimmunology*, **33**, 245–51.

Féry, Y.A., Ferry, A., Vom Hofe, A., and Rieu, M. (1997) Effect of physical exhaustion on cognitive functioning. *Perceptual and Motor Skills*, **84**, 291–8.

Gevins, A. and Smith, M.E. (1999) Detecting transient cognitive impairment with EEG pattern recognition methods. *Aviation Space and Environmental Medicine*, **70**, 1018–24.

Huberman, M., Sredni, B., Stern, L., Kott, E., and Shalit, F. (1995) IL-2 and IL-6 secretion in dementia: correlation with type and severity of disease. *Journal of Neurological Science*, **130**, 161–4.

Kaseda, Y., Jiang, C., Kurokawa, K., Mimori, Y., and Nakamura, S. (1998) Objective evaluation of fatigue by even-related potentials. *Journal of Neurological Science*, **158**, 96–100.

Kato, T., Murashita, J., Shioiri, T., Inubushi, T., and Kato, N. (1999) Relationship of energy metabolism detected by 31P-MRS in the human brain with mental fatigue. *Neuropsychobiology*, **39**, 214–18.

Krupp, L.B. and Elkins, L.E. (2000) Fatigue and declines in cognitive functioning in multiple sclerosis. *Neurology*, **55**, 934–9.

Kurzrock, R., Wetzler, M., Estrov, Z., and Talpaz, M. (1995) Interleukin-1 and its inhibitors: a biologic and therapeutic model for the role of growth regulatory factors in leukemias. *Cytokines and Molecular Therapy*, **1**, 177–84.

Larson, S.J. and Dunn, A.J. (2001) Behavioral effects of cytokines. *Brain Behavior and Immunity*, **15**, 371–87.

Lezak, M.D. (1995) *Neuropsychological Assessment*. Oxford University Press, New York.

Lorist, M.M., Klein, M., Nieuwenhuis, S., De Jong, R., Mulder, G., and Meijman, T.F. (2000) Mental fatigue and task control: planning and preparation. *Psychophysiology*, **37**, 614–25.

Lou, J.S., Kearns, G., Oken, B., Sexton, G., and Nutt, J. (2001) Exacerbated physical fatigue and mental fatigue in Parkinson's disease. *Movement Disorders*, **16**, 190–6.

Lozoff, B. (1988) Behavioral alterations in iron deficiency. *Advances in Pediatrics*, **35**, 331–60.

Marsh, J., Brown, W.E., Wolcott, D., Carr, C.R., Harper, R., Schweitzer, S.V. *et al.* (1991) RhuEPO treatment improves brain and cognitive function of anemic dialysis patients. *Kidney International*, **39**, 155–63.

Martin-Lester, M. (1997) Cognitive function in dialysis patients. *ANNA Journal*, **24**, 359–65.

Masand, P.S. and Tesar, G.E. (1996) Use of stimulants in the medically ill. *Psychiatric Clinics of North America*, **19**, 515–47.

Mendoza, T.R., Wang, X.S., Cleeland, C.S., Morrissey, M., Johnson, B.A., Wend, J.K. *et al.* (1999) The rapid assessment of fatigue severity in cancer patients: use of the Brief Fatigue Inventory. *Cancer*, **85**, 1186–96.

Meyers, C.A. (2000) Neurocognitive dysfunction in cancer patients. *Oncology (Huntington)*, **14**, 75–9.

Meyers, C.A. and Valentine, A.D. (1995) Neurologic and psychiatric adverse effects of immunological therapy. *CNS Drugs*, **3**, 56–68.

Meyers, C.A., Weitzner, M.A., Valentine, A.D., and Levin, V.A. (1998) Methylphenidate therapy improves cognition, mood, and function of brain tumor patients. *Journal of Clinical Oncology*, **16**, 2522–7.

Mock, V. (1998) Breast cancer and fatigue: issues for the workplace. *AAOHN Journal*, **46**, 425–31.

Moss, R.B., Mercandetti, A., and Vojdani, A. (1999) TNF-alpha and chronic fatigue syndrome. *Journal of Clinical Immunology*, **19**, 314–16.

Nissenson, A.R. (1989) Recombinant human erythropoietin: impact on brain and cognitive function, exercise tolerance, sexual potency, and quality of life. *Seminars in Nephrology* (Supplement 2), 25–31.

Nissenson, A.R. (1992) Epoetin and cognitive function. *American Journal of Kidney Disease*, **20**(Supplement 1), 21–4.

Paul, R.H., Cohen, R.A., Goldstein, J.M., and Gilchrist, J.M. (2000) Fatigue and its impact on patients with myasthenia gravis. *Muscle and Nerve*, **23**, 1402–6.

Pentilla, I.A., Harris, R.J., Storm, P., Haynes, D., Worswick, D.A., and Marmion, B.P. (1998) Cytokine dysregulation in the post-Q-fever fatigue syndrome. *QJM—Monthly Journal of the Association of Physicians*, **91**, 549–60.

Plata-Salaman, C.R. and Ffrench-Mullen, J.M. (1992) Interleukin-1 beta depresses calcium currents in CA1 hippocampal neurons at pathophysiological concentrations. *Brain Research Bulletin*, **29**, 221–3.

Pollitt, E. (1993) Iron deficiency and cognitive function. *Annual Review of Nutrition,* **13**, 521–37.

Preti, H.A., Cabanillas, F., Talpaz, M., Tucker, S.L., Seymour, J., and Kurzrock, R. (1997) Prognostic value of serum interleukin-6 in diffuse large cell lymphoma. *Annals of Internal Medicine,* **127**, 186–94.

Schagen, S.B., van Dam, F.S.A.M., Muller, M.J., Boogerd, W., Lindeboom, J., and Bruning, P. (1999) Cognitive deficits after postoperative adjuvant chemotherapy for breast carcinoma. *Cancer,* **85**, 640–50.

Seymour, J.F., Talpaz, M., Hagemeister, F.B., Cabanillas, F., and Kurzrock, R. (1997) Clinical correlates of elevated serum levels of interleukin-6 in patients with untreated Hodgkin's disease. *American Journal of Medicine,* **102**, 21–8.

Sherman, A., Jaeckle, K., and Meyers, C.A. (2002) Pre-treatment cognitive performance predicts survival in patients with leptomeningeal disease. *Cancer,* **95**, 1311–16.

Smets, E.M., Visser, M.R., Garssen, B., Frijda, N.H., Oosterveld, P., and de Haes, J.C. (1998) Understanding the level of fatigue in cancer patients undergoing radiotherapy. *Journal of Psychosomatic Research,* **45**, 277–93.

Sugiyama, H., Inoue, K., Ogawa, H., Yamagami, T., Soma, T., Miyake, S. *et al.* (1996) The expression of IL-6 and its related genes in acute leukemia. *Leukemia and Lymphoma,* **21**, 49–52.

Temple, R.M., Deary, I.J., and Winney, R.J. (1995) Recombinant erythropoietin improves cognitive function in patients maintained on chronic ambulatory peritoneal dialysis. *Nephrology Dialysis Transplantation,* **10**, 1733–8.

Valentine, A.D., Meyers, C.A., Kling, M.A., Richelson, E., and Hauser, P. (1998) Mood and cognitive side effects of interferon-α therapy. *Seminars in Oncology,* **25**(Supplement 1), 39–47.

Vgontzas, A.N., Papanicolaou, D.A., Bixler, E.O., Lotsikas, A., Zachman, K., Kales, A. *et al.* (1999) Circadian interleukin-6 secretion and quantity and depth of sleep. *Journal of Clinical Endocrinology and Metabolism,* **84**, 2603–7.

Waage, A. and Espevik, T. (1988) Interleukin-1 potentiates the lethal effect of tumour necrosis factor alpha/cachectin in mice. *Journal of Experimental Medicine,* **167**, 1987–92.

Wade, D.T. (1992) *Measurement in Neurological Rehabilitation.* Oxford University Press, Oxford.

Wagner, G.J., Rabkin, J.G., and Rabkin, R. (1997) Dextroamphetamine as a treatment for depression and low energy in AIDS patients: a pilot study. *Journal of Psychosomatic Research,* **4**, 407–11.

Walter, T. (1994) Effect of iron-deficiency anaemia on cognitive skills in infancy and childhood. *Baillere's Clinical Haematology,* **7**, 815–27.

Williamson, A.M. and Feyer, A.M. (2000) Moderate sleep deprivation produces impairments in cognitive and motor performance equivalent to legally prescribed levels of alcohol intoxication. *Occupational and Environmental Medicine,* **57**, 649–55.

Wollmann, E.E., Kopmels, B., Bakalian, A., and Dantzer, R.D. (1992) Cytokines and neuronal degeneration. In: *Interleukin-1 in the Brain,* (ed. N.J. Rothwell and R.D. Dantzer), Pergamon Press, New York. pp. 187–203.

World Health Organization (1980) *International Classification of Impairments, Disabilities, and Handicaps.* World Health Organization, Geneva.

Chapter 12

Clinical interventions for fatigue

Emma Ream and Paddy Stone

Introduction

Healthcare professionals are becoming increasingly aware of the difficulties patients with cancer face when they experience fatigue. A growing body of research portrays the relentlessness of this symptom for this group of patients, and describes the challenges associated with its successful management. Clinicians themselves have reported difficulties with assisting patients to cope with fatigue, and allude to their frustration when their intervention fails (Copp and Dunn 1993). Yet it is vital that those caring for patients with cancer continue to support and educate them in its management. Without intervention and guidance from the healthcare team, patients cope with this complex symptom alone. Researchers who have investigated the self-care activities used by patients with cancer to counteract fatigue have reported patients initiating few attempts to alleviate it (Graydon *et al.* 1995; Richardson and Ream 1997; Hamilton *et al.* 2001). Richardson and Ream (1997) investigated this anomaly and suggested that patients delay any response until their fatigue is severe enough to disrupt their daily lives. Actions they do take tend to be sedentary in nature, including resting and sleeping. In the study conducted by Richardson and Ream (1997) resting and napping were employed by 84% of the sample at some stage during data collection. Patients' efforts were generally ineffective, however, providing only partial relief on half of the occasions that they were performed and no relief on 10% of occasions. It appears that whilst reducing activity and increasing sleep can be effective in relieving fatigue in well populations, these actions are generally ineffective for patients with cancer. Indeed, they can lead to further loss of functional capacity and energy reserves (Winningham 2001).

Wherever possible, interventions should be prescribed to treat the underlying cause of fatigue or to boost individuals' functioning. In addition, patients should be guided in the selection of effective and appropriate self-care strategies for its relief. Graydon *et al.* (1995) stressed that patients receiving cancer treatment should be encouraged to employ strategies besides sleep and rest, and in particular active strategies including exercise, doing something different from their normal activity, and talking to friends.

This chapter considers the utility and efficacy of clinical interventions—both pharmacological and non-pharmacological—for the relief of cancer-related fatigue. However, it begins with a section that discusses the purpose of such interventions.

Prior to developing protocols for its management, their purpose needs to be determined. What should we try to achieve when developing an intervention for this symptom?

Purpose of interventions for fatigue

Interventions for fatigue should aim to reduce the actual level of patients' fatigue. This is only possible when the root cause is treated. Although the mechanisms of fatigue are not fully understood as yet, some of the factors that can increase fatigue have been identified, such as poor control of other symptoms, inadequate sleep, the onset of anaemia, and poor nutritional status to name a few (Piper et al. 1987; Winningham 1996; Portenoy and Itri 1999). Thus, it is crucial that initially these contributing factors are managed effectively.

Secondly, any intervention should aim to reduce the impact of fatigue on patients' lives. It should enable individuals to lead a more fulfilling life, where they can engage in the activities that they value and that give their life meaning.

Thirdly, an intervention should aim to reduce the distress associated with fatigue. Fatigue can evoke considerable distress, especially if individuals perceive its onset as a sign that their treatment is failing, their disease progressing, or their treatment ineffective (Ferrell et al. 1996; Hilfinger Messias et al. 1997; Ream and Richardson 1997). If this distress can be alleviated, the quality of the lives of patients with cancer will be greatly enhanced.

Interventions should, however, be realistic. It is likely for the foreseeable future that fatigue will continue to accompany most treatments and increase as patients' disease progresses. Practitioners should accept that fatigue is unlikely to abate completely and aim to facilitate patients' adaptation to, and understanding of, fatigue.

Pharmacological interventions

Before embarking on pharmacological, or indeed non-pharmacological, treatments for cancer-related fatigue it is important to exclude potentially treatable underlying causes of fatigue – for example, metabolic disturbance, anaemia, hypothyroidism, infection, or depression. Thus patients whose fatigue is thought to be secondary to hypercalcaemia should receive the appropriate treatment for their metabolic disturbance (such as intravenous fluids and bisphosphonates), before receiving treatment aimed solely at palliating their fatigue. However, for many patients no specific or treatable cause of fatigue will be identified. In such individuals it may be appropriate to consider less specific treatments aimed at reducing the fatigue without necessarily treating the underlying condition. Unfortunately, the evidence to support the effectiveness of many of these interventions is rather sparse.

Glucocorticoids

Glucocorticoids (for example prednisolone and dexamethasone) have wide therapeutic applications throughout medicine. They are used to treat inflammatory conditions and autoimmune diseases as well as being used in the management of shock and as part of anticancer therapies. In clinical practice they are often prescribed for their non-specific effects on appetite, mood, and energy levels. What is the evidence that they are effective in the management of cancer-related fatigue?

Moertal and co-workers (Moertel *et al.* 1974) undertook a double-blind, randomized placebo-controlled trial in patients with advanced gastrointestinal cancer. A total of 116 patients were randomized to receive either placebo or two different doses of oral dexamethasone (0.75 mg or 1.5 mg four times a day). After 4 weeks of therapy 34% of the treated patients (regardless of dosage) reported an improvement in 'strength' compared with 13% of the placebo group. Unfortunately this difference failed to reach statistical significance ($p = 0.07$). Bruera's group (Bruera *et al.* 1985) studied the effectiveness of oral methylprednisolone (16 mg administered twice daily) for the palliation of symptoms in 40 heterogeneous advanced cancer patients. In a randomized, double-blind, placebo-controlled crossover study they reported an improvement in activity levels in 61% of patients. Activity level was assessed by a nurse using a structured interview. No attempt was made to record self-reported energy levels or subjective fatigue. The largest and best-designed study in this area has been undertaken by Robustelli Della Cuna and colleagues (Robustelli Della Cuna *et al.* 1989). They recruited 403 patients with heterogeneous advanced cancers and randomized them to receive either intravenous methylprednisolone (125 mg daily) or placebo in a blinded parallel groups study design. Although the authors reported an improvement in a number of quality of life measures, they failed to find any improvement in self-reported 'weakness' scores. Rather worryingly, they also reported a larger than expected mortality rate among female subjects receiving the active treatment compared with female subjects receiving the placebo. In order to investigate this excess mortality further Popiela *et al.* (1989) repeated the study in a group of 173 women with advanced cancer. On this occasion, no excess mortality was observed in the methylprednisolone group. Interestingly this study did demonstrate an improvement in self-reported 'weakness' in the steroid treated group after 2 weeks of therapy. However, the improvement was not maintained beyond 2 weeks.

None of these studies specifically investigated the effects of glucocorticoids on subjective fatigue and their conclusions regarding 'weakness', 'strength', and 'activity levels' are somewhat contradictory. Nonetheless, in the absence of any more reliable evidence there is a widespread clinical impression that steroids have a beneficial effect on at least some patients with cancer-related fatigue. Given the uncertainty of their beneficial action but the well-documented existence of potentially severe side-effects, these drugs should only be prescribed in the context of a therapeutic trial. It is the authors' own practice to prescribe oral dexamethasone 4 mg once per day, for a 5 to 7 day period, and then to assess response. If there has been no improvement in fatigue (or other symptoms) then the drug should be stopped immediately. If there has been a clinically significant effect then the dose should be reduced to the lowest dose compatible with a sustained effect.

Progestational steroids

Progestational steroids such as medroxyprogesterone acetate (MPA) or megestrol acetate (MA) are often used as hormone therapy for cancers of the breast, prostate, endometrium, or kidney. However, these drugs have also been used for symptomatic relief of anorexia and cachexia, and a number of randomized controlled trials have demonstrated their effectiveness for this indication (Bruera *et al.* 1990; Tchekmedyian *et al.* 1992; Downer *et al.* 1993; Loprinzi *et al.* 1993; Gebbia *et al.* 1996; Simons *et al.* 1996; Beller *et al.* 1997; De Conno *et al.* 1998; Loprinzi *et al.* 1999; Westman *et al.* 1999). If it is hypothesized that one of the causes of cancer-related fatigue is poor nutritional status then it might be expected that treatments that result in improved appetite and weight gain may also improve fatigue. Unfortunately, most of the studies that investigated the effectiveness of progestational steroids for anorexia/cachexia did not rigorously assess their effects on fatigue. Bruera *et al.* (1990) investigated 40 patients with advanced cancer and cachexia (>10% loss of body weight) in a crossover study comparing MA (480 mg/day) with a placebo. They found a significant difference in self-reported 'energy' levels after MA treatment. In a subsequent study, Bruera *et al.* (1998) undertook a double-blind, randomized crossover study in order to more fully investigate the subjective effects of MA (480 mg/day) in cachectic cancer patients. In this study, the authors reported a significant improvement in 'activity' (measured using a visual analogue scale) and in 'fatigue' (on 2/3 factors measured by the Piper Fatigue Scale). In contrast, most other studies that have specifically measured fatigue have found no improvement in response to either MA or MPA (Downer *et al.* 1993; Simons *et al.* 1996; De Conno *et al.* 1998; Westman *et al.* 1999). Simons *et al.* (1996) undertook a double-blind, randomized placebo-controlled study to evaluate the effects of MPA (500 mg/day) on appetite, weight, and quality of life in 206 patients with advanced non-hormone-sensitive cancers. They measured quality of life using the European Organization for Research and Treatment of Cancer Quality of Life Questionnaire (EORTC QLQc30), which contains a well-validated triple item fatigue sub-scale. Despite reporting beneficial effects of MPA on appetite and weight loss they found no improvement in quality of life or fatigue. Westman and colleagues (Westman *et al.* 1999) undertook a randomized placebo-controlled study to investigate the effects of MA (320 mg/day) on quality of life in 255 patients with advanced cancer. They also measured quality of life using the EORTC QLQc30. They reported that although MA improved appetite, it did not result in any improvement in quality of life or level of fatigue. Indeed, fatigue was significantly worse after eight weeks treatment with either MA or placebo.

Thus, the results of these studies are conflicting. Both studies undertaken by Bruera's group were very short. In the first study (1990) the crossover was made after 7 days' treatment. In the second one (1998), the crossover was made after 10 days. In the studies undertaken by Simons *et al.* (1996) and Westman *et al.* (1999) treatment was given for 12 weeks and the first assessment of response was not made until 4 to 6 weeks after starting therapy. It is possible that the discrepancy between these studies may be attributable to this difference in design. Perhaps there is a very acute effect of progestational steroids on improving fatigue that is lost after 4 weeks of treatment.

Whatever the explanation for this disagreement, the current evidence is not strong enough to recommend the use of progestational steroids for managing cancer-related fatigue. These drugs may have a role in the treatment of patients who are troubled by anorexia/cachexia in addition to fatigue, but further clarification on this point is still required.

Psychostimulants

Psychostimulants are drugs that increase alertness and/or motivation. There have been no randomized controlled trials that have specifically assessed the effectiveness of psychostimulants for the management of cancer-related fatigue. However, the effects of some of these drugs have been studied in patients with HIV disease (Breitbart *et al.* 2001) or multiple sclerosis (Weinshenker *et al.* 1992; Krupp *et al.* 1995). Krupp *et al.* (1995) failed to find any benefit with pemoline in a double-blind randomized placebo-controlled study involving 93 patients with multiple sclerosis. In contrast, Weinshenker's group (Weinshenker *et al.* 1992) reported that pemoline provided good or excellent relief of fatigue in 46% of patients with multiple sclerosis and fatigue compared with 20% of patients receiving the placebo. Breitbart *et al.* (2001) undertook a double-blind randomized placebo-controlled study to compare the efficacy of two psychostimulants (methylphenidate and pemoline) for the treatment of fatigue in patients with HIV disease. They recruited 144 patients with HIV disease and severe, persistent fatigue. Fatigue was measured using both the Piper Fatigue Scale and the Lee Fatigue Scale. After 6 weeks of treatment there was a 'clinically significant' improvement in fatigue in 41% (15/37) of patients receiving methylphenidate, in 36% (12/33) of patients taking pemoline, and in only 15% (6/39) of patients taking the placebo. No similar studies have been undertaken in patients with cancer. However, Bruera's group (Bruera *et al.* 1987) have investigated the role of amphetamines in alleviating the drowsiness associated with the use of opioid analgesics. In one small, randomized placebo-controlled crossover study they found that methylphenidate resulted in an improvement in self-reported activity levels. The same group failed to find any such improvement in a similar study using mazindol (Bruera *et al.* 1986). In neither study was subjective fatigue *per se* one of the end-points.

Current evidence to support the use of psychostimulants in cancer-related fatigue is therefore quite weak and suitably designed placebo-controlled studies with fatigue as a pre-specified end-point are needed.

Antidepressants

A number of studies have demonstrated a close association between fatigue and symptoms of depression in patients with cancer (Bruera *et al.* 1989; Blesch *et al.* 1991;

Morant 1996; Smets *et al.* 1996; Stone *et al.* 2000*a*). For this reason it has been hypothesized that depression and fatigue may share a 'final common pathway' and that treatment of the former may provide relief of the latter. This hypothesis has recently been tested in a large double-blind, randomized, placebo-controlled study (Morrow *et al.* 2001). 738 patients undergoing chemotherapy were randomly assigned to receive either 20 mg paroxetine or placebo. At the end of the study, patients receiving paroxetine reported significantly fewer symptoms of depression but there was no significant effect on fatigue.

Although this is not necessarily the final word on the matter, this study does appear to rule out the use of selective serotonin re-uptake inhibitors for the prevention of chemotherapy-related fatigue. Whether paroxetine may help in other forms of cancer-related fatigue (such as radiotherapy related, hormone-therapy related, or non-treatment related) or whether other classes of antidepressants (for example, Tri-cyclics, Noradrenaline re-uptake inhibitors) may have beneficial effects on fatigue, are still unanswered questions.

Erythropoietin

The association between anaemia and fatigue has long been recognized by clinicians. There have, however, been few studies that have attempted to quantify the strength of this association. A recent study by Cella *et al.* (2002) demonstrated that anaemic cancer patients are more fatigued than non-anaemic cancer patients and that both groups are more fatigued than the general population. Randomized controlled trials (Case *et al.* 1993; Henry and Abels 1994; Littlewood *et al.* 2001) and large open label studies (Glaspy *et al.* 1997; Demetri *et al.* 1998), have shown that treating anaemia with recombinant human erythropoietin results in improvements in energy levels, decreased fatigue and other quality of life benefits. These changes are significantly correlated with increases in haemoglobin level and are independent of tumour response. Improvements have been found to occur across a range of haemoglobin levels, with the maximal incremental gain in quality of life occurring between 11 g/dL and 13 g/dL (Crawford *et al.* 2002). Although statistically significant, the reported increases in quality of life are relatively modest. Lind *et al.* (2002) reported that only 8% of the variation in fatigue scores amongst anaemic cancer patients could be explained by their haemoglobin level. Indeed, one study of fatigue undertaken in patients with advanced cancer (Stone *et al.* 1999*b*), found no association between fatigue levels and anaemia. Other studies have reported statistically significant but weak associations (Stone *et al.* 2000*a*; Crawford *et al.* 2002). To date, erythropoietin has only been investigated in the management of chemotherapy-related anaemia, and its wider role in the management of cancer-related fatigue in the absence of anaemia has not been evaluated. It is also unclear which patients stand to benefit most from therapy, and whether blood transfusion would be equally efficacious. Nonetheless, there is now good evidence that anaemia is a significant contributor to cancer-related fatigue and that erythropoietin is one effective way to improve this.

Other approaches

There are theoretical reasons for believing that a number of other therapeutic approaches may be helpful in alleviating cancer-related fatigue. As yet none of these drugs have been formally investigated.

◆ Carnitine plays a central role in energy metabolism. Chemotherapy can interfere with carnitine metabolism and excretion. In one open-labelled study of patients undergoing palliative chemotherapy, oral levocarnitine supplementation resulted in improvements in fatigue (Graziano *et al.* 2002). The authors commented that further investigation of this compound in a randomized placebo-controlled trial was warranted.

◆ Patients with prostate cancer who receive anti-androgen therapy have been reported to experience increased fatigue (Stone *et al.* 2000*a*). There is also some evidence that hypogonadism is relatively common in cancer patients who are not receiving anti-androgren treatment (Chlebowski and Heber 1982; Stone *et al.* 1999*b*). Taken together these findings suggest that hypogonadism (low serum testosterone) may be a potentially remediable cause of fatigue in cancer patients. In support of this hypothesis Stone (1999*b*) has reported a significant correlation (Rs = −0.35, $p < 0.01$) between serum testosterone levels and fatigue severity in 58 men with a variety of different non-hormone dependent cancers. In contrast, a study by Howell *et al.* (2000) reported that survivors of haematological malignancy who had mild Leydig cell dysfunction were no more fatigued than survivors with normal gonadal function, suggesting that hypogonadism is not a significant cause of fatigue in this population. The relevance of low testosterone to the genesis of fatigue is thus still open to dispute. As yet, no studies have specifically investigated the effects of exogenous testosterone as a treatment for cancer-related fatigue.

◆ Early studies of fish-oil based interventions in cancer cachexia have yielded promising results. The n-3 polyunsaturated fatty acids are immunomodulatory and down-regulate pro-inflammatory cytokine production. In an uncontrolled, open-label study Barber *et al.* (1999) reported that patients gained a median of 2.5 kg of body weight after 7 weeks of consuming a fish-oil enriched nutritional supplement, with a significant improvement in appetite. Body composition analysis suggested no change in fat mass but a significant gain in lean body mass. The functional ability of patients was seen to improve significantly, as measured by the Karnofsky performance score, suggesting that this treatment may also have a beneficial effect on fatigue. In contrast, a more recent study (Bruera *et al.* 2003) failed to find any beneficial effects for fish oil on either appetite or 'tiredness' in patients with advanced cancer. It is possible that these disappointing results may be explained by the short duration of the latter study (2 weeks).

In summary, the current evidence is insufficient to be able to definitively recommend any of the pharmacological approaches discussed in this section for the routine management of cancer-related fatigue. Until more evidence is available regarding the effectiveness/side-effects of these treatments, clinicians should only prescribe them in the context of a therapeutic trial and after non-pharmacological approaches have been considered.

Non-pharmacological interventions

In addition to pharmacological interventions, there are a number of non-pharmacological interventions that can enable patients with cancer to live more effectively with fatigue. For some of these there is a growing body of empirical work supporting their value, whilst for others empirical evidence is scant.

Exercise interventions

Research evidence suggests that exercise reduces the impact of fatigue. The benefits of exercise for patients with cancer were initially identified by Winningham (1983). She investigated the effects of the Winningham Aerobic Interval Training (WAIT) protocol on the quality of life of a group of patients with cancer. Her exploratory study investigated the functional capacity, feelings of control, and emotional response of six patients with breast cancer and receiving chemotherapy that followed a bicycle ergonometry programme based on the tenets of the WAIT protocol. She compared these data with those recorded by six healthy women that exercised and four patients with breast cancer not participating in the cycling programme. This study found that the patients following the WAIT protocol experienced enhanced quality of life, with increased exercise tolerance and functional capacity, and greater feelings of control. Following these preliminary findings, Winningham devised and evaluated further exercise programs for patients with breast cancer (MacVicar and Winningham 1986; MacVicar et al. 1989), thereby testing further the benefits of exercise in this group of patients. Once again, the patients receiving the exercise protocol reported decreased perceptions of fatigue, and confirmed the benefits of aerobic activity for women receiving treatment for breast cancer.

The relationship between exercise and fatigue has been tested further in research evaluating a rehabilitation programme for patients receiving radiotherapy for breast cancer (Mock et al. 1997). This programme incorporated a low-impact exercise component, based on the protocol developed by Winningham. The patients who followed the exercise protocol reported half of the levels of fatigue experienced by those not exercising ($p < 0.05$). Furthermore, those in the exercise group reported additional psychosocial benefits which enabled them to adapt more easily to their breast cancer diagnosis and to their treatment (Mock et al. 1997).

Dimeo and his colleagues have also examined the efficacy of physical activity in reducing fatigue and promoting rehabilitation. They conducted research in heterogeneous groups of patients with both solid tumours and lymphomas receiving both conventional and high-dose chemotherapy (Dimeo et al. 1997, 1999). In both studies, the patients not exercising reported greater fatigue, lower physical performance, and more limitations in daily activities unlike the group exercising who reported enhanced physical performance and improved psychological well-being.

The largest study examining the effect of exercise on physical functioning and other dimensions of health-related quality of life in women with early stage breast cancer (stages I and II) was reported by Segal *et al.* (2001). In this study, participants ($n = 123$) were randomized between usual care (control group), self-directed exercise, or supervised exercise. Women in the self-directed exercise group were prescribed a home exercise programme that required them to exercise 5 times a week for 26 weeks. Those randomized to the supervised intervention attended the local cancer centre where an exercise specialist ran exercise classes 3 times a week for the 26-week period. Further, they were additionally instructed to exercise at home on at least 2 other days in the week. Outcome data collected in this study determined that exercise significantly enhanced physical functioning ($p < 0.05$). Further it determined that self-directed exercise was as, or more, effective at improving physical functioning than supervised exercise in this group of patients with cancer.

The above studies have provided compelling evidence of the benefits of exercise for some patient groups. However, they provide little understanding of the suitability or efficacy of this intervention for those with advanced cancer. Porock *et al.* (2000) has addressed this shortcoming.

They conducted a pilot study to test the efficacy of an exercise intervention in patients with advanced cancer experiencing fatigue. Although of small scale ($n = 9$), their study determined that the 28-day Duke Energising Exercise plan, which was evaluated in this study, enabled individuals to increase their activity levels without compounding their levels of fatigue. In addition, they noted that participants reported increased quality of life and decreased anxiety. Whilst these improvements may not be attributable to the programme, these findings are encouraging. The study supports the suitability of exercise for individuals with advanced cancer and supports the conduct of further research to test the relationship between fatigue and exercise in this population.

A further small scale study ($n = 31$) employed a pre-test/post-test one-group design to explore the pattern of fatigue in women with breast cancer (stages I–IV) who did, and did not, adhere to an 8-week home-based exercise programme (Schwartz 2000). Women recruited to the study were due to undergo chemotherapy and were provided with instructions to follow a low-intensity aerobic programme. The programme was designed to accommodate individual levels of functioning. Participants were directed to exercise for between 15–30 minutes on 3 or 4 occasions during the week. Schwartz determined that whilst some women did not adhere to the exercise programme (40%), those that did had significantly higher functioning ($p < 0.02$) than non-exercisers, and reported decreasing fatigue during the course of their chemotherapy. The non-exercisers in this study also demonstrated a fall in levels of fatigue over time, but the decline in their fatigue was less than that expressed by the exercisers.

Undoubtedly, non-adherence to prescribed programmes can undermine their efficacy. This is likely to be of particular importance with exercise programmes. Many adults in the 21st century have sedentary lifestyles with little enthusiasm for undertaking exercise. Pickett *et al.* (2002) investigated patterns of adherence to a brisk walking programme in women undergoing adjuvant treatment for newly diagnosed breast cancer. 52 women were recruited to this pilot, randomized controlled trial. The study determined that 33% of the exercise group did not exercise at the prescribed levels, whereas 50% of the control group reported maintaining or increasing their physical activity to a moderate intensity. They concluded that those that exercised prior to diagnosis attempted to maintain this, irrespective of the group they were randomized to. Conversely, those that were not exercisers prior to their illness were less willing, or less able, to adopt and maintain exercise programmes. They suggested that these women may benefit from information and support in adherence strategies.

These studies have demonstrated the potential value of prescribed and structured exercise for the management of cancer-related fatigue. Most of the research has been conducted with samples of patients with early stage breast malignancy, although the research conducted recently by Dimeo and his colleagues and Porock have indicated the suitability of exercise interventions for other groups of patients with cancer. However, it must be recognized that prescribed exercise may not be feasible for, or culturally acceptable to, all patients. For such individuals, other methods of managing fatigue must be explored.

Attention-restoring interventions

Fatigue is widely recognized as a multidimensional phenomenon. At least four dimensions are postulated to account for patients' subjective perceptions of fatigue (Piper 1997). Attentional fatigue, an aspect of the sensory dimension, has been defined as a decreased capacity to concentrate or direct attention (Cimprich 1992). This type of fatigue has been evident in patients with breast cancer 3 months following surgery (Cimprich 1992, 1993), and in patients with lymphoma during and after treatment (Cull *et al.* 1996).

Cimprich, a pioneer of research into attentional fatigue, has developed and evaluated attention-restoring interventions (Cimprich 1992, 1993). She devised a protocol that required patients to select and perform a favourite activity for 30 minutes three times a week. This diversional programme promoted enjoyable pastimes and prevented fatigue arising through boredom and under-stimulation. The repeated intervention devised by Cimprich proved effective. The patients who followed the programme displayed enhanced attentional capacity relative to the control group and were able to return to work before them (Cimprich 1993). Although these findings are encouraging, this is the sole published work evaluating an attention-restoring intervention programme. Cull *et al.* (1996) question whether memory and concentration impairments reflect negative affect as opposed to attentional fatigue. Further evaluative studies are required before the effects of this approach can be confirmed and the relationship between under-stimulation and fatigue clarified.

Psychosocial interventions

Psychological distress is frequently reported by patients diagnosed with cancer. Psychological symptoms including depression, anxiety, and anger have been reported in 70% of cancer patient populations (Telch and Telch 1986; Derogatis 1986). These cognitions can alter their perceptions of, and reactions to, both their symptoms and any side-effects of their treatment and can tax their ability to cope with them. Patients frequently find their symptoms distressing, yet symptom distress is often underestimated by nurses caring for them (Vogelzang *et al.* 1997; Tanghe *et al.* 1998). Low mood is not only correlated with fatigue in patients with cancer (Richardson 1995; Blesch *et al.* 1991) but in patients with other chronic diseases (Ream and Richardson 1997) and it can impinge on their ability to perform self-care activities for its relief.

A number of psychological interventions have been implemented to relieve patients' psychological reactions to cancer, and these have been evaluated in literature reviews (Watson 1983; Trijsburg *et al.* 1992; Burish and Tope 1992) and meta-analyses (Smith *et al.* 1994; Devine and Westlake 1995). These interventions were not aimed specifically at reducing fatigue, but they resulted in higher energy levels and reduced feelings of tiredness. Forester *et al.* (1985) evaluated weekly individual psychotherapy sessions for patients receiving radiotherapy and reported significantly reduced emotional and physical symptoms, including fatigue. They proposed that this serendipitous finding occurred either because symptoms like fatigue are essentially of emotional origin, or because emotional state influences perception and reporting of them.

Trijsburg *et al.* (1992) evaluated 22 studies in a review exploring the effectiveness of psychological treatment for populations with cancer. This review concluded that 'tailored counselling', where counselling and support were provided according to patients' needs, was effective not only for the reduction of distress and the enhancement of self-concept, but also for the reduction of fatigue. A further review (Burish and Tope 1992), exploring a decade of research examining the role of progressive muscle relaxation training (PMRT) in the control of the adverse side-effects of chemotherapy, also concluded that this form of psychosocial intervention can be effective in not only reducing the distress of chemotherapy but also the distress of symptoms including fatigue. This has also been evident in research evaluating group psychiatric support for cancer patients (Spiegel *et al.* 1981; Fawzy *et al.* 1990) where the experimental group has shown significantly less depression and fatigue, and significantly greater vigour, than patients in the control group. However, Watson (1983) was more cautious following her review of psychosocial intervention with cancer patients. She suggests that psychological interventions may not be practical or suitable for all and thus a blanket service would be inappropriate. Furthermore, she advocates a selective service targeted at those at risk of psychological morbidity.

These psychosocial studies suggest unequivocally that psychological support should form one aspect of a programme for the management of fatigue. However, it does also raise the point that the programme should be tailored to the needs of individual patients, for otherwise it may prove ineffective. Through further testing of the relationship between mental affect and fatigue, the mechanism associating them will become better understood, furthering understanding of the manifestation of fatigue and the role that psychosocial interventions may play in its management.

Supportive/educative interventions

Patients can be distressed by the manifestation of fatigue during treatment. They may interpret this symptom as an ominous sign, if they perceive it as an indication that their disease has progressed or that their treatment is ineffective (Ream and Richardson 1997). These perceptions, at times inaccurate, can lead to feelings of despondency if patients are unprepared for fatigue and are unaware that it is a common side-effect of treatment. Furthermore, if they are unaware of measures they can take to manage fatigue, they are likely to feel distressed and frustrated when they experience it.

A number of pilot studies have been conducted recently to determine the feasibility and acceptability of a range of different supportive/educative programmes for patients with cancer to enable them to manage fatigue more effectively. Barsevick *et al.* (2002) developed and evaluated an energy conservation and activity management (ECAM) intervention. The ECAM intervention was conducted over the telephone. It comprised of 3 sessions which sought to provide information about fatigue, develop an energy conservation plan, and evaluate that plan's effectiveness. It was evaluated through the conduct of a single group pre-test/post-test study ($n = 80$). Data were compared with those attained from a non-equivalent control group ($n = 182$). The study determined that the programme was suitable for, and relevant to, the target population; the completion rate for the sessions being 100%. This conclusion was endorsed by participants' favourable comments, and assertions that they would continue the plan on their completion of the study. The outcome data were likewise promising; they suggested that the programme moderated the expected rise in fatigue associated with cancer therapy (radio and chemotherapy). However, these pilot data need to be augmented by a larger RCT before firm conclusions can be drawn.

Holley and Borger (2001) developed and evaluated an 8-week rehabilitative group intervention, known as Energy for Living with Cancer, in the south-eastern United States. This programme entailed weekly, structured 90-minute sessions which incorporated educational elements and facility to share experiences of fatigue with others. Whilst the group was facilitated by nurses, a physiotherapist, occupational therapist, and Tai Chi master contributed to the educational sessions. Outcome data have been collected from 20 individuals who have completed the programme to date. These pre-test/post-test data indicated a significant decrease in fatigue ($p = 0.00$). In the absence of a control group it is difficult to conclude that this was due solely to this intervention, but the participants' comments regarding the programme have endorsed its utility. They alluded to the manner in which the intervention allowed them to focus on fatigue, gain needed information about the symptom and accept and adapt to it.

A further intervention programme for patients undergoing chemotherapy has been developed and evaluated in the United Kingdom (Ream et al. 2002; Ream 2002). Known as 'Beating Fatigue', this programme entailed provision of investigator-designed written information prior to treatment, and monthly in-depth assessment of the symptom and coaching in effective self-care for its relief. The intervention was conducted over a 3 month period, and evaluated through the conduct of an RCT ($n = 103$). Preliminary pilot data ($n = 8$) identified the benefits of the approach at the outset, not only in terms of reducing fatigue, but in the psychological benefits it afforded participants. These findings were corroborated in the main study where those in the intervention group reported significantly less fatigue over time ($p < 0.05$) and notably less distress from it ($p < 0.01$) than those in the control group. In addition, they reported that they were more able to engage in hobbies and pastimes ($p < 0.05$).

Two further initiatives have addressed the management of fatigue. One focused on managing fatigue alongside pain (Grant et al. 2000), and the other on managing fatigue along with troublesome symptoms more widely (Given et al. 2002). The former initiative, the 'I Feel Better Programme', was conducted in the community and entailed a double session educational group workshop taught by masters-prepared oncology nurses. Each session lasted 2.5 hours and provided participants with general information about each symptom, advice on methods for their assessment and management, and strategies for communicating effectively with health professionals. This programme was piloted at 4 sites in Southern California, USA, with 73 patients with a variety of diagnoses. Participants' responses to a simple evaluation tool about the effectiveness of the programme indicated that its objectives were met. Their evaluations were positive and supported the content and format of the trialled intervention. However, despite these favourable reports, attendance at the second session was low. Only 31 of the 73 that enrolled on the programme were present at the follow-up session. The reason for this attrition is unclear, as data were not collected from those that did not attend. However it is probable that this occurred where individuals were unable to attend through ill health or fatigue, or where they felt that the programme did not meet their needs or expectations. Conversely, individuals may not have attended if their health and energy levels had improved. In the absence of confirmatory data, one can only surmise. Clearly, further research needs to be conducted to evaluate this approach to managing fatigue and pain, and to determine factors which may hinder its success.

The second programme was developed to assist patients newly diagnosed with cancer to cope with symptoms, notably fatigue and pain, on commencement of chemotherapy. It was evaluated by Given et al. (2002) through the conduct of a randomized controlled trial. The intervention entailed nurses' utilization of intervention software loaded onto a laptop computer. During 10 contacts over a 20-week period, 6 in person and 4 by telephone, the nurse and patient identified problematic symptoms. On their identification, the software was used to select problem-specific, evidence-based interventions which patients could implement on their own behalf to help resolve their symptoms. This approach was evaluated in 4 chemotherapy outpatient departments in the United States ($n = 113$). Findings from this study were encouraging; on its completion, more patients in the experimental group reported neither fatigue nor pain ($n = 10$) than those in the control group ($n = 3$). However, logistic regression failed to identify the effect of the intervention over other factors. The researchers attributed this to lack of study power due to inadequate sample size. Given this, although preliminary findings are favourable, further research needs to be undertaken to enable the benefits of this approach to be clearly determined.

In conclusion, there is a growing body of research that has evaluated different non-pharmacological approaches to managing cancer-related fatigue. Initially, individual strategies were tested, including exercise and distraction. However, most recently clinicians and researchers have tended to adopt programmes incorporating a variety of complementary strategies for the relief of fatigue. Given the multi-causal and multi-dimensional nature of fatigue this would seem more apt. Certainly, the pilot findings reported in the studies above appear most favourable.

Providing patients with the time and the opportunity to discuss fatigue and the meaning that it holds for them could prove a key aspect of any fatigue intervention strategy. Patients' worries and fears are frequently channelled through discussion of fatigue (Krishnasamy 1997). Discussion can be especially important when a patient has recently been diagnosed as having cancer, and can become increasingly important as the patient's disease advances and more active strategies requiring either physical or mental effort become more difficult. Patients could be assisted with prioritizing their daily activities and hobbies, and with pacing their energies, to ensure that valued activities remain possible. Patients' self esteem, confidence, and overall psychological well-being can be enhanced when patients achieve realistic and valued goals, thereby boosting their morale.

Future directions for research

Properly conducted studies of both pharmacological and non-pharmacological interventions for fatigue are urgently needed. Can any general methodological advice be given about the types of study that are required?

◆ It is important that homogeneous groups of patients are studied. At present we do not know enough about the aetiology of cancer-related fatigue to be sure that all patients with cancer and fatigue can be treated in the same way. It may be that interventions that will be effective for patients with non-small cell lung cancer (for instance) may not work for patients with breast cancer. It may be that interventions that are effective for chemotherapy-related fatigue will not work for

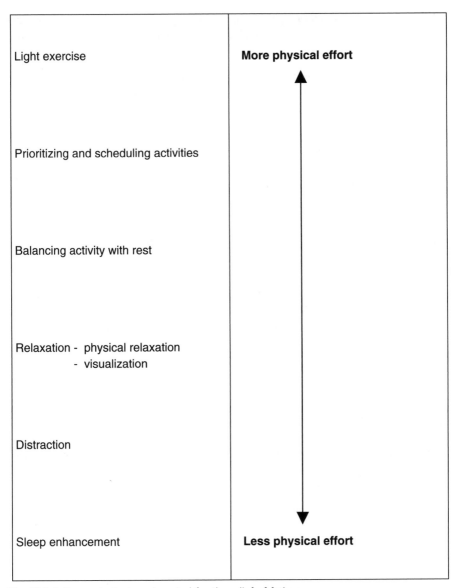

Fig. 12.1 Self-care strategies advocated for the relief of fatigue.

radiotherapy-related fatigue. Moreover, the type of chemotherapy regimen may also be important. For these reasons researchers need to clearly identify which group of patients they are studying.

- It is important that a well-validated fatigue assessment instrument is used as the primary end-point of the study. Given that there is no unanimity as to the best scale to use, researchers would be wise to employ at least two different fatigue measures.

In studies where one is looking for a change in fatigue scores over time, it is particularly important that the instrument chosen should have good test–retest reliability and should be sensitive to change.

♦ Ideally intervention studies should be double-blind, randomized, and placebo-controlled. Although this methodology can usually be attempted in drug trials, it can become almost impossible in studies of non-pharmacological interventions.

♦ Studies should be designed with sufficient statistical power such that 'negative' results can be interpreted as indicating a probable lack of effectiveness rather than an insufficient sample size. In practical terms this will mean that more studies will have to become collaborative and multicentred.

Assuming that an appropriate methodology is used, which are the areas that most deserve attention from researchers (see Box 12.1)?

♦ In terms of pharmacological interventions it is important that the role of corticosteroids is properly defined. These are the most commonly prescribed drugs for cancer-related fatigue but they are not without side-effects. No studies have yet looked specifically at their effectiveness in relieving cancer-related fatigue. A careful comparison between the beneficial and unwanted effects of these drugs is required. It is simply not enough to determine their effect on 'subjective fatigue' in the short term. Other questions also need to be addressed. How long is their effectiveness maintained? What is the optimal dose? Who are the patients most likely to benefit?

Box 12.1 Future areas for research

♦ Evaluation of the role and effectiveness of corticosteriods in the management of cancer-related fatigue.

♦ Evaluation of the effectiveness of exercise as an intervention for fatigue in patients with metastatic disease.

♦ The development and evaluation of educational strategies to promote patients and family members' ability to perform self-care in relation to cancer-related fatigue.

Future studies should incorporate a number of key design issues to overcome weaknesses in current evidence—most notably:

♦ homogeneous samples;

♦ inclusion of two or more well-validated fatigue instruments;

♦ where possible and relevant, do double-blind, randomized, placebo-controlled trials, and

♦ include sufficient numbers to ensure sufficient statistical power.

Is any one steroid superior (in terms of effectiveness or patient acceptability) than any other? Other drugs are also in need of further evaluation particularly erythropoietin, antidepressants, and anabolic steroids.

◆ In terms of non-pharmacological interventions a number of areas deserve further investigation. Exercise has shown itself to be an effective treatment predominantly for patients with early stage cancer. However, there is little evidence to indicate whether this approach could be used successfully in other groups of cancer patients, particularly those with more advanced disease. At what stage should patients be encouraged to exercise? Could exercise be usefully combined with other interventions? Such questions need to be addressed. Furthermore, little is currently known about the optimal way of educating patients about fatigue. Preparatory information will undoubtedly prepare patients for treatments that may cause fatigue, but conventional written information may not be the optimal medium for presenting information to a group characterized by poor concentration. Finally, we do not know which interventions patients find most acceptable or appealing. Undoubtedly, patients may be reluctant to follow protocols or to comply with treatments that they perceive as unappealing or antithetical to their usual mode of coping.

Future directions for practice

There is a growing body of evidence upon which to base interventions for fatigue in patients with cancer. It is important that multidisciplinary teams of healthcare professionals take up the challenge to address the effective management of this most pervasive of symptoms. It is imperative that fatigue is consistently and comprehensively assessed to determine as far as possible its causes and consequences. This will facilitate the selection of appropriate combinations of pharmacological and non-pharmacological support. Given the dynamic nature of fatigue, patients and healthcare professionals will need to adopt a flexible approach to its management. Fatigue will vary in quality and quantity during the course of the disease and its treatment. Healthcare professionals need to appreciate and plan for this.

Conclusion

It is important to recognize that if we raise patients' and healthcare professionals' awareness of fatigue we will also raise their expectations that effective management is available. At present, there are a number of different management strategies with the potential to decrease the impact of fatigue and enhance individuals' adaptation to living with it. The evidence from the research conducted to date provides some evidence of their efficacy. However, further investigation is required, and research into fatigue interventions should be seen as a priority. Researchers and clinicians alike need to constantly appraise the efficacy of clinical interventions. It is likely, given the multifactorial nature of fatigue, that no single treatment will be universally effective. A broad approach looking

Box 12.2 Summary points

- Evidence to support clinical interventions for fatigue remains scarce.
- Given the multifactorial nature of fatigue no single treatment will be universally effective.
- Comprehensive and consistent assessment is essential to advances in appreciation of its causes and consequences.
- A multidisciplinary approach to cancer-related fatigue is imperative if advances in its management are to be achieved.
- Effective management will require a dynamic, flexible approach drawing on both pharmacological and non-pharmacological therapies.

at both pharmacological and non-pharmacological therapies is required. With growing interest in this area it is to be hoped that existing therapies will continue to be evaluated and new therapies developed. Box 12.2 summarizes the points made in this chapter.

Acknowledgement

Some of the material used in this chapter has been previously published in Ream, E. and Richardson, A. (1999). From theory to practice: designing interventions to reduce fatigue in patients with cancer. *Oncology Nursing Forum* **26**: 1295–303.

References

Barber, M.D., Ross, J.A., Voss, A.C., Tisdale, M.J., and Fearon, K.C. (1999) The effect of an oral nutritional supplement enriched with fish oil on weight-loss in patients with pancreatic cancer. *British Journal of Cancer*, **81**(1), 80–6.

Barsevick, A., Whitmer, K., Sweeney, C., and Nail, L. (2002) A pilot study examining energy conservation for cancer-treatment fatigue. *Cancer Nursing*, **25**(5), 333–41.

Beller, E., Tattersall, M., Lumley, T., Levi, J., Dalley, D., Olver, I., *et al.* (1997) Improved quality of life with megestrol acetate in patients with endocrine-insensitive advanced cancer: A randomised placebo-controlled trial. *Annals of Oncology*, **8**(3), 277–83.

Blesch, K., Paice, J., Wickham, R., Harte, N., Schnoor, D., Purl, S. *et al.* (1991) Correlates of fatigue in people with lung and breast cancer. *Oncology Nursing Forum*, **18**(1), 81–7.

Breitbart, W., Rosenfeld, B., Kaim, M., and Funesti-Esch, J. (2001) A randomized, double-blind, placebo-controlled trial of psychostimulants for the treatment of fatigue in ambulatory patients with human immunodeficiency virus disease. *Archives of Internal Medicine*, **161**(3), 411–20.

Bruera, E., Roca, E., Cedaro, L., Carraro, S., and Chacon, R. (1985) Action of oral methylprednisolone in terminal cancer patients: a prospective randomized double-blind study. *Cancer Treatment Reports*, **69**(7–8), 751–4.

Bruera, E., Carraro, S., Roca, E., Barugel, M., and Chacon, R. (1986) Double-blind evaluation of the effects of mazindol on pain, depression, anxiety, appetite, and activity in terminal cancer patients. *Cancer Treatment Reports*, **70**, 295–8.

Bruera, E., Chadwick, S., Brenneis, C., Hanson, J., and MacDonald, R.N. (1987) Methylphenidate associated with narcotics for the treatment of cancer pain. *Cancer Treatment Reports,* **71**(1), 67–70.

Bruera, E., Brenneis, C., Michaud, M., Rafter, J., Magnan, A., Tennant, A., *et al.* (1989) Association between asthenia and nutritional status, lean body mass, anemia, psychological status, and tumor mass in patients with advanced breast cancer. *Journal of Pain and Symptom Management,* **4**(2), 59–63.

Bruera, E., MacMillan, K., Kuehn, N., Hanson, J., and MacDonald, R.N. (1990) A controlled trial of megestrol acetate on appetite, caloric intake, nutritional status, and other symptoms in patients with advanced cancer. *Cancer,* **66**(6), 1279–82.

Bruera, E., Ernst, S., Hagen, N., Spachynski, K., Belzile, M., Hanson, J., *et al.* (1998) Effectiveness of megestrol acetate in patients with advanced cancer: a randomized, double-blind, crossover study. *Cancer Prevention and Control,* **2**(2), 74–8.

Bruera, E., Strasser, F., Palmer, J.L., Willey, J., Calder, K., Amyotte, G., *et al.* (2003) Effect of fish oil on appetite and other symptoms in patients with advanced cancer and anorexia/cachexia: a double-blind, placebo-controlled study. *Journal of Clinical Oncology,* **21**(1), 129–34.

Burish, T. and Tope, D. (1992) Psychological techniques for controlling the adverse side effects of cancer chemotherapy: findings from a decade of research. *Journal of Pain and Symptom Management,* **7**(5), 287–301.

Case, D., Bukowski, R., Carey, R.W., Fishkin, E.H., Henry, D.H., Jacobson, R.J. *et al.* (1993) Recombinant human erythropoietin therapy for anaemic cancer patients on combination chemotherapy. *Journal of the National Cancer Institute,* **85**(10), 801–6.

Cella, D., Lai, J.S., Chang, C.H., Peterman, A., and Slavin, M. (2002) Fatigue in cancer patients compared with fatigue in the general United States population. *Cancer,* **94**(2), 528–38.

Chlebowski, R.T. and Heber, D. (1982) Hypogonadism in male patients with metastatic cancer prior to chemotherapy. *Cancer Research,* **42**(6), 2495–8.

Cimprich, B. (1992) Attentional fatigue following breast cancer surgery. *Research in Nursing and Health,* **15**(3), 199–207.

Cimprich, B. (1993) Development of an intervention to restore attention in cancer patients. *Cancer Nursing,* **16**(2), 83–92.

Copp, G. and Dunn, V. (1993) Frequent and difficult problems perceived by nurses caring for the dying in community, hospice and acute care settings. *Palliative Medicine,* **7**(1), 19–25.

Crawford, J., Cella, D., Cleeland, C.S., Cremieux, P.Y., Demetri, G.D., Sarokhan, B.J., *et al.* (2002) Relationship between changes in hemoglobin level and quality of life during chemotherapy in anemic cancer patients receiving epoetin alfa therapy. *Cancer,* **95**(4), 888–95.

Cull, A., Hay, C., Love, S., Mackie, M., Smets, E., and Stewart, M. (1996) What do cancer patients mean when they complain of concentration and memory problems? *British Journal of Cancer,* **74**, 1674–9.

De Conno, F., Martini, C., Zecca, E., Balzarini, A., Venturino, P., Groff, L., *et al.* (1998) Megestrol acetate for anorexia in patients with far-advanced cancer: a double-blind controlled clinical trial. *European Journal of Cancer,* **34**(11), 1705–9.

Demetri, G., Kris, M., Wade, J., Degos, L., and Cella, D. (1998) Quality-of-life benefit in chemotherapy patients treated with epoetin alfa is independent of disease response or tumour type: results from a prospective community oncology study. *Journal of Clinical Oncology,* **16**(10), 3412–25.

Derogatis, L. (1986) Psychology in cancer medicine. *Journal of Consulting and Clinical Psychology,* **54**(5), 632–8.

Devine, E. and Westlake, S. (1995) The effects of psychoeducational care provided to adults with cancer: meta-analysis of 116 studies. *Oncology Nursing Forum,* **22**(9), 1369–81.

Dimeo, F., Tilmann, M., Bertz, H., Kanz, L., and Mertelsmann, J. (1997) Aerobic exercise in the rehabilitation of cancer patients after high dose chemotherapy and autologous peripheral stem cell transplantation. *Cancer,* **79**(9), 1718–22.

Dimeo, F., Stieglitz, R., Novelli-Fischer, U., Fetscehr, S., and Keul, J. (1999) Effects of physical activity on the fatigue and psychologic status of cancer patients during chemotherapy. *Cancer,* **85**(10), 2273–7.

Dodd, M. (1988) Efficacy of proactive information on self-care in chemotherapy patients. *Patient Education and Counselling,* **11**, 215–25.

Downer, S., Joel, S., Allbright, A., Plant, H., Stubbs, L., Talbot, D. *et al.* (1993) A double blind placebo controlled trial of medroxyprogesterone acetate (MPA) in cancer cachexia. *British Journal of Cancer,* **67**(5), 1102–5.

Fawzy, F., Cousins, N., Fawzy, N., Kemeny, M., Elashoff, R., and Morton, D. (1990) A structured psychiatric intervention for cancer patients. I. Changes over time in methods of coping and affective disturbance. *Archives of General Psychiatry,* **47**(August) 720–5.

Ferrell, B., Grant, M., Dean, G., Funk, B., and Ly, J. (1996) 'Bone tired': the experience of fatigue and its impact on quality of life. *Oncology Nursing Forum,* **23**(10), 1539–47.

Forester, B., Kornfeld, D., and Fleiss, J. (1985) Psychotherapy during radiation: effects on emotional and physical distress. *American Journal of Psychiatry,* **142**, 22–7.

Fredette, S. and Beattie, H. (1986) Living with cancer. A patient education programme. *Cancer Nursing,* **9**(6), 308–16.

Gebbia, V., Testa, A., and Gebbia, N. (1996) Prospective randomised trial of two dose levels of megestrol acetate in the management of anorexia-cachexia syndrome in patients with metastatic cancer. *British Journal of Cancer,* **73**(12), 1576–80.

Given, B., Given, C., McCorkle, R., Kozachik, S., Cimprich, B., Rahbar, M., *et al.* (2002) Pain and fatigue management: Results of a Randomized Clinical Trial. *Oncology Nursing Forum,* **29**(6), 949–56.

Glaspy, J., Bukowski, R., Steinberg, D., Taylor, C., Tchekmedyian, S., and Vadhan-Raj, S. (1997) Impact of therapy with epoetin alfa on clinical outcomes in patients with nonmyeloid malignancies during cancer chemotherapy in community oncology practice. *Journal of Clinical Oncology,* **15**(3), 1218–34.

Grahn, G. (1993) 'Learning to cope'—an intervention in cancer care. *Supportive Care in Cancer,* **1**, 266–71.

Grant, M., Golant, M., Rivera, L., Dean, G., and Benjamin, H. (2000) Developing a community program on cancer pain and fatigue. *Cancer Practice,* **8**(4), 187–94.

Graydon, J., Bubela, N., Irvine, D., and Vincent, L. (1995) Fatigue-reducing strategies used by patients receiving treatment for cancer. *Cancer Nursing,* **18**, 123–8.

Graziano, F., Bisonni, R., Catalano, V., Silva, R., Rovidati, S., Mencarini, E., *et al.* (2002) Potential role of levocarnitine supplementation for the treatment of chemotherapy-induced fatigue in non-anaemic cancer patients. *British Journal of Cancer,* **86**(12), 1854–7.

Hamilton, J., Butler, L., Wagenaar, H., Sveinson, T., Ward, K., McLean, L., *et al.* (2001) The impact and management of cancer-related fatigue on patients and families. *Canadian Oncology Nursing Journal,* **11**(4), 192–8.

Henry, D. and Abels, R. (1994) Recombinant human erythropoietin in the treatment of cancer and chemotherapy induced anaemia: results of double-blind and open-label follow-up studies. *Seminars in Oncology,* **21**(2, Supplement 3), 21–8.

Hilfinger Messias, D., Yeager, K., Dibble, S., and Dodd, M. (1997) Patients' perspectives of fatigue whilst undergoing chemotherapy. *Oncology Nursing Forum,* **24**(1), 43–8.

Holley, S. and Borger, D. (2001) Energy for living with cancer: Preliminary findings of a cancer reha-bilitation group intervention study. *Oncology Nursing Forum*, **28**(9), 1393–6.

Howell, S.J, Radford, J.A, Smets, E.M., and Shalet, S.M. (2000) Fatigue, sexual function and mood following treatment for haematological malignancy: the impact of mild Leydig cell dysfunction. *British Journal of Cancer*, **82**(4), 789–93.

Johnson, J. (1982) The effects of a patient education course on persons with a chronic illness. *Cancer Nursing*, **5**(2), 117–23.

Johnson, J., Nail, L., Lauver, D., King, K., and Keys, H. (1988) Reducing the negative impact of radiation therapy on functional status. *Cancer*, **61**(1), 46–51.

Krishnasamy, M. (1997) Exploring the nature and impact of fatigue in advanced cancer. *International Journal of Palliative Nursing*, **3**(3), 126–31.

Krupp, L.B., Coyle, P.K., Doscher, C., Miller, A., Cross, A.H., Jandorf, L., et al. (1995) Fatigue therapy in multiple sclerosis: results of a double-blind, randomized, parallel trial of amantadine, pemo-line, and placebo. *Neurology*, **45**(11), 1956–61.

Lind, M., Vernon, C., Cruickshank, D., Wilkinson, P., Littlewood, T., Stuart, N., et al. (2002) The level of haemoglobin in anaemic cancer patients correlates positively with quality of life. *British Journal of Cancer*, **86**(8), 1243–9.

Littlewood, T.J., Bajetta, E., Nortier, J.W., Vercammen, E., Rapoport, B., and Epoetin Alfa Study Group. (2001) Effects of epoetin alfa on hematologic parameters and quality of life in cancer patients receiving nonplatinum chemotherapy: results of a randomized, double-blind, placebo-controlled trial [comment]. *Journal of Clinical Oncology*, **19**(11), 2865–74.

Loprinzi, C.L., Michalak, J.C., Schaid, D.J., Mailliard, J.A., Athmann, L.M., Goldberg, R.M., et al. (1993) Phase III evaluation of four doses of megestrol acetate as therapy for patients with cancer anorexia and/or cachexia. *Journal of Clinical Oncology*, **11**(4), 762–7.

Loprinzi, C., Kugler, J., Sloan, J., Mailliard, J., Krook, J., and al Mwe (1999) Randomized comparison of megestrol acetate versus dexamathasone versus fluooxymesterone for the treatment of cancer anorexia/cachexia. *Journal of Clinical Oncology*, **17**(10), 3299–306.

MacVicar, M. and Winningham, M. (1986) Promoting functional capacity of cancer patients. *Cancer Bulletin*, **38**(5), 235–9.

MacVicar, M., Winningham, M., and Nickel, J. (1989) Effects of aerobic interval training on cancer patients' functional capacity. *Nursing Research*, **38**(6), 348–51.

Mock, V., Hassey Dow, K., Meares, C., Grimm, P., Dienemann, J., Haisfield-Wolfe, M. et al. (1997) Effects of exercise on fatigue, physical functioning, and emotional distress during radiation therapy for breast cancer. *Oncology Nursing Forum*, **24**(6), 991–1000.

Moertel, C.G., Schutt, A.J., Reitemeier, R.J., and Hahn, R.G. (1974) Corticosteroid therapy of preterminal gastrointestinal cancer. *Cancer*, **33**(6), 1607–9.

Morant, R. (1996) Asthenia: an important symptom in cancer patients. *Cancer Treatment Reviews* **22** (Suppl A), 117–22.

Morrow, G.R., Hickok, J.T., Raubertas, R., Flynn, P.J., Hynes, H.E., Banerjee, T., et al. (2001) Effect of an SSRI antidepressant on fatigue and depression in seven hundred and thirty eight cancer patients treated with chemotherapy: A URCC CCOP Study. *Proceedings American Society of Clinical Oncology 2001 Annual Meeting*, 1531.

Pickett, M., Mock, V., Ropka, M., Cameron, L., Coleman, M. and Podewils, L. (2002) Adherence to moderate-intensity exercise during breast cancer therapy. *Cancer Practice*, **10**(6), 284–92.

Piper, B. (1997) Measuring fatigue. In: *Instruments for Clinical Health-Care Research*, (ed. M. Frank-Stromborg and S. Olsen) Jones and Bartlett Publishers, Sudbury, MA, pp. 199–208.

Piper, B., Lindsey, A., and Dodd, M. (1987) Fatigue mechanisms in cancer patients: developing a nursing theory. *Oncology Nursing Forum*, **14**(6), 17–23.

Piper, B., Lindsey, A., Dodd, M., Ferketich, S., Paul, S., and Weller, S. (1989) The development of an instrument to measure the subjective dimension of fatigue. In: *Key Aspects of Comfort : Management of Pain, Fatigue and Nausea*, (ed. S. Funk, E. Tornquist, M. Champagne, L. Archer Copp, and R. Wiese), Springer, New York. pp. 199–208.

Piper, B., Lindsey, A., and Dodd, M. (1997) Fatigue mechanisms in cancer patients: developing a nursing theory. *Oncology Nursing Forum*, **14**(6), 17–23.

Popiela, T., Lucchi, R., and Giongo, F. (1989) Methylprednisolone as palliative therapy for female terminal cancer patients. The Methylprednisolone Female Preterminal Cancer Study Group. *European Journal of Cancer Clinical Oncology*, **25**(12), 1823–9.

Porock, D., Kristjanson, L., Tinnelly, K., Duke, T., and Blight, J. (2000) An exercise intervention for advanced cancer patients experiencing fatigue: a pilot study. *Journal of Palliative Care*, **16**(3), 30–6.

Portenoy, R. and Itri, L. (1999) Cancer-related fatigue: Guidelines for evaluation and management. *The Oncologist*, **4**(1), 1–10.

Ream, E. (2002). *Impact of Nursing Intervention on Fatigue in Patients Undergoing Chemotherapy*. PhD Thesis, University of London.

Ream, E. and Richardson, A. (1996) The role of information in patients' adaptation to chemotherapy and radiotherapy: a review of the literature. *European Journal of Cancer Care*, **5**(3), 132–8.

Ream, E. and Richardson, A. (1997) Fatigue in patients with cancer and chronic obstructive airways disease: a phenomenological enquiry. *International Journal of Nursing Studies*, **34**(1), 44–53.

Ream, E., Richardson, A., and Alexander-Dann, C. (2002) Facilitating patients' coping with fatigue during chemotherapy: pilot outcomes. *Cancer Nursing*, **25**(4), 300–9.

Richardson, A. (1995) The pattern of fatigue in patients receiving chemotherapy. In: *Nursing Research in Cancer Care* (ed. A. Richardson and J. Wilson-Barnett), Scutari Press, London. pp. 225–45.

Richardson, A. and Ream, E. (1997) Self-care behaviours initiated by chemotherapy patients in response to fatigue. *International Journal of Nursing Studies*, **34**(1), 35–43.

Robustelli Della Cuna, G., Pellegrini, A., and Piazzi, M. (1989) Effect of methylprednisolone sodium succinate on quality of life in pre-terminal cancer patients: a placebo-controlled, multicenter study. *European Journal of Cancer Clinical Oncology*, **25**(12), 1817–21.

Schwartz, A. (2000) Daily fatigue patterns and effect of exercise in women with breast cancer. *Cancer Practice*, **8**(1), 16–24.

Segal, R., Evans, W., Johnson, D., Smith, J., Colletta, S., Gayton, J., *et al.* (2001) Structured exercise improves physical functioning in women with stages I and II breast cancer: Results of a randomised controlled trial. *Journal of Clinical Oncology*, **19**(3), 657–65.

Simons, J.P., Aaronson, N.K., Vansteenkiste, J.F., ten Velde, G.P., Muller, M.J., Drenth, B.M., *et al.* (1996) Effects of medroxyprogesterone acetate on appetite, weight, and quality of life in advanced-stage non-hormone-sensitive cancer: a placebo-controlled multicenter study. *Journal of Clinical Oncology*, **14**(4), 1077–84.

Smets, E.M., Garssen, B., Cull, A., and de Haes, J.C. (1996) Application of the multidimensional fatigue inventory (MFI-20) in cancer patients receiving radiotherapy. *British Journal of Cancer*, **2**, 241–5.

Smith, M., Holcombe, J., and Stullenburger, E. (1994) A meta-analysis of intervention effectiveness for symptom management in oncology nursing research. *Oncology Nursing Forum*, **21**(7), 1201–9.

Spiegel, D., Bloom, J., and Yalom, I. (1981) Group support for patients with metastatic cancer: a randomised prospective outcome study. *Archives of General Psychiatry*, **28**, 527–33.

Stone, P. (1999*a*) Fatigue in patients with cancer. *MD Thesis.* London University. London.

Stone, P., Hardy, J., Broadley, K., Tookman, A.J., Kurowska, A., and A'Hern, R. (1999*b*) Fatigue in advanced cancer: a prospective controlled cross-sectional study. *British Journal of Cancer,* **79**(9–10), 1479–86.

Stone, P., Hardy, J., Huddart, R., A'Hern, R., and Richards, M. (2000*a*) Fatigue in patients with prostate cancer receiving hormone therapy. *European Journal of Cancer,* **36**(9), 1134–41.

Stone, P., Richards, M., A'Hern, R., and Hardy, J. (2000*b*) A study to investigate the prevalence, severity and correlates of fatigue among patients with cancer in comparison with a control group of volunteers without cancer. *Annals of Oncology,* **11**(5), 561–7.

Tanghe, A., Evers, G., and Paridaens, R. (1998) Nurses' assessments of symptom occurrence and symptom distress in chemotherapy patients. *European Journal of Oncology Nursing,* **2**(1), 14–26.

Tchekmedyian, N.S., Hickman, M., Siau, J., Greco, F.A., Keller, J., Browder, H., *et al.* (1992) Megestrol acetate in cancer anorexia and weight loss. *Cancer,* **69**(5), 1268–74.

Telch, C. and Telch, M. (1986) Group coping skills instruction and supportive group therapy for cancer patients: a comparison of strategies. *Journal of Consulting and Clinical Psychology,* **54**(6), 802–8.

Trijsburg, R., van Knippenberg, F., and Rijpma, S. (1992) Effects of psychological treatment on cancer patients: a critical review. *Psychosomatic Medicine,* **54**, 489–517.

Vogelzang, N., Breitbart, W., Cella, D., Curt, G., Groopman, J., Horning, S. *et al.* (1997) Patient, caregiver, and oncologist perceptions of fatigue: results of a tripart assessment survey. *Seminars in Hematology,* **34**(3, Supplement 2), 4–12.

Watson, M. (1983) Psychosocial intervention with cancer patients: a review. *Psychological Medicine,* **13**, 839–46.

Weinshenker, B.G., Penman, M., Bass, B., Ebers, G.C., and Rice, G.P.A. (1992) A double-blind randomised crossover trial of pemoline in fatigue associated with multiple sclerosis. *Neurology,* **42**, 1468–71.

Westman, G., Bergman, B., Albertsson, M., Kadar, L., Gustavsson, G., Thaning, L., *et al.* (1999) Megestrol acetate in advanced, progressive, hormone-insensitive cancer. Effects on the quality of life: a placebo-controlled, randomised, multicentre trial. *European Journal of Cancer,* **35**(4), 586–95.

Winningham, M. (1983) Effects of a bicycle ergometry program on functional capacity and feelings of control in women with breast cancer. Dissertation. The Ohio State University, Columbus, OH.

Winningham, M. (1996) Fatigue. In: *Cancer Symptom Management* (ed. S. Groenwald, M. Hansen-Frogge, M. Goodman, and C. Henke Yarbro), Jones and Bartlett Publishers, Sudbury, MA, pp. 42–58.

Winningham, M. (2001) Strategies for managing cancer-related fatigue. A rehabilitation approach. *Cancer,* **92**(4) (Suppl.), 988–97.

Chapter 13

Fatigue and everyday function in people living with cancer

Trudy Mallinson and David Cella

Introduction

> I could not get out of bed and walk into the bathroom and I would have to sit down, go to the shower, take a shower, but then I would have to sit down, put my clothes on, then I would have to sit down—I would have to rest between each activity. If I just walked out to my car, I would have to sit in the car for a few minutes and rest because I had no energy left.

(Rhodes *et al.* 1988, p. 191)

Fatigue is becoming recognized as one of the most common and most devastating side-effects from cancer treatment. Previous research has identified that 70–80% of cancer patients will experience debilitating fatigue during the course of treatment (Portenoy *et al.* 1994). Further, fatigue does not always resolve with the termination of cancer therapy (Ferrell *et al.* 1996). Its impact on patients' daily lives can range from difficulty completing simple tasks such as shopping, to resuming productive roles such as working and childcare (Messias *et al.* 1997). The impact of fatigue on daily life activities may be overlooked since the person does not generally lack the physical capacity to perform the activity but rather lacks the energy to complete tasks at a usual pace or for a usual duration (Persson *et al.* 1997).

In an attempt to describe and quantify the various manifestations of fatigue, a range of assessment tools and interviews have been developed to help clinicians and researchers evaluate it. These assessments examine the impact of fatigue in a person's life on a variety of dimensions. One dimension is the experience of the symptom of fatigue, that is, about the severity and intensity of the fatigue. Another dimension includes the impact of fatigue on a person's capacity for action. That is, how weak the person feels, how much endurance the person has, or if the person has memory or attention problems. Yet another dimension is concerned with the person's ability to, or difficulty with, carrying out everyday activities. Some instruments include several of these dimensions in a single scale, which may obscure what it is that the assessment is really measuring (Leidy 1994). Whilst it is certainly the case that fatigue is multidimensional (Aistars 1987; Piper *et al.* 1987; Ferrell *et al.* 1996), the inclusion of multiple dimensions within a single scale clouds distinctions between how a person experiences fatigue, his or her underlying capacity, and what he or she actually does on a day-to-day basis. In her discussion of a theoretical framework for describing everyday functioning, Leidy (1994) has argued that this lack of distinction between experience, capacity, and performance limits our progress in understanding. She notes that mixing dimensions within a single scale results in confounding between dependent and independent variables and limits comparison of findings amongst studies, since it is unclear how the content of various scales are or are not comparable.

As a further complication, these assessments utilize a variety of approaches to data collection. For example, many use patient self-report, while others utilize interview, and some require that clinicians score items following observation of performance. Unfortunately, little is known about the similarities and differences that arise when data are gathered using various approaches, making the investigation of relationships amongst variables more difficult. However, when dealing only in the realm of self-report, the relationship amongst symptom experience, capacity, and performance may be too high to support interpretable differentiation. Of greater interest is the relationship between self-reported (subjective) fatigue and observable (objective) behaviour that is presumed to be related to fatigue.

Consequently, little is known to date about the relationship between a person's experience of fatigue as a symptom, his or her capacity for action, and performance in everyday activities. Of particular concern is that we do not know what a particular score on any given assessment of fatigue means for a patient's future functional performance. For example, does a certain score mean a person is able to return to work or does it mean they will require daily assistance with everyday activities? Such relationships to external criteria of functional ability have not been established for measures of self-reported fatigue. In addition, since a given score does not tell us about a person's ability to do everyday activities, we cannot easily determine who might be most appropriate for intervention programmes such as energy conservation and exercise programmes. Finally, since we do not know how a particular score relates to a particular level of daily functioning, we cannot easily determine what represents a *meaningful* change in a fatigue score. For example, has a patient who reports a reduction of five points in fatigue on a certain assessment, also experienced a meaningful improvement in functional ability?

A model of the relationship between capacity and performance

Figure 13.1 presents the hypothesized relationships between fatigue as a symptom experience, capacity for action, and functional performance. The symptom experience of fatigue refers to the intensity, severity, and duration of fatigue. Capacity for action includes, but is not limited to, the motor and cognitive components necessary for functional performance. Motor components include range of motion, muscle strength,

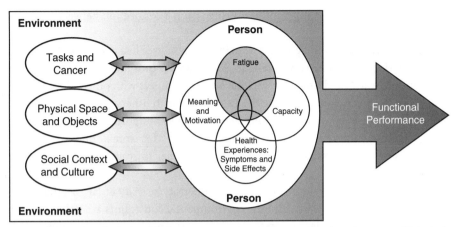

Fig. 13.1 Conceptual relationship between person, environment, and performance. (Adapted from Kielhofner (1995).) Permission sought.

and endurance. Cognitive components include attention, concentration, and memory. As such, motor and cognitive components provide the person with the *potential* to engage in everyday activities. Functional performance refers to a person's actual ability to do everyday tasks and activities, and is, in part, the result of the coordination of various motor and cognitive components within the context of a particular environment, in order to meet the demands of a particular task or activity (Kielhofner 1995).

Although simplified, the figure depicts how the experience of fatigue is a confluence of one's physical and cognitive capacity for action with the motivation and personal meanings one assigns to the experience. The cancer disease process and its treatments can influence capacity, motivation, and meaning. The environment, consisting of the everyday task and activities available to the person, the physical space and objects, and the social space in which the person performs the everyday activities, influence the many dimensions of the person.

An example may be illuminating. The second author recently treated a gentleman who worked as writer and was experiencing significant fatigue following chemotherapy. The man's writing studio was located on the upstairs floor of his house, while his living spaces (kitchen, living room) were located on the ground floor and he was becoming increasingly fatigued walking up and down the stairs between these rooms. He found he was writing less and less during the day and becoming increasingly depressed about his lack of productivity. One obvious solution might be to simply move his computer, books etc to the ground floor so that his work and living areas were all on the same level. Ergonomically, this is the most efficient solution. However, this man was reluctant to pursue this option. He had worked in his studio for many years; some of his best works had been created there. For him, it was more than simply a room and equipment; it was life space, a connection between past and present literary works.

We can contrast this by imagining a woman, who also lives in a two-storey house and who is experiencing cancer-related fatigue. She views her computer as a form of access to the outside world, and uses it to 'surf the net' and connect with others through chat rooms. For this person, maintaining the connection with others is what is important and satisfying, the environment in which she works is less important, since her focus is on being able to communicate with her friends online. This woman finds moving the computer downstairs a satisfying solution, enabling her to continue the activity she finds most meaningful.

These two people illustrate that knowing the intensity/severity of fatigue, the capacity to walk up and down stairs, and the environmental constraints are not enough to understand the impact of fatigue on functional status. That is, the whole activity experience is more than the sum of the parts. Rather, it is the combination of the environmental supports and constraints, the demands of the task, the individual capacities of the person, *and* the meaning of the activity for the person at this point in their life story that mediate the influence of fatigue on *actual* performance of the task. That is, while underlying capacity is necessary for functional performance, it is not sufficient. For example, there is only a moderate correlation between capacity for action and functional performance (Leidy 1990; Roth *et al.* 1998). Therefore, an important distinction must be made between the *potential* for performance and the *actual* performance of everyday activities—that is, the person's functional performance.

One attempt to account for the relationship between capacity and performance is provided by Leidy (1994). She describes four dimensions of functional status: functional capacity, functional reserve, functional performance, and functional capacity utilization. Functional capacity is a person's maximum potential (physical, psychological, social, and spiritual) to perform everyday activities. Functional performance refers to the activities that a person actually does in the course of daily life. Functional reserve is the difference between capacity and performance, reflecting that performance of everyday activities does not always take a person's full capacity. Functional capacity utilization refers to the percentage of capacity that is used in any given performance. These concepts are not interchangeable, rather the distinctions are helpful in highlighting what a person is capable of doing, can do, and actually does.

In a similar vein, Glass (1998) notes that the investigation and study of functional performance requires further clarification. He distinguishes between hypothetical, experimental, and enacted tenses. In the hypothetical tense, function is that which is typically obtained through pencil-and-paper surveys whereby the person (or proxy) reports what activities they can or cannot do, but this 'doing' is devoid of context. In the experimental tense, functional performance is observed under controlled or unusual circumstances and may or may not reflect what the person actually does in his or her own home or community. In the enacted tense, functional performance is 'the end result of the confluence of situational and ecological factors which shape the moment-to-moment performance of functional tasks in the real world' (Glass 1998, p. 103).

Why distinguish between capacity and performance?

This distinction between capacity and functional performance provides several important advantages. First, it makes clear the difference between the *potential* for action and the *realization* of that potential in the performance of everyday activities. Second, it highlights the indirect relationship between capacity and performance and, in doing so, may account for research findings where capacity explains only a small portion of the variance in functional performance (Roth *et al.* 1998). Third, it demonstrates that the study of the impact of fatigue on daily life must take into account the notion that capacity alone is insufficient to explain/understand functional performance.

Three issues seem relevant to understanding the relationship between capacity and performance. These include the quality or effectiveness of performance, the role of the environment in constructing performance, and the impact of motivation and meaning on performance.

Quality and effectiveness of performance

While components such as range of motion, muscle strength, endurance, memory, and attention describe the capacity for performance, they do not say anything about 'how *effective* an action is in accomplishing a functional purpose' (Fisher and Kielhofner 1995, p. 114). This is because there are many ways in which underlying capacities can be 'assembled' in order to complete an everyday activity. As such, underlying capacity is related to, but does not predict, successful functional performance since 'one cannot know ahead of time how one will use one's capacities in a given task and context' (Fisher and Kielhofner 1995, p. 115). There is a growing appreciation that motor control (the production of movement) is not under the executive control of the central nervous system, but rather it 'emerges' from the coalescence of the person (including their past motor learning), the demands of the particular task, and the supports (affordances) within the environment. For example, Ma *et al.* (1999) found that when people learned a new skill such as using chopsticks, the actual kinematic quality of performance differed when learning in real life versus simulated settings, even though the motions required to perform the task were identical.

Impact of environment on task performance

Dynamical systems theorists have been instrumental in developing the idea that performance of everyday activities results from a confluence of the person, task, and environment (Kamm *et al.* 1990; Mathiowetz and Haugen 1994). Current research is enhancing our understanding of this notion. For example, in a series of studies looking at the impact of home versus clinic on the performance of everyday activities, Fisher and colleagues (Nygard *et al.* 1994; Park *et al.* 1994; Darragh *et al.* 1998) found that, in general, patients perform the same activities better at home than in the clinic. This appeared to be due in part to observable improvement in the performance of cognitive aspects of the task. Familiarity with the home environment, as well as psychological factors such as motivation and comfort, probably also play a role. For example, a patient may drag him/herself to the clinic for treatment, may complain bitterly about the expenditure of energy required just to receive medical care, and yet may be able to sustain productivity in a sedentary job from his/her home office.

Impact of personal meaning on task performance

Ability (capacity) to perform does not necessarily result in actual performance. For example, Helfrich and Kielhofner (1994) describe a patient who is competent and active in everyday activities in the inpatient setting but who resorts to an inactive life once at home. In a randomized, controlled study Murphy *et al.* (1999) found that when people performed activities they found personally meaningful, their endurance for activity was significantly greater than those who performed activities they found meaningless.

The observation of skilled performance

Both conceptually in the work of Leidy (1994) and Glass (1998) and empirically in the work of Trombly and others (Ma *et al.* 1999; Murphy *et al.* 1999) it is apparent that capacity is not sufficient to understand functional performance. However, observable functional performance has rarely been assessed in the nursing literature. In general, clinicians have evaluated functional status using coarse observer rating scales, such as the Zubrod Performance Status Rating Scale (Zubrod *et al.* 1960) or the Karnofsky Performance Status Rating Scale (Karnofsky *et al.* 1948). These seldom capture the more subtle impact of fatigue on functional performance, such as decreased speed and endurance.

However, if, as Leidy argues, the field is to 'have a better understanding of the functional status of clients in order to design interventions and evaluate outcomes appropriately' (Leidy 1994, p. 202) some observable evaluation of functional performance within a task context will be needed. A concept now widely used in the field of occupational therapy is that of skilled performance. In skilled performance, the focus is on how effectively and efficiently a person actually performs daily tasks within the constraints of the environment. The unit of analysis is skilled action. One asks how well an action served to move the activity towards completion. Skills are observable units of behaviour in three domains: motor, process, and communication (Fisher and Kielhofner 1995). Skills are not steps, or even sequential actions, in fact several skills may be reflected in a single action, but are observable behaviours that facilitate, or interfere with, the completion of the task. As an example, consider reaching to take a can of beans from an overhead cupboard while cooking a meal. Knowing that a person has a particular amount of range of motion in their shoulder or a certain amount of grip strength will not adequately predict whether they will complete the task. This is because it is not always possible to know how large or heavy the can of beans will be, how high the cupboard shelf is, and how near or far from the front of the shelf the can has been placed. A can placed on a high shelf may require a person to retrieve a chair, mount the chair, retrieve the can, bend to place it on the counter top, get down from the chair, and return the chair to its place. A person with fatigue may require several rest stops during this activity, which significantly delays its completion. Two well-developed instruments for the assessment of skilled performance are the Assessment of Motor and Process Skills (Fisher 1997) and the Assessment of Communication/ Interaction Skills (Forsyth *et al.* 1995). These assessments require that the person perform activities that she or he finds personally meaningful so that lack of motivation or desire does not have a negative impact on performance.

The immediate benefit this perspective provides for studying the impact of fatigue in cancer patients is that one can directly observe the more subtle but significant impact that fatigue has on actual performance. For example, does the person prop him/herself against the counter or lean on his/her elbows so that performance is slowed down? Does the person move and reach slowly, delaying completion of the task? Does the person have difficulty starting the next step or stop part way through to rest?

Implications for the evaluation/measurement of fatigue and function

Historically, studies in oncology examining functional status or the impact of fatigue in patients with cancer have relied on self-report (Cella *et al.* 1993; Yellen *et al.* 1997; Mendoza *et al.* 1999). Consequently, little is known about how similar or divergent are patients' reports of functional impairment and therapists' observations of patients' functional performance. For example, a study of injured workers suggests that the more disabled a patient is, the more divergent patient and therapist ratings may be. As the functional status of a patient improved, so patient and therapist ratings became increasingly similar (Gerardi and Eckberg 1995). Patient self-reports of functional status are convenient and often-used methods of capturing change in functional status due to fatigue. While such approaches offer valuable insights into patient perceptions of performance, clinical observation provides an alternative 'outsider' view of performance, i.e. performance as it is observed by others. However, observation of performance, while providing an alternative viewpoint, is hardly objective. For example, it has been shown that, using the Functional Independence Measure, therapists (occupational therapists, physiotherapists) rate the same patients differently from nurses (Bode and Heinemann 1997). Rather than sending us on searches for unexplained error,

Box 13.1 Summary points

- ◆ The performance of everyday activities results from a confluence of the person, task, and the environment.
- ◆ The meaning an activity holds for an individual and how motivated they are to do it plays an important role in its subsequent performance.
- ◆ Little is known about the relationship between a person's experience of fatigue, his/her capacity for action, and performance in everyday activities.

or engaging in debates on the relative merits of 'objective' versus 'subjective' views, differences between clinician and patient perspectives can be a fruitful source of understanding of the impact cancer-related fatigue has on everyday life. This suggests that to understand the impact of fatigue on functional performance will require that evaluations intersect both person and environment, utilizing both emic and etic perspectives. Box 13.1 summarizes the points made in this chapter.

Importance for developing effective intervention strategies

Understanding the impact of fatigue on daily living activities is central to providing effective interventions, including both remediation and compensatory strategies (see Chapter 12). Research suggests that remediation strategies such as engagement in planned exercise (Mock *et al.* 1997) and activities such as gardening and walking (Winningham *et al.* 1986; Cimprich 1993) may relieve fatigue. Compensatory strategies, such as energy conservation techniques, have been used successfully with patients with diagnoses of chronic fatigue syndrome, chronic obstructive airway disease, and arthritis (Furst *et al.* 1987; Hubsky and Sears 1992; Welham 1995; Rashbaum and Whyte 1996; Brus *et al.* 1998). Whilst this approach is being advocated as a technique for managing cancer-related fatigue there is little systematic evaluation of its effectiveness. As patients live longer with cancer and experience ongoing fatigue, efficacious interventions that assist patients in lifestyle changes will become increasingly important.

The model presented in this chapter implies that it is not simply enough to give patients advice regarding energy conservation techniques, or to use interventions that only focus on restoration of underlying capacity. Consideration must be given in rehabilitation programmes to the impact that performing everyday activities differently may have on a person's motivation. For example, does rearranging a person's environment or daily schedule call attention to or accentuate, rather than minimize, someone's disability? If reduction in fatigue intensity or restoration of underlying capacity will take a long time, what might help a person commit long-term to exercise or energy conservation programmes? Having committed to a programme, what changes in

Box 13.2 Implications for research and practice

- ◆ Clinicians should ensure that they consider and address the motivational and meaning aspects of functional performance when discussing this with patients.

- ◆ Clinicians and research studies need to distinguish between capacity for action and actual performance in the assessment of functional capabilities.

- ◆ In order to understand the impact of fatigue on functional performance evaluations should be made of the person in their own environment using subjective and objective rating.

- ◆ Measures of skilled performance should be included in future studies exploring the impact of fatigue on the performance of everyday activities.

actual performance can be detected in both the short and long term? These are important questions if the field is to develop effective behavioural interventions for cancer-related fatigue. Clearly understanding the relationships amongst conceptual components will be central to this endeavour (see Box 13.2).

References

Aistars, J. (1987) Fatigue in the cancer patient: a conceptual approach to a clinical problem. *Oncology Nursing Forum,* **14**(6), 25–30.

Bode, R.K. and Heinemann, A.W. (1997) An exploration of interdisciplinary ratings of functional assessment items. [Paper presented at the First International Outcome Measurement Conference, co-sponsored by Rehabilitation Foundation Inc., and the MESA Psychometric Laboratory at the University of Chicago.] In: *Physical Medicine and Rehabilitation: State of the Art Reviews.* 11(2), 407–24.

Brus, H.L., van de Laar, M.A.F.J., Taal, E., Rasker, J.J., and Wiegman, O. (1998) Effects of patient education on compliance with basic treatment regimens and health in recent onset active rheumatoid arthritis. *Annals of Rheumatic Disease,* **57**(3), 146–51.

Cella, D.F., Tulsky, D.S., Gray, G., Sarafian, B., Linn, E., Bonomi, A. *et al.* (1993) The Functional Assessment of Cancer Therapy scale: development and validation of the general measure. *Journal of Clinical Oncology,* **11**(3), 570–9.

Cimprich, B. (1993) Development of an intervention to restore attention in cancer patient. *Cancer Nursing,* **16**(2), 83–92.

Darragh, A.R., Sample, P.L., and Fisher, A.G. (1998) Environment effect on functional task performance in adults with acquired brain injuries: use of the assessment of motor and process skills. *Archives of Physical Medicine and Rehabilitation,* **79**(4), 418–23.

Ferrell, B., Grant, M., Dean, G., Funk, B., and Ly, J. (1996) 'Bone tired': the experience of fatigue and its impact on quality of life. *Oncology Nursing Forum,* **33**, 1539–47.

Fisher, A., and Kielhofner, G. (1995) Skill in occupational performance. In: *A Model of Human Occupation: Theory and Application* (ed. G. Kielhofner), Williams and Wilkins, Baltimore, MD, pp. 113–38.

Fisher, A.G. (1997) *Assessment of Motor and Process Skills* (2nd edn), Three Star Press, Fort Collins, CO.

Forsyth, K.A., Salamy, M., Simon, S., and Kielhofner, G. (1995) *A User's Guide to the Assessment of Communication and Interaction Skills (ACIS)* (4th edn). Chicago, IL: Model of Human Occupation Clearinghouse, University of Illinois at Chicago.

Furst, G.P., Gerber, L.H., Smith, C.C., Fisher, S., and Shulman, B. (1987) A program for improving energy conservation behaviors in adults with rheumatoid arthritis. *American Journal of Occupational Therapy*, 41(2), 102–11.

Gerardi, S. and Eckberg, S. (1995) Clients vs. therapists. *Rasch Measurement Transactions*, 8(4), 399.

Glass, T.A. (1998) Conjugating the 'tenses' of function: discordance among hypothetical, experimental, and enacted function in older adults. *Gerontologist*, 38(1), 101–12.

Helfrich, C. and Kielhofner, G. (1994) Volitional narratives and the meaning of therapy. *American Journal of Occupational Therapy*, 48(4), 319–26.

Hubsky, E.P. and Sears, J.H. (1992) Fatigue in multiple sclerosis: guidelines for nursing care. *Rehabilitation Nursing*, 17(4), 176–81.

Kamm, K., Thelen, E., and Jensen, J.L. (1990) A dynamical systems approach to motor development. *Physical Therapy*, 70(12), 763–75.

Karnofsky, D.A., Abelmann, W.H., Craver, L.F., and Burchenal, J.H. (1948) The use of nitrogen mustards in the palliative treatment of carcinoma. *Cancer*, 1, 634–66.

Kielhofner, G. (1995) *A Model of Human Occupation: Theory and Application* (2nd edn), Williams and Wilkins, Baltimore, MD.

Leidy, N.K. (1991) Survey measures of functional ability and disability of pulmonary patients. In B. Metzger (ed.), *Altered functioning: impairment and disability*. Center Nursing Press of Sigma Theta Tau International, Indianapolis, IN, pp. 52–79.

Leidy, N.K. (1994) Functional status and the forward progress of merry-go-rounds: toward a coherent analytical framework. *Nursing Research*, 43(4), 196–202.

Ma, H., Trombly, C.A., and Robinson-Podolski, C. (1999) The effect of context on skill acquisition and transfer. *American Journal of Occupational Therapy*, 53(2), 138–44.

Mathiowetz, V. and Haugen, J.B. (1994) Motor behavior research: implications for therapeutic approaches to central nervous system dysfunction. *American Journal of Occupational Therapy*, 48(8), 733–45.

Mendoza, T.R., Wang, X.S., Cleeland, C.S., Morrissey, M., Johnson, B.A., Wendt, J.K. *et al.* (1999) The rapid assessment of fatigue severity in cancer patients: use of the Brief Fatigue Inventory. *Cancer*, 85(5), 1186–96.

Messias, D.H., Yeager, K., Dibble, S., and Dodd, M. (1997) Patient perspectives of fatigue while undergoing chemotherapy. *Oncology Nursing Forum*, 24, 43–8.

Mock, V., Dow, K.H., Meares, C.J., Grimm, P.M., Dienemann, J.A., Haisfield-Wolfe, M.E. *et al.* (1997) Effects of exercise on fatigue, physical functioning, and emotional distress during radiation therapy for breast cancer. *Oncology Nursing Forum*, 26(6), 991–1000.

Murphy, S., Trombly, C., Tickle-Degnen, L., and Jacobs, K. (1999) The effect of keeping an end-product on intrinsic motivation. *American Journal of Occupational Therapy*, 53(2), 153–8.

Nygard, L., Bernspang, B., Fisher, A.G., and Winblad, B. (1994) Comparing motor and process ability of persons with suspected dementia in home and clinic settings. *American Journal of Occupational Therapy*, 48(8), 689–96.

Park, S., Fisher, A.G., and Velozo, C.A. (1994) Using the assessment of motor and process skills to compare occupational performance between clinic and home settings. *American Journal of Occupational Therapy*, 48(8), 697–709.

Persson, L., Hallberg, I.R., and Ohlsson, O. (1997) Survivors of acute leukaemia and highly malignant lymphoma—retrospective views of daily life problems during treatment and when in remission. *Journal of Advanced Nursing, 25, 68–78.*

Piper, B.F., Lindsey, A.M., and Dodd, M.J. (1987) Fatigue mechanisms in cancer patients: developing nursing theory. *Oncology Nursing Forum, 14*(6), 17–23.

Portenoy, R.K., Thaler, H.T., Kornblith, A.B., Lepore, J.M., Friedlander-Klar, H., Coyle, N. *et al.* (1994) Symptom prevalence, characteristics and distress in a cancer population. *Quality of Life Research, 3,* 183–9.

Rashbaum, I. and Whyte, N. (1996) Occupational therapy in pulmonary rehabilitation: energy conservation and work simplification techniques. *Physical Medicine and Rehabilitation Clinics of North America, 7*(2), 325–40.

Rhodes, V.A., Watson, P.M., and Hanson, B.M. (1988) Patients' descriptions of the influence of tiredness and weakness on self-care abilities. *Cancer Nursing, 11*(3), 186–94.

Roth, E.J., Heinemann, A.W., Lovell, L.L., Harvey, R.L., McGuire, J.R., and Diaz, S. (1998) Impairment and disability: their relation during stroke rehabilitation. *Archives of Physical Medicine and Rehabilitation, 79*(3), 329–35.

Welham, L. (1995) Occupational therapy for fatigue in patients with multiple sclerosis. *British Journal of Occupational Therapy, 58*(12), 507–9.

Winningham, M.L., MacVicar, M.G., and Burke, C.A. (1986) Exercise for cancer patients: guidelines and precautions. *The Physician and Sportsmedicine, 14*(10), 125–34.

Yellen, S.B., Cella, D.F., Webster, K., Blendowski, C., and Kaplan, E. (1997) Measuring fatigue and other anemia-related symptoms with the functional assessment of cancer therapy (FACT) measurement system. *Journal of Pain and Symptom Management, 13*(2), 63–74.

Zubrod, C.G., Schneiderman, M., and Frei, E. (1960) Appraisal of methods for the study of chemotherapy of cancer in man: comparative therapeutic trial of nitrogen mustard and triethylene thiophosphoramide. *Journal of Chronic Disability, 11,* 7–33.

Chapter 14

The therapeutic effects of exercise on fatigue

Davina Porock and Mei Fu

Introduction

Fatigue has been identified as the most distressing and prevalent cancer-related symptom in a variety of cancer populations. Incidence of cancer-related fatigue ranges from 40% to 100%, depending on cancer diagnoses, treatment modalities, and disease stages (Berger 1998; Fu *et al.* 2002; Hickok *et al.* 1996; Hinds *et al.* 1999; Schag *et al.* 1994; Porock *et al.* 2000; Winningham *et al.* 1994). People with cancer describe their fatigue experience as being different from the fatigue that healthy people experience. Cancer-related fatigue has usually been described as being more intense, severe, chronic, debilitating, distressing, and less likely to be relieved by rest (Andrykowski *et al.* 1998; Fu *et al.* 2002; Glaus *et al.* 1996; Porock *et al.* 2000; Schwartz 1998). Unlike cancer-related fatigue, acute fatigue in healthy people is usually an expected tiredness with rapid onset and short duration. Acute fatigue in healthy people serves as a protective function that signals people to take a rest to restore energy. Generally, a good night's sleep or a few hours of rest will restore a healthy individual to a normal level of functioning. However, cancer-related fatigue often imposes a persistent or relapsing, unpleasant, distressing, and debilitating sensation on individuals with cancer. For many patients, cancer-related fatigue is a common and significant contributor to decreased quality of life (Aistars 1987). It exerts a great impact on an individual's sense of well-being and usual functioning, including daily performance, activities of daily living, relationships with family and friends, and compliance with treatment (Glaus 1993; Pickard-Holley 1991).

Despite the prevalence of fatigue in individuals with cancer and the extent to which it can interfere with daily activities, intervention research designed to prevent or ameliorate fatigue has only begun to emerge. Rest is still the most frequently recommended intervention in practice (Nail *et al.* 1991; Ream and Richardson 1996). However, it is now accepted in the research community that rest alone is generally not effective in returning the cancer patient with chronic fatigue to their previous level of functioning (Winningham 1991). Unnecessary bedrest and prolonged sedentariness can contribute significantly to the development of fatigue and weakness that may result in rapid and potentially irreversible losses in energy and functioning.

Since the mid 1980s exercise has been recognized as a promising strategy for managing and ameliorating fatigue in individuals with cancer and other chronic illness. Research suggests that physical exercise is an effective strategy for reducing cancer-related fatigue, by maintaining or restoring functional capacity, improving depression and anxiety, as well as enhancing quality of life in individuals with cancer (Dimeo *et al.* 1997; MacVicar *et al.* 1989; Mock *et al.* 1997; Porock *et al.* 2000).

Winningham's psychobiological entropy model (Winningham 1992) provides a theoretical framework for exercise as an intervention for managing cancer-related fatigue. This model seeks to link activity, fatigue, symptoms, and functional status, and is based on the clinical observation that individuals who become less active as a result of disease- and/or treatment-related symptoms lose energizing metabolic resources. According to the model, fatigue fulfils a unique and substantial role in the origin of disability that sets it apart from other symptoms. Decreased physical activity, regardless of the cause, leads to decreased energetic capacity (measured in terms of respiratory oxygen uptake or its correlate, calories consumed) for activity. This, in turn, is responsible for increasing fatigue, further decreasing activity, and, subsequently resulting in functional disability.

Five propositions are derived from Winningham's model:

◆ Too much as well as too little rest contributes to feelings of fatigue.

◆ Too little as well as too much activity contributes to feelings of fatigue.

◆ A balance between activity and rest promotes restoration; an imbalance promotes deterioration.

◆ Any symptom that contributes to decreased activity will lead to increased fatigue and decreased functional status.

◆ Any intervention providing relief of a symptom that contributes to decreased activity may also serve to mitigate fatigue, and promote functioning, providing that intervention does not have a sedating or catabolic effect.

The physiological effects of exercise

Defining exercise

Exercise can be defined as episodic performance of repetitive bodily movements produced by skeletal muscles that requires energy expenditure. In the healthy population, exercise with a duration of 30–45 min for each episode and a frequency of at least three times a week is advocated in order to produce cardiovascular benefits. Cancer-related fatigue is characterized by a persistent, intense, and chronic sense of tiredness and exhaustion that interferes with usual functioning. Therefore the duration, intensity, and frequency of exercise aimed at managing and ameliorating cancer-related fatigue is expected to be different from that of the healthy population. To help us understand the physiological effects of exercise in populations of cancer patients a review of the physiological effects of exercise in the healthy population is outlined in Table 14.1.

Table 14.1 Phases of exercise in a healthy population

Phases of exercise	Physical and chemical response of human body to the severity and duration
Phase I: the phosphagenic energy phase	The preexisting stores of high-energy compounds (such as adenosine triphosphate (ATP) and phosphocreatine (PCr)) can be depleted within a few seconds under maximal exercise effort The high-energy compounds can be rapidly replenished in the aerobic energy phase
Phase II: the aerobic energy phase	The process of oxidative phosphorylation is the important mechanism for rapid repletion of the high-energy compounds During oxidative phosphorylation, glycogen, serum glucose, and serum fatty acids are denatured to acetyl coenzyme A and fed into the citric acid cycle, with the ultimate production of carbondioxide (CO_2) and water (H_2O) The process of oxidative phosphorylation leads to either the energy being stored as ATP and PCr or energy release as heat. It can provide the needed energy as long as the level of the activity remains less than 70% of the maximum rate of ATP breakdown The aerobic metabolism cannot always cope in time, especially with heavy exercise workload
Phase III: the anaerobic phase	An alternative energy-producing mechanism to prevent individuals from energy depletion Pyruvic acid is formed from glycogen and transformed into lactic acid (lactate), this process is not economic and only yields enough energy to form 2 moles of ATP, comparing to 38 moles of ATP via the aerobic phase Lactic acid accumulation leads to a continuous fall in blood pH, thus an individual has to stop the exhausting exercise More depletion of oxygen may result from the process in which oxygen is needed to reconvert the lactic acid into pyruvic acid in the liver and muscles Individuals may experience soreness or even pain in the muscle for up to several days following the specific exercise activity The more oxygen that can be delivered for the oxidative phosphorylation, the less will be the need to rely on anaerobic metabolism

Individual maximal oxygen uptake

The amount of oxygen carried and delivered to contracting muscle is called the maximal oxygen uptake ($VO_{2\,max}$) or maximum aerobic power. Maximum aerobic power refers to the highest oxygen uptake attained during physical work (activity or exercise), breathing air at sea level (Astrand 1973). $VO_{2\,max}$ has become the 'gold standard' for measuring an individual's capacity to supply energy aerobically during physical activity and exercise (Glaser 1997). It is directly related to the functional capacities of the cardiovascular, pulmonary, and muscular systems. The higher an individual's $VO_{2\,max}$, the greater is the physiological reserve and the lower will be the relative stress experienced for performing certain given activities. In addition, a high correlation exists between cardiac output and oxygen uptake; thus measurement of oxygen uptake not only reveals the capacity to yield aerobic energy, but also the load on the heart (Astrand 1973).

Training effects

It is common knowledge that after a period of training exercise becomes easier and progressively greater loads can be tolerated. This training effect results from physical and chemical changes which occur as muscle contracts, and implies an increased $VO_{2\,max}$ resulting from increased oxygen delivery due to the increased cardiac output, and by more efficient use of oxygen via contracting muscle cells (Morris 1975). Training not only improves left ventricular performance leading to increased cardiac output, but also enhances elimination of lactate by trained muscles, resulting in lower blood lactate levels (Morris 1975). Consequently, increased cardiac output and efficient elimination of lactate results in an increase in maximum aerobic power. As oxygen uptake reaches maximal levels the cardiac output and stroke volume are also maximal. A further increase in work intensity is possible because of an anaerobic energy yield, but the cardiac output and stroke volume may be somewhat reduced. Certainly the work becomes very exhausting and straining (Astrand 1973).

Physical activity

Physical activity is defined as bodily movement produced by skeletal muscles that require energy expenditure (NIH Consensus Development Panel on Physical Activity and Cardiovascular Health 1996). Physical activity ranges from repeated work periods from a few seconds' duration up to hours of continuous work, creating a major load on the oxygen-transporting organs, and thereby inducing a training effect. The total amount of physical activity may be as important as episodic exercise in producing important outcomes relating to health and well-being (King 1994; O'Neill and Reid 1991). Increasing physical activity in people with cancer may be an effective intervention for reducing fatigue, promoting functional independence, and physical functioning. The rationale for increasing physical activity in people with cancer is:

◆ The training effect of physical activity that forms part of everyday functioning may be more effective in relieving fatigue and improving physical functioning than episodic exercise.

◆ Physical activity can be carried at any time and in any setting (home, street, gym), an encouraging factor for individuals affected by cancer to engage in activities they enjoy and tolerate.

◆ Unlimited types and durations of physical activity permit individuals with cancer to perform physical activities according to their preference, thus reducing the possibility of boredom.

Beneficial effects of exercise in individuals with cancer

The benefits of exercise are the same for people with cancer as for healthy people. Research on the impact of exercise and physical activity on cancer-related fatigue has been undertaken with patients receiving, or those who have completed, treatment.

Most intervention studies have been conducted with patients undergoing treatment for breast cancer and/or receiving bone marrow transplantation (MacVicar and Winningham 1986; Mock *et al.* 1994, 1997; Schwartz 2000). All of these studies used different types of aerobic exercise: a walking programme (Mock *et al.* 1994, 1997, 1998), cycling (Dimeo *et al.* 1997), patients' own choices of type and time of exercise (Schwartz 2000). In a study conducted by Porock *et al.* (2000), a range of physical activity was prescribed to people with advanced cancer. For example, an individual might walk for 5 min, perform arm exercises with a resisted rubber band in a chair, march on the spot in the kitchen, or dance to favourite music. The duration of exercise regimes in these studies varied from 6 weeks for patients undergoing radiation to 6 months for breast cancer patients undergoing chemotherapy and bone marrow transplantation, respectively. Some of the exercise regimes in the studies were under supervision in a laboratory whilst others were home-based. All of the studies demonstrated that exercise significantly reduces fatigue in patients undergoing cancer treatment. Specific benefits that have been evaluated with cancer patients are summarized in Table 14.2.

Fatigue is recognized as a significant correlate of impaired functional activity among patients receiving radiation and chemotherapy treatment (Irvine *et al.* 1994). Moreover, research indicates an inverse relationship between levels of physical activity and fatigue (Mock *et al.* 1994, 1997; Porock *et al.* 2000). Although the mechanism of how exercise reduces fatigue and increases energy remains unclear, research shows that exercise, particularly aerobic exercise, may be beneficial in relieving fatigue and

Table 14.2 Summary of the research on the benefits of exercise in patients with cancer

Benefit	Study findings	Reference
Relieves fatigue and enhances energy	Studies in women with breast cancer, bone marrow transplantation, and people with metastatic cancer all benefited in terms of perception of fatigue and feelings of enhanced energy. None of these studies were able to isolate the mechanism(s) by which fatigue was relieved	Berger (1998), Dimeo *et al.* (1998), MacVicar *et al.* (1989), Winningham (1996), Mock *et al.* (1997), Porock *et al.* (2000), Schwartz (1998)
Improves physical functioning	Exercise helps to break the cycle of deconditioning	Mock *et al.* (1994, 1997), Porock *et al.* (2000)
Improves mood	Exercise is associated with elevated levels of beta-endorphins and increased brain serotonin levels after acute exercise	Artal and Sherman (1998), Chaouloff (1997)
Weight control	Women receiving adjuvant chemotherapy for breast cancer who did not exercise gained an average of 3.2 kg, while those in the exercise group maintained their pretreatment weight	Schwartz (2000)

enhancing energy. Two hypotheses have been proposed:

- The training effect of aerobic exercise increases cardiac output and thus oxygen perfusion, as long as the individual sustains physical activity (Astrand 1973).
- Exercise induces increased levels of beta-endorphins and their euphoric effect elicits the perception that one is less fatigued (Kennedy and Newton 1997).

In addition to extreme muscular deconditioning related to cancer disease and treatment modalities, cancer-related fatigue is worsened by prolonged rest and inactivity, contributing to muscular catabolism. As a result patients need a higher degree of effort to carry out normal activities. A consequence of this is a persistent and self-perpetuating condition of diminished activity caused by easy fatigability for many weeks and even months post-treatment (Dimeo *et al.* 1997; Winningham 1992). Aerobic exercise may reduce fatigue and improve physical functioning by breaking the cycle of lack of exercise, impaired functioning, and easy fatigability.

The psychological effects of exercise

Cancer diagnosis, treatment, and uncertainty of reoccurrence is a chronic and dynamic process that exerts a great deal of emotional stress on individuals with cancer. Depression may be a co-morbid and disabling syndrome that elicits anxiety, sadness, and fatigue. It is difficult to differentiate whether fatigue causes depression or vice versa. Both fatigue and depression are strong predictors of quality of life in cancer patients (Hopwood and Stephens 2000) and depression is more likely than fatigue to cause emotional distress in family caregivers. Thus, it is important to manage depression not only for the comfort of the patient, but also in order to reduce distress in the family.

Psychological effects of exercise on depression

The psychological effects of exercise refer to what individuals feel psychologically and emotionally when the human body exercises. Currently, most psychopharmacological agents relieve depression by restoring a balance between neuroreceptors and neurotransmitters. Antidepressant medications, including the selective serotonin re-uptake inhibitors (SSRIs), are believed to ameliorate depression by increasing the availability of neurotransmitters at receptor sites (Artal and Sherman 1998). The biological mechanism of exercise in reducing depression still needs clarification. However, there is a body of evidence to suggest that exercise may exert antidepressant effects by influencing the metabolism and availability of central neurotransmitters (Artal and Sherman 1998), and by increasing levels of brain serotonin (Chaouloff 1997). Despite evidence that exercise leads to increased levels of beta-endorphins, it is questionable whether this increase is sufficient to reduce depression (Artal and Sherman 1998). The action of elevated levels of beta-endorphins remains unclear, but its ability to induce euphoria and thus reduce the perception of pain might exert an antidepressant effect by changing the perception of depression.

Research on the psychological effects of exercise in individuals with cancer is limited. Nevertheless, the results of existing studies have demonstrated that exercise does benefit individuals with cancer both psychologically and emotionally, including increased self-concept, improved self-esteem, increased self-control, feeling of decreased depression and anxiety, as well as overall improved quality of life (Courneya and Friedenreich 1997, 1999; Mock *et al.* 1997; Winningham *et al.* 1994). The psychological mechanism of exercise may play the most important role in reducing depression and anxiety by bringing about positive changes in mood states, changes shown to occur in young and older healthy adults and in a variety of patients (Table 14.3).

In one study assessing the effectiveness of an aerobic exercise programme in older patients with depression (Blumenthal *et al.* 1999), aerobic capacity was found to have statistically significant correlation with improved depression. The authors suggested that improved aerobic capacity might account for at least part of the reduction in depression.

Table 14.3 Summary of the research on the psychological effects of exercise

Psychological effects of exercise	Populations	Types of exercise	References
Reduces tension, anger and depression, enhances feelings of vigour	Healthy male and female	Aerobic dance	Kennedy and Newton (1997)
Enhances positive emotions and reduces negative emotions; reduces anxiety	Healthy undergraduate students	Pedalling a stationary bicycle (bicycle ergometer)	Petruzzello *et al.* (1997)
Reduces clinical signs and symptoms of depression	Male and female older patients (aged 50–77 years) with diagnosis of depression	Walking or jogging	Blumenthal *et al.* (1999)
Decreases tension/anxiety, reduces depression/dejection, enhances feelings of vigour	Breast cancer patients	Walking	MacVicar and Winningham (1986)
Reduces anxiety	Stage I or II breast cancer survivors	Pedalling a stationary bicycle (bicycle ergometer)	Blanchard *et al.* (2001)
Enhances sense of well-being, improves self-efficacy in controlling pain and fatigue, reduces depression	Fibromyalgia patients	Walking/jogging/side-stepping/arm exercise against water resistance in a warm therapeutic pool	Gowans *et al.* (1999)

Porock *et al.* (2000) hypothesized that improvement of any aspect of physical, social, and mental well-being will be reflected in an overall improvement in reported quality of life.

Forms of exercise

Theoretically exercise type, intensity, frequency, and duration, are vital in producing effective psychological effects. Activities that are aerobic, non-competitive, predictable, and rhythmical, such as walking, cycling, swimming, aerobic dancing, running (Barabasz 1991; Berger and Owen 1983; Blumenthal *et al.* 1999; Kennedy and Newton 1997; McMurdo and Burnett 1992; Courneya and Friedenreich 1997, 1999; MacVicar and Winningham 1986; Mock *et al.* 1997; Porock *et al.* 2000; Winningham *et al.* 1994), have been shown to produce psychological benefit (Kennedy and Newton 1997).

The intensity of exercise is measured by the amount of exertion. For healthy adults, both high- and low-intensity exercise are thought to lead to positive changes in mood and have positive psychological impact (Kennedy and Newton 1997). However, in an early study comparing high- and low-intensity exercise by Steptoe and Cox (1988), only subjects who exercised at low-intensity demonstrated positive mood change. Research on the intensity of exercise in people with cancer shows that a low to moderate intensity of exercise produces both physical and psychological effects on reducing fatigue, depression, and anxiety (Courneya and Friedenreich 1999; MacVicar and Winningham 1986; Mock *et al.* 1997; Porock *et al.* 2000; Winningham *et al.* 1994).

The duration of exercise refers to both the time for which each episode of exercise lasts and the time frame (usually weeks, months, or years) in which the exercise behaviour lasts. The majority of studies examining aspects of psychological well-being using exercise sessions of at least 20 min duration have obtained positive results on psychological measures (Kennedy and Newton 1997). Blumenthal *et al.* (1999) found that exercise was equally as effective as medication after 16 weeks of an aerobic exercise programme in older patients diagnosed with depression. Most studies employing exercise with a duration from 6 weeks to 6 months in people with cancer have revealed findings of positive psychological changes, such as decreased depression and anxiety, reduced fatigue, increased self-esteem, increased sense of self-control, as well as improved overall well-being and quality of life (Mock *et al.* 1994, 1997, 1998; Dimeo *et al.* 1997, 1999).

Implications for practice and research

More in-depth research still needs to be conducted on the physiological and psychological effects and mechanisms of exercise on fatigue. Nevertheless, the existing literature has revealed that exercise and physical activity are vital aspects of fatigue management at a physical and psychological level. Exercise and physical activity should be encouraged whatever the level of capability the patient or cancer survivor may have, from bed/chair exercises through to fitness training.

Implications for practice

Fatigue assessment and prescriptions for managing fatigue should be a vital aspect of care for cancer patients and survivors during treatment and follow-up care. Exercise and physical activity should be considered as an important fatigue management strategy. Prescription of exercise or physical activities should consider individual health status, exercise type, intensity, duration, frequency, and progression. Table 14.4 lists suggested considerations when prescribing exercise and physical activities (Winningham 1999).

It should be noted that exercise and physical activity are one of several possible interventional strategies for managing fatigue. The multidimensionality of cancer-related

Table 14.4 Prescriptions of physical exercise and activity

Prescription	Rationale/explanation
Status of the individual	Exercise should be tailored to age, gender, condition, risk factors, disease, and treatment
Type of exercise	Should encourage rhythmic, repetitive movement of large muscle groups such as walking, swimming, cycling, dancing, or stretching. Walking and cycling are the most appropriate because they are safe and easily tolerated by cancer patients and survivors. Exercise should be modified based on treatment modalities and disease progression
Intensity of exercise	Low to moderate exercise should be encouraged depending on patient's current fitness level and treatment modalities. Exercise or physical activities should never be so hard that the person is out of breath. Winningham's (1991) half rule of thumb can be an excellent reference, especially for individuals with cancer who are under active treatment and evident disease progression. The half rule of thumb involves finding out how much activity the patient can comfortably tolerate and then instructing them to begin with half that much several times daily, with rest periods between. Instead of a single type, a variety of exercise or physical activities should be prescribed
Frequency of exercise	For moderate exercise or activity (walking or cycling), three to five times per week is sufficient. For low-intensity and shorter-duration exercise and physical activities (stretching or marching in the room), a few minutes two or three times a day is beneficial
Duration of exercise	For cancer survivors and patients with stable conditions, 20–30 min of continuous exercise should be encouraged. For patients who are undergoing treatment and evident disease progression, 3–5 min short exercise bouts with rest intervals are preferable
Progression of exercise	Cancer patients and survivors should be instructed to increase exercise intensity until they meet the frequency and duration prescribed. Long-term exercise from months to a lifetime should be encouraged. A general rule of thumb is starting with what the person can do comfortably and working up very gradually from there

fatigue needs an integrative approach. Exercise and physical activity should be integrated with other fatigue management strategies, including modifying dietary needs, relieving other symptoms, practicing progressive muscle relaxation, and assessing/meeting emotional and spiritual needs. Cognitive therapy focusing on increasing individuals' self-efficacy can be an effective motivational intervention to encourage individuals with cancer to participate in exercise and physical activity (Haas 2000). It can be assumed that an integrative approach to fatigue management will improve the ability of cancer patients and survivors to manage their fatigue.

Implications for research

Although fatigue has been studied from the point of view of many health-related disciplines, its nature and characteristics are not well recognized or widely accepted (Aaronson et al. 1999; Ream and Richardson 1996; Tiesinga et al. 1996). The effectiveness of each individual intervention has not been rigorously researched. Future study should focus on establishing intensity, frequency, duration, and progression of exercise or physical activities for each intervention as well as its effectiveness. Determining the optimal exercise prescription for cancer patients and survivors for various treatment modalities and at various disease stages is an important focus for future research.

Using a cognitive approach to motivating individuals with cancer to participate in exercise or physical activities is an important direction for future research. Cognitive intervention focusing on increasing individuals' self-efficacy beliefs holds promise in motivating individuals to engage in exercise or physical activity. Self-efficacy belief, a component of social cognitive theory, has been found to be the strongest predictor of exercise behaviour among diverse populations (Conn 1997; Bandura 1997; King et al. 1992). Self-efficacy beliefs are personal assessments of one's ability to successfully perform a given behaviour (Bandura 1989, 1997). Research using self-efficacy in cancer patients has focused on disease prevention and early detection behaviours (Lev 1997). To date, no research has been conducted to establish the relationship between self-efficacy beliefs and the motivation of individuals with cancer to participate in exercise or physical activity. In addition, addressing self-efficacy may enhance smoking cessation, adoption of a healthy diet, and relaxation techniques (Haas 2000).

Fatigue is a multidimensional phenomenon and its management necessitates an integrative approach (Fu et al. 2001, 2002; Porock 1999). To date, there is still a lack of a systematic and integrative programme for fatigue management. Future fatigue research should focus on providing systematic and integrative management programmes based on strategies of energy conservation, effective energy use, and energy restoration (Piper et al. 1989). Such a systematic and integrative programme should encompass a variety of interventions, such as planned rest/sleep periods during the day, scheduled aerobic exercise and progressive muscle relaxation, provision of an adequate diet, and assessing/meeting emotional and spiritual needs. As future research documents the effectiveness of intervention programmes in managing fatigue, the quality of life in patients with metastatic disease will be improved.

Conclusion

Fatigue is a complex, subjective symptom that is very prevalent at all stages of the cancer trajectory. Although for many years fatigue was a hidden and ignored symptom of cancer and its treatment, recent focus and research efforts have provided a scientific basis for understanding fatigue, its impact, and management; a foundation that is acknowledged and used by all the health professions. Despite incomplete understanding of the mechanisms of fatigue, several research-based interventions have been tested with encouraging results. Exercise should be encouraged. Careful assessment and treatment of depression needs to be pursued in conjunction with exercise in managing fatigue.

Fatigue is one of a constellation of symptoms that can adversely affect individuals with cancer and their families. It is not an easy symptom to manage; nevertheless its complexity requires the listening empathic ear of health providers to ensure that whatever the outcome, the patient and family feel they have had the best of care possible.

References

Aaronson, L.S., Teel, C.S., Cassmeyer, V., Neuberger, G.B., Pallikkathayil, L., Pierce, J. *et al.* (1999). Defining and measuring fatigue. *Image: Journal of Nursing Scholarship*, **31**(1), 45–50.

Aistars, J. (1987) Fatigue in the cancer patient: a conceptual approach to a clinical problem. *Oncology Nursing Forum*, **14**(6), 25–30.

American Psychiatric Association (1994) *Diagnostic and Statistical Manual of Mental Disorders* (4th edn), American Psychiatric Press, Washington, DC.

Andrykowski, M.A., Curran, S.L., and Lightner, R. (1998) Off-treatment fatigue in breast cancer survivors: a controlled comparison. *Journal of Behavior Medicine*, **21**(1), 1–18.

Artal, M. and Sherman, C. (1998) Exercise against depression. *Physician and Sportsmedicine* **26**(10), 55–60, 70, 74–6.

Angst, J. (1997) Depression and anxiety: implications for nosology, course, and treatment. *Journal of Clinical Psychiatry*, **58**(Supplement 8), 3–4.

Astrand, P.O. (1973) Physiology of exercise and physical conditioning in normals. *Schweizerische Medizinische Wochenschrift*, **103**(2), 41–5.

Bandura, A. (1989) Human agency in social cognitive theory. *American Psychologist*, **44**(9), 1175–84.

Bandura, A. (1997) *Self-efficacy: The Exercise Control*. Freeman and Co, New York.

Barabasz, M. (1991) Effects of aerobic exercise on transient mood state. *Perception and Motivation Skills*, **73**, 657–58.

Beliles, K. and Stoudemire, A. (1998) Psychopharmacologic treatment of depression in the medically ill. *Psychosomatics*, **39**, S2–S19.

Berger, A. (1998) Patterns of fatigue and activity and rest during adjuvant breast cancer chemotherapy. *Oncology Nursing Forum*, **25**(1), 51–62.

Berger, B.G. and Owen, D.R. (1983) Mood alteration with swimming: swimmers really do feel better. *Psychosomatic Medicine*, **45**, 425–33.

Berger, B.G. and Owen, D.R. (1992) Mood alteration with yoga and swimming: aerobic exercise may not be necessary. *Perceptual Motor and Skills*, **75**(3, part 2), 1331–43.

Blanchard, C.M., Courneya, K.S., and Laing, D. (2001) Effects of acute exercise on state anxiety in breast cancer survivors. *Oncology Nursing Forum*, **28**(10), 1617–21.

Blumenthal, J.A., Babyak, M.A., Moore, K.A., Craighead, W.E., Herman, S., Khatri, P. *et al.* (1999) Effects of exercise training on older patients with major depression. *Archives of Internal Medicine*, **159**, 2349–56.

Bower, J.E., Ganz, P.A., Desmond, K.A., Rowland, J.H., Meyerowitz, B.E., and Belin, T.R. (2000) Fatigue in breast cancer survivors: occurrence, correlates, and impact on quality of life. *Journal of Clinical Oncology*, **18**(4), 743–53.

Byrne, A. and Byrne, D.G. (1993) The effect of exercise on depression, anxiety and other mood states: a review. *Journal of Psychosomatic Research*, **37**(6), 565–74.

Chaouloff, F. (1997) Effects of acute physical exercise on central serotonergic systems. *Medical Science on Sports Exercise*, **29**(1), 58–62.

Conn, V. (1997) Older women: social cognitive theory correlates of health behavior. *Women and Health*, **26**, 71–85.

Courneya, K.S. and Friedenreich, C.M. (1997) Relationship between exercise during treatment and current quality of life among survivors of breast cancer. *Journal of Psychosocial Oncology*, **15**(3/4), 35–57.

Courneya, K.S. and Friedenreich, C.M. (1999) Physical exercise and quality of life following cancer diagnosis: a literature review. *Annals of Behavioral Medicine*, **21**(2), 171–9.

Cramer, S.D., Neiman, D.C., and Lee, J.W. (1991) The effects of moderate exercise training on psychological well-being and mood state in women. *Journal of Psychosomatic Research*, **35**, 437–49.

Delgado, P.L., Charney, D.S., Rice, L.H., Aghajanian, G.K., Landis, H., and Heninger, G.R. (1990) Rapid serotonin depletion as a provocative challenge test for patients with major depression: relevance to antidepressant action and the neurobiology of depression. *Archives of General Psychiatry*, **47**, 411–18.

Dimeo, F. (1999) Strategies in managing cancer fatigue. *Rehabilitation Oncology*, **17**(3), 27–8.

Dimeo, F., Fetscher, S., Lange, W., Merfelsmann, R., and Keul, J. (1997) Effects of aerobic exercise on the physical performance and incidence of treatment-related complications after high-dose chemotherapy. *Blood*, **90**, 3390–4.

Dimeo, F., Rumberger, B.G., and Keul, J. (1998) Aerobic exercise as therapy for cancer fatigue. *Medicine & Science in Sports & Exercise*, **30**, 475–8.

Dinan, T.G. (1996) Noradrenergic and serotonergic abnormalities in depression: stress-induced dysfunction? *Journal of Clinical Psychiatry*, **57**(Supplement 4), 14–18.

Doyne, E.J., Osip-Klein, D.J., Bowman, E.D., Osbron, K.M., McDougall-Wilson, I.B., and Neimeyer, R.A. (1987) Running versus weight-lifting in the treatment of depression. *Journal of Consultancy Clinical Psychology*, **55**, 748–54.

Fu, M.R., LeMone, P., McDaniel, R., and Bausler, C. (2001) A multivariate validation of the defining characteristics of fatigue. *Nursing Diagnosis: International Journal of Nursing Language and Classification*, **12**(1), 15–27.

Fu, M.R., Anderson, C.M., McDaniel, R., and Armer, J. (2002) Patients' perception of fatigue in response to biochemotherapy as a treatment for metastatic melanoma. *Oncology Nursing Forum*, **29**(6), 961–6.

Glaser, R. (1997) An evolution of exercise physiology: effects of exercise on functional independence with aging and physical disabilities. *Journal of Rehabilitation Research and Development*, **34**(3), vi–viii.

Glaus, A. (1993) Assessment of fatigue in cancer and non-cancer patients and in healthy individuals. *Supportive Care in Cancer,* **1**(6), 305–15.

Glaus, A., Crow, R., and Hammond, S. (1996) A qualitative study to explore the concept of fatigue/tiredness in cancer patients and in healthy individuals. *European Journal of Cancer Care,* **5**(Supplement 2), 8–23.

Gowans, S.E., deHueck, A., Voss, S., and Richardson, M. (1999) A randomized, controlled trail of exercise and education for individuals with fibromyalgia. *Arthritis Care and Research,* **12**(2), 120–8.

Haas, B.K. (2000) Focus on health promotion: self-efficacy in oncology nursing research and practice. *Oncology Nursing Forum,* **27**(1), 89–97.

Henriksson, M.M., Isometsa, E.T., and Hietanen, P.S. (1995) Mental disorders in cancer suicides. *Journal of Affective Disorders,* **36**(1–2), 11–20.

Hickok, J.T., Morrow, G.R., and McDonald, S. (1996) Frequency and correlates of fatigue in lung cancer patients receiving radiation therapy: implications for management. *Journal of Pain and Symptom Management,* **11**(6), 370–7.

Hinds, P.S., Hockenberry-Eaton, M., Quargnenti, A., May, M., Burleson, C., Gilger, E. *et al.* (1999) Fatigue in 7- to 12-year-old patients with cancer from the staff perspective: an exploratory study. *Oncology Nursing Forum,* **26**(1), 37–45.

Hopwood, P. and Stephens, R.J. (2000) Depression in patients with lung cancer: prevalence and risk factors derived from quality-of-life data. *Journal of Clinical Oncology,* **18**(4), 893–903.

Irvine, D.M., Vincent, L., Graydon, J.E., Bubela, N., and Thompson, L. (1994) The prevalence and correlates of fatigue in patients receiving treatment with chemotherapy and radiotherapy. *Cancer Nursing,* **17**, 367–78.

Keltner, T.A., Flockhart, D.A., Post, R.M., Denicoff, K., Pazzaglia, P.J., Marangell, L.B. *et al.* (1995) The emerging role of cytochrome P450 #A in psychopharmacology. *Journal of Clinical Psychopharmacology,* **15**, 387–98.

Kennedy, M. M. and Newton, M. (1997) Effects of exercise intensity on mood in step aerobics. *Journal of Sports Medicine and Physical Fitness,* **37**, 200–4.

King, A. (1994) Clinical and community interventions to promote and support physical activity participation. In: *Advanced in Exercise Adherence* (ed. R. Dishman), Human Kinetics, Champaign, IL, pp. 183–211.

King, A., Blair, S., Bild, D., Dishmna, R., Dubbert, B., Neil, M. *et al.* (1992) Determinants of physical activity and interventions in adults. *Medicine and Science in Sports and Exercise,* **24**(6S), S221–S236.

Lev, E.L. (1997) Bandura's theory of self-efficacy: applications to oncology. *Scholarly Inquiry for Nursing Practice,* **11**, 21–37.

Lovejoy, N.C., Tabor, D., and Deloney, P. (2000) Continuing education: cancer-related depression: Part II—Neurologic alterations and evolving approaches to psychopharmacology. *Oncology Nursing Forum,* **27**(5), 795–807.

Lydiard, R.B. and Brawman-Mintzer, O. (1998) Anxious depression. *Journal of Clinical Psychiatry,* **59**(Supplement 18), 10–17.

Massie, M.J. and Shakin, E.J. (1993) Management of depression and anxiety in cancer patients. In: *Psychiatric Aspects of Symptom Management in Cancer Patients* (ed. W. Breitbart and J.C. Holland), American Psychiatric Press, Washington, DC, pp. 1–22.

MacVicar, M.G. and Winningham, M.L. (1986) Promoting the functional capacity of cancer patients. *Cancer Bulletin,* **38**, 235–9.

MacVicar, M.G., Winningham, M.L., and Nickel, J.L. (1989) Effects of aerobic interval training on cancer patients' functional capacity. *Nursing Research*, **38**, 348–51.

McMurdo, M.T. and Burnett, L. (1992) Randomized controlled trial of exercise in the elderly. *Gerontology*, **38**, 292–8.

Mock, B., Burke, M.B., Sheehan, P.K., Creaton, E., Watson, P.G., Winningham, M.L. *et al.* (1994) A nursing rehabilitation program for women with breast cancer receiving adjuvant chemotherapy. *Oncology Nursing Forum*, **21**(5), 899–907.

Mock, V., Dow, K., Meares, C.J., Grimm, P.M., Dienemann, J.A., Haisfield-Wolfe, M.E. *et al.* (1997) Effects of exercise on fatigue, physical functioning, and emotional distress during radiation therapy for breast cancer. *Oncology Nursing Forum*, **24**(6), 991–1000.

Mock, V., Ropka, M.E., Rhodes, V.A., Pickett, M., Grimm, P.M., McDaniel, R., *et al.* (1998) Forum focus. Establishing mechanisms to conduct multi-institutional research-fatigue in patients with cancer: an exercise intervention. *Oncology Nursing Forum*, **25**(8), 1391–7.

Morris, R.W. (1975) The physiology of exercise and its clinical implications in coronary heart disease. *South African Medical Journal*, **14**(June), 999–1004.

Murphy, D.L., Andrews, A.M., Wichems, C.H., Li, Q., Tohda, M., and Greenberg, B. (1998) Brain serotonin neurotransmission: an overview and update with emphasis on serotonin subsystem heterogeneity, multiple receptors, interactions with other neurotransmitter systems, and consequent implications for understanding the actions of serotonergic drugs. *Journal of Clinical Psychiatry*, **59**(Supplement 15), 4–12.

Nail, L.M., Jones, L.S., and Geene, D. (1991) Use and perceived efficacy of self-care activities in patients receiving chemotherapy. *Oncology Nursing Forum*, **18**, 883–7.

Nayak, D. (1998) In defense of polypharmacy. *Psychiatric Annals* **28**, 190–6.

Nierenberg, A.A., Alpert, J.E., Pava, J., Rosenbaum, J.F., and Fava, M. (1998) Course and treatment of atypical depression. *Journal of Clinical Psychiatry*, **59**(Supplement 18), 5–9.

NIH Consensus Development Panel on Physical Activity and Cardiovascular Health (1996) Physical activity and cardiovascular health. *Journal of the American Medical Association*, **276**(3), 241–5.

O'Neill, K. and Reid, G. (1991) Perceived barriers to physical activity by older adults. *Canadian Journal of Public Health*, **82**(6), 392–6.

Petruzzello, S.J., Jones, A.C., and Tate, A.K. (1997) Affective responses to acute exercise: a test of opponent-process theory. *Journal of Sports Medicine and Physical Fitness*, **37**(3), 205–12.

Petty, F., Davis, L.L., Kabel, D., and Kramer, G.L. (1996) Serotonin dysfunction disorders: a behavioral neurochemistry perspective. *Journal of Clinical Psychiatry*, **57**(Supplement 8), 11–16.

Pickard-Holley, S. (1991) Fatigue in cancer patients: a descriptive study. *Cancer Nursing*, **14**(1), 13–19.

Piper, B.F., Rieger, P.T., Brothy, L., Haeuber, D., Hood, L.E., Lyver, A. *et al.* (1989) Recent advances in the management of biotherapy-related side effects: fatigue. *Oncology Nursing Forum*, **16**(6, Supplement), 27–34.

Porock, D. (2001) Fatigue. In: *Palliative Care Nursing: a Guide to Practice*, 2nd edn (ed. S. Aranda and M. O'Connor) AUSMED Publications, Melbourne, pp. 137–52.

Porock, D., Kristjanson, L., Tinnelly, K., and Blight, J. (2000) The effect of exercise on fatigue in patients with advanced cancer: a pilot study. *Journal of Palliative Care*, **16**(3), 30–6.

Ream, E. and Richardson, A. (1996) Fatigue: a concept analysis. *International Journal of Nursing Studies*, **33**(5), 519–29.

Richardson, A. and Ream, E. (1997) Self-care behaviours initiated by chemotherapy patients in response to fatigue. *International Journal of Nursing Studies*, **34**, 35–43.

Rosenbaum, J.F., Fave, M., Nierenberg, A.A., and Sachs, G.S. (1995) Treatment-resistant mood disorders. In: *Treatment of Psychiatric Disorders* (ed. G.O. Gabbard) (2nd edn), American Psychiatric Press, Washington, DC, pp. 1275–328.

Schag, C.A.C., Ganz, P.A., Wing, D.S., Sim, M-S., and Lee, J.J. (1994) Quality of life in adult survivors of lung, colon, and prostate cancer. *Quality of Life Research, 3*, 127–50.

Schwartz, A. (1998) Patterns of exercise and fatigue in physically active cancer survivors. *Oncology Nursing Forum, 25*(3), 485–91.

Schwartz, A. (2000) Exercise and weight gain in breast cancer patients receiving chemotherapy. *Cancer Practice, 8*(5), 231–7.

Simpson, S., Baldwin, R.C., Jackson, A., and Burns, A.S. (1998) Is subcortical disease associated with poor response to antidepressants? Neurological, neuropsychological and neuroradiological findings in late-life depression. *Psychological Medicine, 28*, 1015–26.

Steptoe, A. and Cox, S. (1988) Acute effects of aerobic exercise on mood. *Health Psychology, 7*, 329–40.

Stoudemire, A., Bronheim, H., and Wise, T.N. (1998) Why guidelines for consultation-liaison psychiatry patients? *Psychosomatics, 39*, S3–S7.

Tiesinga, L., Dassen, T.W.N., and Halfens, R.J.G. (1996) Fatigue: a summary of the definitions, dimensions, and indicators. *Nursing Diagnosis, 7*(2), 51–62.

Winningham, M.L. (1991) Walking program for people with cancer. *Cancer Nursing 14*, 270–6.

Winningham, M.L. (1992) The role of exercise in cancer therapy. In: *Exercise and Disease* (ed. R.R. Watson and M. Eisinger), CRC Press, Boca Raton, FL, pp. 71–88.

Winningham, M. (1996) Fatigue. In: *Cancer Symptom Management* (ed. S. Groenwald, M. Hansen Frogge, M. Goodman, and C.H. Yarbro), Jones and Bartlett, Boston, MA, pp. 42–58.

Winningham, M.L. (1999) Fatigue. In: *Cancer Symptom Management*, 2nd edn (ed. C. Henke-Yarbo, M. Hansen Frogge, and M. Goodman). Jones and Bartlett, Philadelphia, pp. 58–76.

Winningham, M., Nail, L., Burke, M., Brophy, L., Cimprich, B., Jones, L. *et al.* (1994) Fatigue and the cancer experience: the state of the knowledge. *Oncology Nursing Forum, 21*, 23–36.

Index